HOLISTIC HEALTH SECRETS FOR WOMEN

Discover your unique path to health, healing and happiness

Dr Mark Atkinson

PIATKUS

First published in Great Britain in 2009 by Piatkus Books

Copyright © 2009 by Dr Mark Atkinson

The moral right of the author has been asserted

A CIP catalogue record for this book
is available from the British Library

ISBN 978-0-7499-2824-7

Design by Paul Saunders
Typeset in ITC Stone Serif by Phoenix Photosetting, Chatham, Kent
www.phoenixphotosetting.co.uk
Printed and bound in the UK by CPI William Clowes, Beccles NR34 7TL

Papers used by Piatkus Books are natural, renewable and recyclable
products made from wood grown in sustainable forests and certified
in accordance with the rules of the Forest Stewardship Council

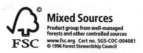

Mixed Sources
Product group from well-managed
forests and other controlled sources
www.fsc.org Cert no. SGS-COC-004081
FSC © 1996 Forest Stewardship Council

Piatkus Books
An imprint of
Little, Brown Book Group
100 Victoria Embankment
London EC4Y 0DY

An Hachette Livre UK Company
www.hachettelivre.co.uk

www.piatkus.co.uk

Acknowledgements

First, my heartfelt thanks to my wife Serena for your patience, support and love. I am so grateful to you for helping me find the time and space to write this book. Your courage and commitment to love and truth continue to inspire me in so many ways; I am blessed to be your life partner. To my daughter Annabelle – I am in awe of your zest for life! You have helped me get in touch with the child within me and my life is so much richer for that. I will do everything I can so that you continue to shine brightly in this world. Mum, Dad and Carl, thank you so much for your loving support over the last year – it has meant so much to me.

I also want to thank my agent David for your support and my editors Helen, Gill and Jillian – your patience and creative input has been wonderful, and you are a delight to work with!

And finally I want to thank my patients. I have learnt so much from you over the years and I continue to be touched by the courage, commitment and honesty that so many of you have. I will do my best to serve you as you continue your healing journeys.

Contents

About Dr Mark Atkinson

Dr Mark Atkinson MBBS BSc (HONS) FRIPH is one of the UK's leading integrated medical doctors and a recognised expert in drug-free approaches to women's health problems, depression, psychosomatic illness and trauma/PTSD.

In 1997 he qualified as a medical doctor from St Mary's Hospital Medical School (now known as the Imperial College School of Medicine) in London. While working as an NHS hospital doctor, Dr Atkinson took the decision to build on his traditional medical education by exploring a variety of complementary and alternative approaches to healing. He subsequently received training in a variety of disciplines, including nutritional medicine and mind–body medicine, and psychological models, such as the Human Givens Approach and Acceptance and Commitment Therapy.

Dr Atkinson now practises integrated medicine as a 'whole-person' approach to health and healing. Unlike Western medicine, which tends to treat symptoms using drugs and/or surgery, integrated medicine provides individuals with a personalised combination of psychological, nutritional, medical and complementary health treatments designed to identify and address the underlying barriers to health and wellbeing.

In addition to his clinical work, Dr Atkinson is the founder of The British College of Integrated Medicine, Chairman of The British Society of Integrated Medicine, founder of The Academy of Human Potential and a fellow of the Royal Institute of Public Health. He is also an award-winning writer, author of *The Mind–Body Bible* and an experienced lecturer and workshop facilitator.

Foreword

Conventional medicine as it is currently practised fails to meet the needs of women. Research shows that the medical system and the doctors who practise within it are ill-equipped to recognise and respond effectively to women's specific health challenges and requirements. For example, most doctors don't know that women who are depressed are much more likely than men to report fatigue, sleep and appetite disturbances, so these symptoms often go unrecognised as the distress signals of an underlying depression. Even when an accurate diagnosis is made, women are usually treated without regard for the abundance of evidence that shows they respond to medications in a different way to men. What's more, when women present with generalised symptoms such as fatigue and moodiness, doctors often dismiss them as trivial, even though they matter a great deal to the patients.

However, a new era is dawning in which increasing numbers of doctors, clinics and hospitals are embracing a new medicine committed to providing women with the very best, personalised holistic care. It is integrated medicine, a healing-orientated system that takes account of the whole person – body, mind and spirit – as well as all aspects of lifestyle. It makes use of all therapies – conventional, complementary and alternative – and places great emphasis on the relationship between the patient and doctor. This partnership approach is designed to empower women to take charge of their health and to live life in a way that fosters harmony of body, mind and spirit. It is an exciting and deeply fulfilling way of practising medicine that is starting to transform healthcare as we know it.

Dr Mark Atkinson is one of a new generation of doctors who is leading the effort to establish integrated medicine in the UK. In addition to helping his patients, and training doctors and nurses in the principles and practices of integrated medicine, he is dedicated to making this approach available to as many people as possible and that is the motivation behind *Holistic Health Secrets for Women*. At the heart of his approach, an approach which I and many integrated medical doctors share, is an emphasis on attending to the needs of the body, mind, heart and soul. He encourages you to walk the path to better health, healing and happiness with mindfulness and self-acceptance. Living mindfully means bringing your alert presence to whatever is arising in the moment; doing so allows you to experience the fullness of life and your connection to it. Self-acceptance brings a deep peace-of-mind in which you are able to celebrate who you are, just as you are. Both are powerful tools for healing and emotional growth.

I now hand you over to Dr Mark Atkinson and wish you a fruitful journey. You are in safe hands.

Dr Andrew Weil

Introduction

I have written this book in order to give you the knowledge and tools to take charge of your health and life using the very best approaches from the worlds of Western, complementary and alternative medicine. I want to share with you five of the most important secrets to lasting health, healing and happiness, and show you how to use the holistic health tools that I teach my patients. I would also like to introduce you to the principles of a revolutionary new approach to healthcare called integrated medicine, and give you complete integrated holistic programmes for the most common health problems faced by women today.

As an integrated medical doctor specialising in holistic approaches to women's health and healing, I have helped over a thousand women transform their lives and I know that one of the key factors in achieving your health goals is for the information that you read to be tailored to you as a woman *and* as an individual. This is what *Holistic Health Secrets for Women* offers and it's one of the reasons why this book is unique. While medicine has traditionally neglected the needs of women and over-focused on the disease or 'problem' at the expense of you as an individual, I, like an increasing number of health professionals, embrace a more personalised approach that concentrates on identifying and resolving the issues that prevent you from thriving and flourishing as a woman. For me, this is one of the key differences between conventional medicine and the new integrated medicine.

Integrated medicine

Because so much of the information in this book has been inspired by integrated medicine, I want to tell you how I became involved with it. About ten years or so ago I was working as a hospital-based doctor, but I had begun to feel increasingly disillusioned with the over-emphasis on diseases and drugs, and the almost complete neglect for the person being treated. Of the hundreds of patients that I was responsible for during this time, I probably got to know less than ten of them on a personal level.

What's more, many of my patients were telling me how diet, nutritional and herbal supplements, stress management and complementary therapies had helped them not only reduce their various symptoms, but also experience greater levels of health and even happiness. However, none of these approaches had been mentioned in my six years at medical school! I remember one lady telling me how excluding wheat from her diet and taking fish oil and a glucosamine sulphate supplement had alleviated her arthritis, meaning that she didn't have to take painkillers, which gave her constipation. I felt deeply embarrassed because I had no idea what she was talking about and, as a result, vowed to teach myself complementary and alternative approaches to health and healing.

While continuing to practise as a doctor I studied nutrition and meditation, took courses in hypnotherapy, emotional healing, psychotherapy, breathwork and guided imagery, and explored how intention, beliefs, awareness and conditioning influence health and healing. Once I felt competent in these areas I started using them with my patients and quickly found that they not only got better results, but that my patients were becoming healthier and happier, because they felt more empowered and in control of their life and health.

At a personal and professional level my passion for medicine began to return and I developed a deep desire to help people flourish – emotionally and spiritually, as well as physically. Initially I felt alone in practising medicine this way, but I came across a book by a doctor called Andrew Weil. It was about an emerging approach called integrated medicine – or integrative medicine as it's known in the US – and it articulated everything that I was starting to discover for myself, and more.[1]

I discovered that integrated medicine is concerned with honouring and addressing the whole person – body, mind, emotions, spirit, environment and community – because all these influence and contribute to health, healing and happiness. I read about how integrated medical doctors use the safest and most effective combination of conventional and complementary medicine to help their patients, prescribing healthy eating programmes, exercise, supplements, meditation and relaxation alongside medications. Rather than doctors telling patients what to do, which was certainly the way I was used to practising medicine, integrated medicine focused more on helping individuals access their own inner wisdom and take charge of their own health and life. Rather than just helping individuals *recover* from ill-health, I realised that integrated medicine was about helping them to *discover* how to live a healthy and fulfilling life.

The word 'integrate' sounds a little like to move 'into greatness' and that for me captures the essence of what integrated medicine does – it empowers you to develop your physical, emotional, psychological and spiritual potential in a way that brings you greater health, happiness and wholeness. The ideas and principles first put forward by Dr Weil and other authors within this field resonated so strongly with me that I knew that this was the way I *had* to practise medicine. That was eight years ago.

The present

I now teach doctors and nurses about integrated medicine, present lectures throughout the UK on the subject and run a busy integrated medical clinic, where 90 per cent of my patients are women. In fact, women are the principal champions of integrated medicine. There are numerous reasons for this, including women's traditional responsibility for health and caring within the family, your ability to see and think about life in a holistic way, your greater awareness of your physical and emotional needs (at least when compared with men!), as well as the aversion some women have to the male-dominated medical system.

Indeed, many of the women who come to see me feel that the medical system has let them down. Some have asked their GP for advice and have been offered medication, even though they instinctively knew that drugs were not the answer. Others find that their doctors don't respect their perspective, insight and experience or simply don't listen to them. Either way, increasing numbers of women (and to a lesser degree men) are calling for an approach that helps them achieve the best possible level of health in a way that is safe, effective and empowering. This is what integrated medicine can provide.

How to use this book

Regardless of whether you have a specific health problem or want to know how to improve your general health, I encourage you to read parts one, two and three of *Holistic Health Secrets for Women,* rather than going directly to the sections on the health problems you know or suspect you may have. I find that those patients who are willing to learn about the fundamentals of health and healing, and then incorporate them into a new way of being and living, while also treating their specific health problem, do much better in the long term than those who focus exclusively on dealing with their disease or symptoms.

Part one, section one, looks at the way in which women's health, and your unique physical and psychological needs, have traditionally been neglected by conventional medicine. I then go on to describe how integrated medicine is different and I explain the principles upon which it is built and upon which most of my patients transform their health.

Part one, section two, is very important, because it allows you, through the use of a series of self-assessment questionnaires, to identify what barriers might be preventing you from experiencing your fullest potential for health, healing and happiness. For me, this process of individualised assessment and care is at the heart of integrated medicine. Your questionnaire scores will then help you to decide which other parts of the book to focus on.

Part two features the five secrets of health, healing and happiness. I encourage you to read them all, even if you have completed the questionnaires and already identified those that are particularly relevant to you. These secrets are the real foundation for my work with my patients, and once you embrace them and incorporate them into your life, they will not only help you recover from existing health problems, but also help you flourish physically, emotionally and spiritually.

Part three outlines the five main holistic health tools that I teach to my patients. Please read through them all as I refer to them throughout the book. While you certainly don't need to *learn* all of them, I encourage you to choose two or three and to try them on real-life issues.

Part four features my step-by-step integrated medical approach to a wide variety of women's health problems, ranging from PMS and fibroids to infertility and menopause. Using your secrets as the foundations, I will show you how to build a programme that incorporates the medical, nutritional, psychological, self-help and complementary therapy treatment options that I recommend in my medical practice.

Part five provides my integrated medical prescription for 25 of the most common health problems experienced by women, ranging from acne and constipation to depression and rheumatoid arthritis. While these conditions also affect men, my experience is that women really need an approach that is specific to them as women and as individuals, and this part provides you with that.

I sincerely hope that this book gives you the support you need to recover from illness, transform your health and create a deeply fulfilling life. I wish you every success.

Dr Mark Atkinson

Part One

~

You are unique

In this first part of the book I outline how and why mainstream medicine has, to date, been unable to meet the needs of women and how integrated medicine is changing that. You will learn about the principles and practices of integrated medicine upon which this book is based and I'll provide plenty of suggestions to really help you get the most out of the information and ideas that I offer.

To aid that process there is a series of questionnaires that will help you work out exactly what is stopping you from optimising your potential for health, healing and happiness.

Women and the new medicine

~

I am not alone in believing that the old medicine – Western medicine – continues to fail to meet the needs of women and is limited in its ability to treat and prevent chronic disease. However, the inadequacies of Western medicine have given birth to a new, common sense way of delivering healthcare that is orientated towards helping the whole person to heal. Although still in its embryonic stages here in the UK, this new integrated medicine is taking root and it is women who are driving the demand for it. Women like you want healthcare that not only meets your needs and honours your uniqueness, but also celebrates who you are as women and as individuals. Women like you are demanding a system with more heart and soul and, as a result, you are changing the face and shape of medicine and health. These are exciting and challenging times and over the next couple of decades integrated medicine will transform our healthcare system as we know it.

The old medicine – Western medicine

Antibiotics, vaccinations, improved surgical procedures, cardiac medications, analgesics, diagnostics and health screening are all medical advances that have enriched and enhanced the quality of life of millions of women throughout the world. On average, women are living longer, and surviving cancer and heart disease better, than at any other time in history. At face value all is well. However, if we scratch the surface it's clear that things are not quite as they seem. Despite increases in wealth, technology and access to health services, women are nonetheless experiencing increased levels of health problems such as obesity, asthma, osteoporosis, chronic fatigue syndrome, autoimmune disease and diabetes, and rising levels of stress and mental illness. Some experts consider depression and anxiety amongst women to be at almost epidemic levels.[1] Happiness levels are also falling. One poll, for example, found that the proportion of people saying they are 'very happy' has fallen from 52 per cent in 1957 to just 36 per cent in 2005.[2] So while on the face of it things appear better, the reality is that the health of women, particularly at an emotional and psychological level, is deteriorating rather than improving.

The causes of disease and dis-ease

Why are women's overall health and happiness declining? I believe it is because most women are living a life that they are not genetically designed to live. Humankind's genetic make-up has hardly changed in the last 30,000 to 40,000 years – you and I are still hardwired to eat fresh, local produce; keep physically active; get plenty of rest and stay socially connected through community-orientated living.[3] This is a far cry from the reality for most women today. In fact, most women are likely to experience many of the following:

- A diet high in sugar and processed foods and low in nutrient-dense wholefoods

- Nutritional deficiencies

- Exposure to un-natural light and radiation

- Exposure to hormone-disrupting toxins

- Lack of physical activity

- Disconnection from nature

- Long working hours

- Excessive time pressure

- Sleep deprivation

- Lack of role models

- Role confusion

- The breakdown of the family unit

- Being a sole carer

- Financial debt

- Increasing levels of isolation

- Cultural and societal focus on appearance, weight and socio-economic status

- Sex and gender discrimination

- High risk of sexual and physical abuse

- Increasing levels of fear and insecurity

- A healthcare system based on the needs of men not women

- The over-prescription of medications

- Disempowerment

The truth is most women struggle to cope with the physical, emotional, psychological and social changes that have taken place in the last 50 years. This failure to adapt to the demands of 21st-century life is making it progressively more difficult for women to meet the physical and emotional needs that are so essential for health and happiness. Those physical needs include a healthy diet, sleep and rest, touch, physical activity and a healthy environment. The emotional needs include receiving and giving positive attention, love, safety, meaning and purpose, a sense of competence and stress resilience, and a connection to family, friends, community and nature. The failure to meet these needs in a healthy and balanced way sows the seeds of physical disease and mental 'dis-ease', and, in my opinion, is at the heart of the health and wellbeing crisis that so many women are experiencing.

It's not all bad news, though. Women have a primary impulse to survive and thrive. The challenge is to listen to that instinct and take action, which is exactly what increasing numbers of women are doing. I believe that the reason more women are turning to complementary and now integrated medicine is they instinctively know that, for women especially, Western medicine is limited in what it can offer. Its detached, mechanistic approach to disease, which focuses on fixing and eradicating symptoms, and its failure to empower you with the knowledge and tools to create health and support your own healing, is simply not enough to help you flourish in today's challenging environment. While I don't wish to minimise modern-day medicine's achievements, I feel it is important to acknowledge the truth – that orthodox medical practice has failed and continues to fail to meet the needs of women.

How Western medicine has let women down

A recent example of the way in which the Western medical system has ignored the knowledge women have about their own bodies is the routine prescription of Hormone Replacement Therapy (HRT). Touted as a panacea for all the problems related to the menopause, HRT did seem to alleviate hot flushes and mood swings, and it was also claimed it reduced the risk of heart disease and osteoporosis. However, from the perspective of integrated medicine HRT only worked by aggressively suppressing the symptoms of the menopause, rather than helping women to cope with an entirely natural process, and there was a lack of evidence to substantiate its beneficial effects on heart disease and osteoporosis.

One of my patients told me how, back in 1995, her doctor said she would be silly not to take HRT, because it was entirely safe. She took it for two years, but all along intuitively felt it wasn't right to be artificially suppressing her hormones. Eventually she stopped taking it and by changing her diet and lifestyle was able to pass through the menopause without any problems. Her intuition was, of course, absolutely correct, as HRT was subsequently found to increase the risk of cancer, as well as stroke, heart disease and blood clots.[4]

Another significant contributor to the substandard care women have received from the medical system has been that, as recently as the mid 1990s, the use of women in clinical trials involving drugs and medical technology was a rarity.[5] This was not simply down to male chauvinism or the fact that most scientists were men. The primary reason was that, with the exception of your reproductive system, it was *assumed* that women are physiologically and psychologically the same as men. Eventually this complacency was addressed and in the last ten years solid evidence has emerged to confirm what women instinctively know – that many approaches, treatments and medications affect them differently to the way they affect men. For example, if I prescribed you steroids for an inflammatory condition such as rheumatoid arthritis, you would be much more likely to experience weight gain, fluid retention and fluctuations in your mood than a man taking the same dose. However, a doctor would rarely take this into account.[6]

Inequality of treatment

Women also receive different treatment to men. If you had a heart attack in the next hour and were admitted to hospital, when compared with a man who was also having a heart attack, on average you would have to wait longer to receive medical attention, you would be less likely to undergo a diagnostic test such as cardiac catheterisation (failure of which is linked to a higher risk of death from heart attack), you would receive clot-busting drugs less quickly and be less likely to be discharged home on aspirin, a drug that has been shown to reduce complications relating to heart attacks. Astonishingly, when compared to the man with a heart attack, your doctor would be 26 per cent *more* likely to assign a do-not-resuscitate (DNR) order to you.[7] This means that, should your heart stop beating, the medical team would not attempt to revive you. I don't mean to be sensationalist here, but my point is this – men are treated differently to women and in the majority of cases it is women who suffer as a consequence.

Ignorance

Ignorance and lack of knowledge by the medical profession is also a factor in the substandard care of you as a woman. The majority of doctors simply aren't taught anything about sex differences and their relevance to your health and treatment. For example, few doctors would know that when compared to men women are more likely to:

- Complain of bodily symptoms such as fatigue, sleep disturbance or changes in appetite when depressed[8]

- Develop post-traumatic stress disorder (PTSD) following a traumatic experience[9]

- Have a heart attack, stroke, cancer or diabetes when they smoke cigarettes[10]

- Fail to stop smoking and have more severe withdrawal symptoms[11]

- Take medications such as non-steroidal anti-inflammatory painkillers and take them for longer, putting them at higher risk of side effects such as bleeding and gastritis[12]

The lack of awareness of the different health challenges facing women is also surprising. For example, one in three doctors surveyed in 1995 did not know that cardiovascular disease (CVD) is the leading cause of death among women in the US[13] and fewer than one in five doctors surveyed in 2004 knew that more women than men die of CVD each year.[14]

Ignorance, lack of adequate training concerning sex differences, societal bias, economics, the status quo and a long history of disregard for women and women's health, combined with little or no training in nutrition, stress resilience, exercise and complementary medicine, has lead to a health system that does not yet adequately meet women's needs. That, combined with spiralling healthcare costs, increasing levels of disillusionment with the medical profession, a reductionist approach to treating illness and the increasing burden of chronic disease, necessitates a new, sustainable approach to health and healing that meets the needs of the people it serves, and restores heart and pride to the practice of medicine. The good news is that a new medicine is already here and it's starting, albeit slowly, to alter healthcare worldwide.

The new medicine – integrated medicine

Integrated medicine is a modern-day approach to health and healing that has its roots in common sense. Rather than taking a one-size-fits-all approach to treating disease, integrated medicine recognises that the most effective way to support you through a health problem – or to help you improve your health and prevent disease – is to provide you with a personalised programme of care that combines the best of conventional, nutritional, psychological, self-help and complementary medicine.

Integrated medicine as it is practised in the UK involves doctors and nurses trained in the principles and practices of integrated medicine, working as part of a team of diagnosticians (for example, a radiologist, a practitioner of traditional Chinese medicine or a specialist in nutritional and hormonal assessment), therapists (for example, an acupuncturist, healer, massage or nutritional therapist), doctors and relevant professionals or organisations (for example, self-help or support groups, local NHS services, private treatment facilities or a life coach specialising in health). All these people and agencies work together to support you in achieving your health and life goals. It is very much a partnership-based model of health, with you at the helm.

Whereas in my pre-integrated medicine days I would have met you, delivered a diagnosis and told you what medications to take, my intention now as an integrated medical doctor is for us to work together to identify and then address what is preventing you from experiencing your fullest potential for health, healing and happiness. That might involve us exploring your diet, your past, getting an idea about how you manage your stress and emotions, understanding your life situation, relationships and environment, and talking about meaning, purpose and spirituality. At the heart of this relationship is mutual respect, genuine care and a real desire to support you in achieving your goals.

The following are the main core principles upon which integrated medicine is being established and upon which this book is written. Don't be tempted to skip this part as it sets the stage for the suggestions that I make later on in the book.

The principles of integrated medicine

Get to the heart of the problem

Integrated medicine attempts to identify and address the root causes and contributors to your health problem. This includes physical, emotional, psychological, environmental, social and spiritual factors. For example, having arranged the appropriate investigations and tests, the cause of one of my patient's fatigue and weight gain was found to be a low functioning thyroid, nutritional deficiencies and adrenal fatigue, whereas another patient with similar symptoms had mercury toxicity and constipation. Despite having the same problem they had very different reasons for feeling tired and therefore very different treatment programmes.

Honour your preferences

Integrated medicine is individualised to you as a person, in that it takes account of underlying causes (as in the examples above), but also your needs, insights, beliefs, past experiences, preferences and life circumstances. For example, following a consultation with me, we might agree that a stress-resilience training programme would be of benefit. If you had previously enjoyed and had a positive experience of yoga, then we would probably agree on you using yoga rather than, for example, meditation or t'ai chi.

Support the inner healer

Integrated medicine acknowledges that there is an inner healer within you, an intelligence that is programmed to heal and repair your body given the right conditions. Helping you to increase your level of awareness of, and communication with, the inner healer and to learn how to respond to its cues and messages is part of the integrated medicine process. Learning how to become an expert on yourself is one of the goals of integrated medicine.

Tap into the healing power of happiness

Experiencing genuine happiness and contentment with one's life not only feels good, but is also good for your health. Happy people tend to be healthy people; happiness and health go hand-in-hand – they feed off each other. A nine-year Dutch study into the elderly found that those who were happy, optimistic or generally satisfied with life had around 50 per cent less risk of dying over the period of the study than those who were unhappy or pessimistic.[15] Other research has found that people who are happy and contented seem to be at less risk from conditions such as hypertension, heart disease, diabetes, colds and upper respiratory infections.[16] When they receive a flu vaccine, people who are rated as very happy by psychologists develop around 50 per cent more antibodies than the average.[17] The other side of the coin is that depression can exacerbate the impact of a wide range of illnesses.

Creating happiness is not, however, about doing things that are pleasurable and avoiding things that cause pain – far from it. Happiness comes from living a meaningful and fulfilling life in which you have the presence and skills to respond effectively to whatever comes your way, and do so from a place of authenticity, awareness and acceptance. Each of the five secrets is designed to create not only better health and support the process of healing, but also to increase your experience of authentic happiness.

Supporting you in being in charge

Integrated medicine empowers you wherever possible to take an active role in your own healing by providing you with the knowledge and skills to meet your physical and emotional needs, and actively manage your own health. Rather than a 'pill for every ill', I use the phrase a 'skill for every ill'. I teach most of my patients skills and tools that they can use to manage their own health. The five I use most are featured in part three.

Safety first

Integrated medicine uses the safest, most effective and least invasive procedures wherever possible. In the case of arthritis, for example, this can mean removing sugar and processed foods, checking for food intolerances, losing excess fat and taking natural supplements, *before* resorting to anti-inflammatory medications (which are associated with bleeding from the gut, gastritis and an increased risk of heart problems).

Utilise the best of all worlds

Integrated medicine harnesses the best combination of available conventional and non-conventional treatments. For example, if you were diagnosed with heart disease, it might be recommended that in addition to taking aspirin and cholesterol-lowering medications, you switch to a diet high in vegetables and wholefoods and low in sugar and processed foods, start exercising for 30 minutes a day, learn stress-resilience skills, receive support to help heal emotional trauma from the past and be encouraged to strengthen your social connections and relationships.

Prioritise evidence-informed treatments

Wherever possible integrated medicine takes into account the available evidence on the effectiveness of a particular therapy in treating the condition you have. For example, we know that osteopathy can be helpful for back pain and acupuncture for nausea.[18]

Harness the mind

Integrated medicine harnesses the healing power of the mind by teaching you how to use your intention, beliefs, awareness and imagination to support your healing. For example, you might be invited to listen to a guided imagery CD, learn how to meditate or explore and change your belief systems.

Encourage healthy relationships

Integrated medicine places a central emphasis and importance on the quality of your relationships. This includes your relationships with yourself, your family, friends, health team, and with your community and nature as well. I might suggest – and I do this a lot with my patients – that you work on developing greater self-acceptance and perhaps learn ways to deepen intimacy and resolve conflict with partners, because if you don't address it this can be a significant source of stress.

Focus on health, vitality and happiness

Rather than being exclusively focused on disease and problems, a health professional using an integrated medical approach will be very keen to support you in creating a vision for the level of health and quality of life that you desire for yourself. This might involve helping you identify and pursue goals rooted in your values, teaching you mindfulness-based meditation, which can help to increase your level of awareness and ability to respond, rather than react, to life, and taking measures to increase the probability of you living as long and healthy a life as possible.

If I had to capture the essence of integrated medicine and identify what its ultimate aim is I would say it is about supporting people to experience a greater level of wholeness, integration, acceptance and inner peace. It's about helping you to realise your health and healing potential and thrive and flourish as a woman.

SUMMARY

- Despite improvements in wealth and technology, the physical and mental health of many women is deteriorating not improving.

- Western medicine's depersonalised and mechanistic approach to dealing with disease, along with its lack of respect for women's health needs and issues, has driven many women to seek help outside Western medicine.

- You know yourself better than anyone, and by tuning into your body and allowing yourself to be led by your intuition, your inner healer will guide you to better health and happiness.

- Integrated medicine is a common-sense approach to health and healing that is designed to help you recover from disease, and discover how to live a healthy and fulfilling life.

Your personal health, healing and happiness programme

One of the key differences between the approach of Western medicine and that of integrated medicine is that with the latter the recommendations and suggestions are tailored to you as an individual. The personalisation is vitally important if you are to achieve lasting health and happiness. This is clearly illustrated by the example of the varying approaches to the treatment of depression.

The traditional medical model says that depression is caused by a biochemical imbalance and that the solution, once an individual has been 'diagnosed' with depression, is to treat that person with medication (although the evidence for effectiveness of antidepressants in treating people with mild to moderate depression is unconvincing) and/or talking therapy such as Cognitive Behavioural Therapy (CBT). At one level this all sounds good – the doctor makes the diagnosis and you get the appropriate treatment. However, from an integrated medicine perspective depression is not a diagnosis, but a label to describe someone who has a certain pattern of body, mind and behavioural symptoms. The label – depression – tells us nothing about what is causing the depression or what is preventing the person from recovering from it.

CASE STUDY

Three patients of mine, Marcia, Stella and Jane, came to see me for help with their depression. After consulting with them and arranging the appropriate assessments and investigations, it became clear that each of them had a very different reason for experiencing depression. Marcia's depression was related to a combination of blood-sugar imbalances and hypothyroidism. Stella was experiencing a 'hole in the soul', the chronic low-grade depression associated with untreated addictions and codependency (blocked emotional and psychological development due to early childhood trauma). Jane's depression was related to the loss of meaning and purpose following her retirement from a job that she'd done for 40 years.

Here were three women with seemingly the same problem – depression – but they needed three very different solutions. The solution for Marcia was to avoid sugar and caffeine, and to start taking some supplements to balance her blood-sugar levels and support her thyroid and adrenal function. I also taught her some basic stress reduction techniques, including mindfulness meditation and guided imagery. Her depression lifted within four weeks and stayed away.

Stella's route to health was much more challenging. It involved her committing to an addiction recovery programme which included nutritional repair work; emotional healing; attending a 12-step programme; learning how to create healthy physical, emotional, intellectual and spiritual boundaries; and being taught a variety of stress reduction techniques. Stella's depression took six months to lift, but because she had the courage to face reality and do the necessary inner recovery work she is now living an incredibly rich and meaningful life. She describes her depression and addictions as the gift that brought her home to her true, authentic self.

The approach I took with Jane was again completely different. Her recovery involved her identifying what her values were and using them as a compass in deciding what actions and activities to follow. Within a couple of weeks she was training in aromatherapy (something she had always wanted to do), volunteering at a local charity shop, and practising mindfulness and compassionate self-acceptance throughout the day. Her depression lifted in two weeks and since that time, like the other two patients, she has gone on to create a healthy and fulfilling life.

Getting to the heart of the problem, and then using our heart and head to guide us in our decisions and actions, is what integrated medicine aspires to facilitate with women, men, children, families and communities.

In this section I show you how you can create your own personalised health, healing and happiness programme. However, please note that:

- If you are reading this book to learn how to create higher levels of health and happiness you will just need to follow steps one and two (pages 16–26)

- If you have a specific health problem that you want to treat and resolve you should follow steps one to three (pages 16–36)

Step 1 – Create Your Foundation Programme This involves completing five self-assessment questionnaires, each of which relates to one of the five secrets of health, healing and happiness. I regard each of these as the building blocks of good health and happiness.

Step 2 – Become Your Own Detective Part of my work as an integrated medical doctor is to help you identify the principal barriers that are preventing you from reaching your full potential for health and happiness. While there are many, including those covered in step one, I find in my own medical practice that there are seven barriers that are frequently missed, but which are, in fact, relatively common. I have provided a questionnaire for each of them and I encourage you to complete them all.

Step 3 – Maximise Your Healing and Recovery Having completed steps one and two, and prior to following the instructions for the specific health problem that you have, I strongly encourage you to read through the advice that I have provided in this step. It shows you how to enhance your recovery from a specific illness using an integrated medicine approach.

At this point I do want to emphasise that if you are at all unsure as to the cause of your symptoms, are overwhelmed, confused or experiencing a number of different health problems, it is much safer and effective to work with an integrated medical doctor or a combination of health professionals, such as a GP and nutritional therapist. Because supplements can interact with drugs and also occasionally interfere with medical treatment, it's important that you follow my recommendations, particularly where I ask you to check with you own doctor. In addition, you can check yourself for any possible adverse interactions between drugs and supplements – see www.wholehealthmd.com.

Create your personalised programme

Step 1 • Create your foundation programme

Each of the following questionnaires relates to one of the five secrets in part two and will help you identify the secrets that are most relevant to you. As you go through the questionnaires give yourself plenty of time and try not to rush your answers. Breathing deeply and slowly will help you to get in touch with the truth of the situation. Having completed the questionnaires, fill in the score table.

QUESTIONNAIRE ONE: Nurture your physical body

---

no = 0, occasionally = 1, yes = 2

Do you:

- Feel that your diet is in any way negatively affecting your health and energy levels? ☐

- Suffer from insomnia or get less than eight hours of quality sleep most nights? ☐

- Exercise or keep physically active for less than 30 minutes most days? ☐

- Love eating sweet foods or experience cravings for sugar and/or carbs? ☐
- Use food to change the way you feel? ☐
- Ignore certain aspects of your health and wellbeing? ☐
- Abuse or neglect your physical body? ☐
- Expose yourself to toxic personal care products or household products? ☐

Total score ☐

QUESTIONNAIRE TWO: De-stress and relax

no = 0, occasionally = 1, yes = 2

Do you:

- Feel stressed most of the time? ☐
- Find it hard to cope with stressful situations? ☐
- Find it hard not to worry about things? ☐
- Struggle to manage your stress? ☐
- Find it difficult to relax and enjoy life? ☐
- Think or know that stress is negatively affecting your health or life? ☐
- Manage stress through the use of food, drink, smoking, gambling, drugs or sex? ☐
- Get easily irritated, depressed, upset and/or anxious? ☐

Total score ☐

QUESTIONNAIRE THREE: Face and embrace your emotions

no = 0, occasionally = 1, yes = 2

Do you:

- Feel that you in any way repress, suppress, deny or control your emotions?

- Feel numb or emotionally neutral?

- Have a history of trauma, abuse, neglect, hurt or heartbreak?

- Deny your anger or get back at others using passive-aggressive tactics?

- Hold on to resentments?

- Find that fear holds you back from living life fully?

- Get overwhelmed by your emotions?

- Find it hard or uncomfortable to be emotionally vulnerable and honest?

Total score

QUESTIONNAIRE FOUR: Accept yourself

no = 0, occasionally = 1, yes = 2

Do you:

- Have a strong inner judge – an internal voice that gives you a hard time?

- Push yourself hard?

- Have a strong perfectionist personality?

- Know that you are, or have you been told that you are, overly controlling?

- Dislike or disapprove of yourself in any way?

- Fail to completely appreciate your inner beauty and preciousness? ☐
- Tell yourself that you should be different to how you are? ☐
- Judge others or compare yourself to others? ☐

Total score ☐

QUESTIONNAIRE FIVE: Develop and deepen your relationships

no = 0, occasionally = 1, yes = 2

Do you:

- Have few friends? ☐
- Lack someone that you can be completely open and honest with? ☐
- Feel disconnected from yourself and others? ☐
- Deliberately avoid or feel uncomfortable in social situations? ☐
- Struggle to receive and experience compliments and love? ☐
- Tend to keep your guard up and reveal little about yourself to people you know? ☐
- Think that your relationship with your partner could be better? ☐
- Feel uncomfortable talking about issues to do with intimacy and love? ☐

Total score ☐

Score chart

Having completed the questionnaires, the next step is to transfer your scores to the chart below or, if you prefer, to a notebook or journal. A score of six or more on any questionnaire suggests that you would benefit from reading about the related secret, but, as I've said before, I would like you to make yourself familiar with all five secrets. Even if you scored low on the questionnaire related to a secret you may feel intuitively drawn to it and you should trust your intuition.

Secret		Your score
One:	Nurture Your Physical Body	☐
Two:	De-Stress and Relax	☐
Three:	Face and Embrace Your Emotions	☐
Four:	Accept Yourself	☐
Five:	Develop and Deepen Your Relationships	☐

Step 2 • Become your own detective

Having discovered which of the five secrets are particularly relevant to you, the next step is to identify if any of the following health problems or imbalances are restricting your health and level of happiness. In my experience most people with chronic health problems have at least two that are relevant. If you score highly on any of these questionnaires, read parts two and three first, then turn to the relevant section in part five of the book.

Are you depressed?

During the last month, have you often:

- Felt down, depressed or hopeless? ☐
- Had little interest or pleasure in doing things? ☐
- Experienced fatigue or low energy? ☐

If you have experienced at least one of these, most days, most of the time, for at least two weeks, then depression might be contributing to your symptoms. For more information see page 316.

Do you have metabolic syndrome?

no = 0, occasionally = 1, yes = 2

Do you:

- Struggle with your weight despite watching what you eat?

- Experience forgetfulness, poor memory or mental confusion, particularly after eating?

- Store most of your body fat around your middle?

- Crave sugary or starchy foods?

- Have a waist size of more than 86cm (34in)? (give yourself a score of 6 here)

- Experience drowsiness or a drop in energy or mood after meals?

- Regularly feel tired, despite having had a good night's sleep?

- Have high blood pressure or high cholesterol?

- Have a history of early heart disease or diabetes in your family?

Total score

A score of six or more suggests that you might have metabolic syndrome, a condition associated with an increased risk of diabetes, cancer and heart disease. For more information see page 368.

Food intolerances

no = 0, occasionally = 1, yes = 2

Do you:

- Currently suffer from ear infections, eczema or asthma or had these, colic or glue ear as a child?

- Experience excess mucus or catarrh formation in the throat, nose or sinuses? ☐

- Have cravings for certain foods, such as chocolate, cheese or doughy foods? ☐

- Experience irritable bowel syndrome? ☐

- Suffer from migraines or regular headaches? ☐

- Have recurrent, unexplained symptoms? ☐

- Have fluid retention? ☐

- Have dark circles under your eyes and/or facial puffiness? ☐

- Feel lethargic soon after eating? ☐

Total score ☐

A score of six or more suggests that your symptoms might be related to food intolerances. For more information see page 344.

Adrenal fatigue

no = 0, occasionally = 1, yes = 2

Do you:

- Experience light-headedness on standing? ☐

- Feel more awake at night? ☐

- Crave salty food, sugar or liquorice? ☐

- Feel stressed, restless, overwhelmed and/or exhausted? ☐

- Tremble when under stress? ☐

- Have dark circles under your eyes or your eyes are sensitive to bright lights? ☐

- Spend the whole day rushing from one thing to another? ☐

- Experience anxiety, irritability, nervousness, phobias or panic attacks? ☐

- Get absent-minded or feel that your short-term memory lets you down? ☐
- Keep yourself going on sugar, caffeine and/or nicotine? ☐

Total score ☐

A score of six or more suggests that your symptoms might be related to adrenal fatigue. For more information see page 267.

Addictions

no = 0, occasionally = 1, yes = 2

Do you:

- Have an addiction? (give yourself a score of 6 here) ☐

- Find that your tolerance for a particular substance, substances or activity (food, drink, drug, sex, gambling, taking care of others, obsessing, smoking) is increasing? ☐

- Become unsettled at the thought of not being able to have the substance(s) or activity, if I told you that you couldn't have it or them? ☐

- Find yourself giving up or reducing important social, occupational, or recreational activities because of this substance(s) or activity? ☐

- Continue with the substance(s) or activity despite the knowledge that a persistent or recurrent physical or psychological problem is likely to be caused or exacerbated by it? ☐

- Have a persistent desire or a history of unsuccessful attempts to cut down or to control a particular substance(s) or activity? ☐

- Become jittery or anxious without a coffee, cigarette or something sweet? ☐

- Smoke cigarettes? □

- Experience withdrawal symptoms from the substance(s) or activity? □

Total score □

A score of six or more suggests that your symptoms might be related to undiagnosed or untreated addictions. For more information see page 260.

Codependency

no = 0, occasionally = 1, yes = 2

Do you:

- Tend to assume responsibility for other people's feelings and/or behaviours? □

- Have difficulty in identifying what feelings you are experiencing? □

- Have difficulty expressing your feelings? □

- Have difficulty establishing intimacy in your relationships? □

- Feel uncomfortable receiving praise, gifts or affection? □

- Rarely ask others to meet your needs and wants? □

- Fear rejection? □

- Judge yourself harshly and/or are you a perfectionist? □

- Have difficulty making decisions? □

- Tend to put other people's wants and needs before your own? □

- Tend to value other people's opinions more than your own? □

- Get your feelings of worth from other people's opinions and/or by what you do? □

- Find it difficult to be vulnerable and ask for help? □

- Try to be in control of your feelings and the situations that you are in? □

- Need to be in relationships in which you feel needed?

- Do you suppress your thoughts or feelings only to 'explode' in anger later? □

- Do you feel rejected or angry when another person does not want your help? □

Total score □

A score of 12 or more suggests that your happiness and emotional health might be limited due to the presence of codependency. For more information see page 307.

Dysbiosis

no = 0, occasionally = 1, yes = 2

Do you:

- Have any food allergies or intolerances? □

- Have constipation or diarrhoea? □

- Experience indigestion? □

- Experience digestive problems, such as wind, bloating or irregular bowels? □

- Have or suspect that you have candida and/or parasites? □

- Feel tired and fatigued for no apparent reason? □

- Have unexplained skin rashes, joint pain, headaches and/or foggy thinking? □

- Have bad breath? □

Total score □

A score of six or more suggests that your symptoms might be related to dysbiosis (an imbalance of the bacteria in the gut). For more information see page 334.

Step 3 • Maximise your healing and recovery

The following recommendations are designed to support you to do everything you can to successfully recover from a particular health problem.

Identify the level of healing that you are focused on

When working with my patients I find it extremely useful for both my patients and I to talk about the three levels of healing. I do this because it helps us to agree on our aims. Having a clear intention – one that is revisited and tuned into every day – provides the firm foundations, energy and direction for making the necessary changes to the body, mind, heart and soul for whole-person healing. I find that the majority of women coming to me for help and guidance wish to work at one of the three levels of healing.

Level One is driven by the intention to remove symptoms using natural approaches (usually as quickly as possible). This is usually done either as a complement to, or as an alternative to, Western medicine. About 20 per cent of my patients come to me at this level of healing. An example of this was a patient called Tracy, who wanted nothing more than for me to recommend some supplements and herbs for her to take in order to treat and eliminate her PMS symptoms.

Level Two is driven by the intention to get to the heart of what is causing the symptoms and then follow an integrated holistic health programme to address those issues. About 30 per cent of my patients come to me at this level. Amanda also had PMS but, in contrast to Tracy, was keen and willing to delve deeper. In doing so we identified stress, undiagnosed anxiety and unhealthy eating habits as contributors to her symptoms. Her programme involved a combination of self-acceptance mind training, stress reduction exercises, supplements and herbs, and a healthy eating programme.

Level Three is driven by the intention and commitment to use the experience of illness as an invitation to grow emotionally and spiritually. This accounts for about 50 per cent of my patients. This level of work is focused on reconnecting to what I refer to as the true self – the wellspring of joy, aliveness and inspiration that resides at the heart of our being. This spiritually focused work involves a number of integrated approaches, including mindfulness (bringing awareness to the present moment), compassionate self-acceptance (cultivating an attitude of loving kindness to yourself no matter what), facing reality (looking at the facts of your total life situation as they are) and emotional release work (releasing trauma and unprocessed emotions from the bodymind, the entity that is mind and body).

It's challenging work, but the rewards are considerable. A good example of this was Gwendoline who, like Tracy and Amanda, had moderately severe PMS symptoms. Gwendoline was able to see how her symptoms reflected the disharmony that she had in relationship to herself, her partner and indeed to life itself. By using her illness as an invitation to re-assess her life and priorities, using some of the approaches I mentioned above, she not only experienced complete relief of her symptoms, but she emerged from the experience a more enlightened and 'authentic' person.

What differentiates levels two and three from level one is that someone who is working with their symptoms at level one will return to the same patterns of being, living, eating and relating that created the health challenge in the first place. Their level of consciousness remains the same and no shifts in perspective take place. Someone working at level two will usually change the way they live their life not only to ensure that the symptoms don't come back, but also to experience a much higher level of health and wellbeing. Someone working at level three will almost always experience a shift in consciousness and emerge from the illness as someone who is much more in touch with their authentic self, and more equipped to bring their unique gifts and talents into the world. For individuals working at level three, illness (or indeed a major life challenge) can trigger a whole new way of being and living rooted in heartfelt values, self-awareness and self-acceptance. It is a privilege to witness the transformation that occurs at level three.

While level three healing sounds better than levels two and one, each of these levels of healing is neither better nor worse than the other; they are simply what they are. Before you decide which level is appropriate for you, I encourage you to be clear about why you are doing what you are doing, what your intentions are and also to be open to the possibility that a deep experience of transformation is available to you, one that can help you thrive and flourish as you walk your unique path to health, healing and happiness.

Create and embody your intention

Once I know which level of healing my patients are focused on, I invite them to consider the following questions, which I would like you to answer too:

- What is it you want to achieve?

- Are you looking to reduce or eliminate your symptoms?

- Are you hoping to identify the roots of your health or life challenges?

- Are you looking to make positive changes in your health, life and/or relationships? Are you looking for more balance or fulfilment?

- Are you on a spiritual quest – a search for your true self?

- Are you looking for a cure?

- Are you looking for an alternative to conventional medicine or a complement?

Once my patients have clarified their intention I invite them to write it down and then, at the start of each day, for a minimum of two weeks, to do the following exercise.

EXERCISE: Embody your intention

Upon waking up in the morning, or whenever you can, spend a couple of minutes focusing on everything that you have to be grateful for, allow those feelings to build and become strong inside you.

When you sense that you are filled with gratitude, focus on your intention and say it aloud once, as though it is already happening. So, for example, rather than saying, 'I am getting better and healing' you would say 'I am whole, healthy and healed.'

Now imagine, see or feel the words of your intention moving to the area where your physical heart is. Breathe into that area and allow the vibration or essence of that intention to move throughout your body. Embody your intention. Once you can really feel this, focus on the day ahead and infuse that day with your intention. Continue with this until you feel it is done.

Many of my patients regard this very simple exercise as one of the keys to their recovery or achieving their health and life goals, because it keeps their choices and actions connected to their intention. The key is to repeat it every day, otherwise it wears off. I invite you to put it to the test by trying the exercise for a couple of weeks.

Make healthy self-care a priority

Healthy self-care – the intuitive, ongoing process of taking care of your health and self – is at the heart of good health. It's about being in tune with the wisdom of your bodymind, in which your thoughts and emotions are in constant dialogue with your physical body, and responding in an appropriate way to the messages it provides. For example, a patient of mine, Denise, was so caught up in the toxic combination of excessive worrying and busyness she was simply not in touch with her bodymind's need to rest and eat healthy foods. By the time she finished her day at 8pm and sat down in front of the TV, she felt absolutely exhausted and starving.

Another patient of mine, Sandra, a mother of four, rushed around all day tending to the needs of her children and husband, at the expense of her own needs. This inevitably led to adrenal fatigue, sleep deprivation and high levels of stress. Another patient, Florence, ignored the feelings of heaviness and aching in her breast for two years. With some reluctance she eventually went for some tests, which confirmed that she had breast cancer.

So what would have provided Denise and Sandra with a solution to their predicament? What could have prevented Florence's breast cancer from advancing? One answer is healthy self-care. If they had been willing to acknowledge and respond appropriately to the early, subtle warning signs of bodymind distress – Denise by taking regular breaks and seeking help for her compulsive busyness and worrying; Sandra by eating at meal times, having time to herself and getting as much sleep as she could; and Florence by seeking medical help earlier on – I'm convinced that they could not only have prevented their respective distress and disease, but that they would now be experiencing greater levels of health than they actually are.

Become knowledgeable about your disease

One of the challenges faced by anyone with a health issue, whether high blood pressure, pain, endometriosis or cancer, is the fact that whatever advice your health professional shares with you is their perspective, not 'the truth'. This is really important to acknowledge. When a medical doctor tells you that the only treatment available for your back is painkillers or surgery, what she is really saying is that, according to her experience, beliefs and training, the only things conventional medicine has to offer you are painkillers or surgery. Her recommendations don't take into account the many other approaches that might help, from osteopathy and the herb devil's claw, to acupuncture, the Alexander technique and microcurrent therapy devices.

In a nutshell, when you go to your doctor you will only ever get a medical perspective. When you go to a nutritional therapist you'll get a nutritional perspective, and so on. These are valid and important views, but ultimately incomplete. Because of that, and to fill in the gaps, I encourage my patients to read about their disease and to research different approaches, although it's important to strike a balance, as too much information can be overwhelming. See Resources for details of websites and books that I recommend.

Create a support team

One of the most significant factors in a healthy and happy life is the existence of a network of people – professionals, friends and family – who support you and to whom you feel connected. I explore this in some detail in Develop and Deepen Your Relationships (see page 127), but essentially many patients find that it is important to surround themselves with life-affirming people, while also limiting their exposure to life-denying people (this is particularly important for those dealing with life-threatening illnesses such as cancer). Of course, this is easier said than done, but it can make a difference to your healing and mood.

I do appreciate that you may not always have a choice, but whenever possible find a health professional who is positive, caring and open-minded enough to support your exploration of holistic approaches. Having such a practitioner or team of practitioners on your side can make such a difference, particularly if you are facing a serious illness.

Illness as teacher

I have seen in my own medical practice how many health and life experiences, especially those that we experience as significant, *can* provide a wake-up call that causes us to re-evaluate the meaning of our life and the way we live it. Although this is certainly not the case for everyone, when the experience of illness is viewed as an opportunity to learn and grow, that shift in attitude, from perceiving illness as an adversary to seeing it as a friend, can trigger an awakening in which previously dormant talents, gifts and insights begin emerging from within. If you have the courage to take charge of your health and life, along with a willingness to learn how to deal effectively with distressing feelings and start living according to what is most meaningful to you, you can really thrive and flourish, especially if you are well supported.

Watch out for your blind spots

One of the biggest barriers to overcoming any health problem is focusing on a particular aspect of your life, such as diet, supplements or exercise, to the exclusion of the areas that really need to be attended to, for example, stress, trauma, relationships or lack of meaning in life. As humans we have an inbuilt tendency to avoid those areas of our life that cause us distress. In other words, we turn a blind eye to things that are often blindingly obvious to others.

An example of this is Marjorie, who came to me with a long history of abdominal pain and bloating. She was taking over 12 supplements and had tried more than five types of diet in an attempt to 'correct the problem'. Now as a general rule of thumb (and the exception is if the person is under the care of a nutritional therapist) if someone is taking five or more supplements I have a strong suspicion that stress or some emotion-related situation is at play. After talking to Marjorie for 20 minutes it became apparent what was at the heart of her symptoms – her stress at being in an emotionally abusive relationship with her husband, her spiralling debts, a lack of emotional management skills and her very strong inner judge. We put together a programme to address these and within three months her pain disappeared and she started experiencing much more joy and fulfilment in her life. She left her husband, started a debt reduction self-help programme, and learnt some emotional processing skills and how to reduce the power that her inner judge had over her.

In contrast to this, some people, especially those with a strong spiritual belief system, have a tendency to put everything down to emotions, but fail to acknowledge the role that toxicity, nutritional deficiencies, poor diet and lack of exercise can have in ill-health. It's all about balance and seeing the bigger picture.

Explore the complementary and self-help options

If you go to a doctor with a particular health problem, it's unlikely that they will recommend any complementary or self-help approaches, usually because they know very little about them. Personally I am all for exploring complementary and alternative medicine (CAM) as a means of either enhancing the effectiveness of conventional medical treatment or as a safer alternative. Of course, working out which approach is best for you is not that straightforward. Having asked my own patients how they select CAM I have concluded that most people either use a head- or heart-based approach.

The head-based approach looks at the evidence relating to a particular complementary medicine's effectiveness, as well as cost factors and the experience of the practitioner. If you went down this route you might, for example, take St John's wort for depression, use acupuncture to help relieve nausea, meditation for anxiety, osteopathy for acute back pain and massage for chronic non-specific back pain.

The heart-based approach is very different and tends to focus on trying approaches that *feel* right or whose principles resonate with your own values and beliefs. For example, you might be drawn to Reiki or some other form of healing approach because you believe in the principle of universal energy or *qi*. Other people are passionate proponents of homeopathy or traditional Chinese medicine (see Resources).

My advice to my patients and to you is to use your head *and* heart when deciding on which CAM approaches to take, and if at all possible work with an integrated medical doctor or team who can support you in your decisions. This is particularly important if you are treating serious diseases such as cancer. My advice on CAM is to know what you are treating, so always get an accurate diagnosis. Research the different CAM options (see Resources), tell your GP if you want to use CAM and if possible get a recommendation-based referral to a CAM practitioner. Speak to them beforehand to make sure you feel comfortable with them and that they are going to be able to help you, and make sure that your CAM approach, supplements or self-help don't interfere with any medical drugs you might be taking. To check for interactions between supplements, herbs and medications please see Resources.

Keep things simple and realistic

One of the reasons my own patients sometimes fail to make the necessary changes in their life is because they, and I, sometimes over-complicate things, either by trying to do too much too soon or by not taking time to focus on what is most important. For example, a patient consulted with me about five years ago with chronic fatigue syndrome. In my over-enthusiasm to help her I started her on five different supplements, a special diet, a programme of mindfulness training (a type of meditation), exercises for emotional release, guided imagery and gratitude. While all of these are an important part of my programme I simply overloaded her with information and 'things' to do. Within two days she was on the phone feeling completely overwhelmed. I learnt a big lesson that day, and one of the most important factors in healing and recovery is to agree on a manageable level of approaches that, wherever possible, fit into the existing routine. Put another way, I learnt how important it is to keep things simple. Now, and this comes with experience, I usually recommend a maximum of two, maybe three, emotional or psychological exercises to do at any one time and I alter them when appropriate to stop boredom creeping in, as well as in response to the patient's progress.

My advice is to be easy on yourself and to keep things simple. For example, if you are going to improve your diet, rather than completely overhauling it by throwing out all processed foods and eating only vegetables, fruits and rice (and then probably reverting back to your old diet within a few days or weeks), start by increasing your intake of fruit to two portions a day during the first week and then in the second week halve the number of chocolate bars and desserts you eat. Of course, some people do best with more dramatic approaches, but my point is that you should do whatever is realistically going to help you achieve your goals. When we are unrealistic and end up faltering, it only proves to our inner judge that we can't do it and that we are a failure. It becomes a self-fulfilling prophecy.

Keep a journal

I'm a big fan of journaling (yes, I know it sounds very American, but it's the easiest way to describe it!). Journaling is one of the most potent tools that I teach my patients. It can be used to off-load worries, vent emotions and thoughts, gather insights into challenging situations and help you to process events and experiences from the past and present. I find journaling is one of the most important contributing factors in the recovery of patients with emotionally induced illness and for supporting personal growth and development. If you are new to it don't worry about getting it right, just go easy on yourself and you will soon get into a way of journaling that feels right for you. Here are some suggestions to get you started:

- Most people find that a personal diary dedicated to journaling is ideal. It should be for your own eyes only and kept with you wherever you go. This allows you to record insights as they come up.

- It doesn't matter what you write, how you write it or whether it's grammatically correct or punctuated; anything you write is an expression of your reality. Try not to judge what you write. If you find yourself judging yourself take a look at secret four – Accept Yourself.

- Try writing in your journal at least once a day. This might be on waking up or just before you go to bed. Discover what works for you.

There are no strict guidelines for what you do and don't write, but in the early days it's a good idea to stick to some kind of format until you've found out what works for you. The things you can include are:

- The key events of the day

- How you feel about a certain issue that happened to you

- Any thoughts, insights or new perspectives that you have had

Get committed

I was once asked in an interview what I thought was the key to creating lasting health and happiness. My response was unequivocal – commitment. In my experience, if someone doesn't prioritise their health, isn't really committed to their health and happiness, *and* isn't addressing their own personal barriers to commitment, the likelihood of them succeeding in achieving their health and life goals is greatly diminished. While most people tend to start out with good intentions, after a couple of days and weeks, old habits kick in, the new way of living grinds to a halt and they are back where they started. Is this your experience? The reason why wholehearted commitment is so important is because the act of committing to whatever it is you desire taps into the resources, energy, clarity, motivation and insight that helps you to achieve your goals. By committing to your health and happiness, and addressing the barriers to that commitment, you access the inner power that will help make your desires a reality.

Prior to starting your health, healing and happiness programme, write down with absolute honesty the likely factors that will come between you and your goals. This might, for example, include fear, getting distracted, forgetting to take supplements, low energy levels, habits and so on. Having written them down, write next to them what proactive action you can take to address them. If you get stuck ask a friend for help. Doing this can really make a difference to your ability to stay on track.

Go with the flow

As things change – your health, circumstances, life situation and so on – re-evaluate what you are doing and why you are doing it. Any health, healing and happiness programme should have flexibility built into it, enabling you to address the demands that are being placed on you. For example, you might start your health programme by focusing on reducing stress. Then, after a couple of months, once you're feeling relatively stress free, it might be appropriate to focus on a certain difficult relationship or to consider the possibility of changing your job or work role. If you follow the guidelines in secrets one, two and, in particular, three you will become increasingly sensitive and attuned to what you need physically and emotionally. You will naturally feel uncomfortable watching certain types of TV programme or eating certain types of food. You might be much more sensitive to certain environments or people. Acknowledging this and taking action to meet your needs is an important part of the process of emerging more fully into your potential.

SUMMARY

- Labelling your symptoms as a specific disease rarely tells you what is actually causing or contributing to your symptoms.

- For optimum health it is more important to discover what is preventing you from fulfilling your health and happiness potential. The personalised approach, in which you identify and address your unique barriers to health and healing, is at the heart of integrated medicine.

- Regardless of whether you have a specific health problem or wish to improve your health and happiness, deciding which of the five secrets is relevant to you is vital to building a healthier and happier life.

- If you have a particular health problem you can enhance your chances of making a full and deep recovery by identifying which level of healing you are focused on, creating your intention and then embodying it at the start of every day, making sure you have a team of supportive people around you and by becoming an expert in your own disease. Keep things as simple as you can and remember that commitment is the key to success.

Part Two

~

The five secrets of health, healing and happiness

In this section I provide you with what I consider to be the five most important secrets or foundations upon which health, healing and happiness are created. Following these will not only help you enjoy better energy and wellbeing, and help prevent future health problems, but they will also support your recovery from any illness that you currently have. It is my experience that most diseases and health problems will improve just by making positive changes to your diet, getting regular physical activity, restful sleep, managing your stress and learning how to be easier on yourself.

My five secrets to health, healing and happiness are:

Secret One   Nurture Your Physical Body
Secret Two   De-Stress and Relax
Secret Three   Face and Embrace Your Emotions
Secret Four   Accept Yourself
Secret Five   Develop and Deepen Your Relationships

I suggest you read all the secrets; although you may not think all of them are necessarily relevant to you, you may just discover something revelatory. And if you haven't done so already I encourage you to fill in the questionnaires in part one, section two, as they will help guide you to the secrets that are most appropriate to you.

Secret One
Nurture your physical body

How well do you take care of your body? Do you nourish it daily with high-vitality foods such as fresh fruits, vegetables and whole grains, or do you tend to fill up on sugary, processed foods and snacks? Do you keep your body hydrated with plenty of fresh water, or pour in copious amounts of caffeine and alcohol? Do you exercise your body daily and keep yourself fit and well toned, or are you carrying excess fat around your middle? Are you in tune with the messages and rhythms of your body, or do you feel detached from your body? Overall, do you accept, honour and nurture your body or do you abuse and neglect it?

If you are like most women, the chances are high that you will say yes to the latter. Failing to nurture and take care of the physical body is at epidemic levels in Western society: 21 per cent of women smoke, 7 per cent of women have used illicit drugs in the last year and 13 per cent of women regularly drink over the recommended weekly alcohol limit of 14 units per week.[1] While most women know that they need to eat a minimum of five portions of fruit and vegetables each day, on average most women manage just 2.7 servings.[2] Women, like men, are piling on weight. During the last 25 years, the rate of obesity has quadrupled in the UK. In England alone, 25 per cent of women were classified as clinically obese in 2005 and 32 per cent of women were overweight.[3]

It's not just what you do to your body that counts, it's also about how you feel about your body. For example, one survey found that women are up to ten times more likely than men to be unhappy with their body image.[4] Another survey found that 66 per cent of women felt depressed about the shape and size of their body.[5]

CASE STUDY

Mary-Anne, a 38-year-old mother of two children, came to me for guidance on how to resolve her tiredness. Like many mothers, Mary-Anne's attention and energy was focused on taking care of her children, who were aged one and three. Unlike most mothers, however, Mary-Anne was completely lost in the role of motherhood and was neglecting to take care of herself. Although she was looking for a supplement to 'fix the tiredness', I explained to her that to feel better (and prevent future health problems) she must make her own health and wellbeing a priority, and that the best way to do this was to take care of the body's basic needs – sleep, rest, physical activity, relaxation, healthy diet, sunlight and a healthy environment.

While making changes for her was not easy or straightforward, within four months she had introduced a new routine which meant that she always sat down to eat at meal times, rather than snacking on the go, she swapped chocolate and crisps for fruit and wholegrain snacks, she had started to ask for help and support with the children, which she had not done previously, and she took time to rest and sleep whenever she could. By prioritising the care of her physical body, and intuitively responding to its need for food, rest, sleep and exercise she found that she was able to deal with the demands of motherhood so much more effectively and without losing sight of herself.

So why are the majority of women failing to consistently nurture and take care of their physical bodies? In a nutshell, it comes back to what I said in part one; that most women are failing to cope with the physical, psychological and social demands being placed upon them and this stress results in them returning to their default settings of putting others – and other priorities – before their own self-care. For most this means getting inadequate amounts of sleep and rest, failing to get enough exercise, eating foods that promote disease and inhibit health and healing, and exposing themselves unnecessarily to toxic chemicals.

Get the basics right

Good health and happiness is built on the foundations of adequate sleep and rest, healthy eating, daily physical activity and living in a healthy, low toxicity environment. In addition to this I would also add preventative healthcare, such as having regular medical check-ups with your doctor or nurse; knowing about illnesses that are common to your family; stopping smoking; maintaining your optimum weight; receiving appropriate immunisations; getting pre-conception advice; knowing your cholesterol, homocysteine and blood pressure measurements; and brushing your teeth twice a day and seeing a dental hygienist every six months. I continue to be amazed at how symptoms such as fatigue, skin rashes, pain, bloating, headaches and even depression resolve when my patients start to nurture and take care of their physical bodies.

The following mini-questionnaires are designed to help you identify which of the following physical needs you should be attending to. If you answer yes to one or more of the questions within each of the four categories then I strongly encourage you to follow my suggestions on that particular topic (these begin on page 45).

PHYSICAL NEEDS QUESTIONNAIRES

Physical need 1 – rest and sleep

- Do you sleep less than seven hours a night on more than three nights a week?

- Do you feel that you are sleep deprived in any way?

- Do you rarely take time to just sit and do nothing?

- Do you feel tired most of the time?

- To you ever nod off when driving? ☐
- Do you drink alcohol on most evenings? ☐
- Do you have insomnia? ☐

Physical need 2 – healthy diet

- Do you eat less than five servings of fruit and vegetables a day? ☐
- Do you feel that your diet is in any way negatively impacting on your health? ☐
- Do you eat sugary snacks more than once a day? ☐
- Do you have cravings for certain foods? ☐
- Do your energy levels dip at certain times of the day? ☐
- Do you eat more processed food than fresh food? ☐
- Are you overweight or obese? ☐

Physical need 3 – physical activity and touch

- Do you get less than two and a half hours a week of aerobic exercise? ☐
- Do you tend to avoid or have an aversion to physical activity or exercise? ☐
- Are you overweight or obese? ☐
- Do you rarely do strength training exercises or flexibility exercises? ☐
- Do you feel that your lack of physical activity is in any way negatively impacting on your health? ☐
- Do close friends or family tell you that you should exercise more? ☐
- Do you have any chronic health problems, such as heart disease or depression? ☐

Physical need 4 – healthy environment and sunlight

- Do you use non low-toxicity household cleaning materials? ☐

- Do you smoke? ☐

- Do you drink chlorinated and/or fluoridated tap water? ☐

- Do you have an alarm clock radio next to your bed or an electrical blanket under it? ☐

- Do you spend most of your time indoors? ☐

- Do you have a weakened immune system? ☐

- Do you suffer from a change in mood during the months prior to and immediately after winter? ☐

Rest and sleep

When I explain the concept of rest to my patients I tend to get a lot of puzzled looks because it's such as foreign concept to most people. Rest is simply not-doing; it's a passive state of open receptivity to what is, ideally, in an environment of low or zero stimulation. Unlike relaxation (which I cover in secret two), which is an active process designed to trigger the relaxation response in the body, rest is passive. For example, if I look out of the window and just sit without thinking about anything in particular I am resting. If I sit in a coffee shop and get engrossed in a good novel then I am resting. However, if I watch a TV programme that is highly stimulating or emotionally charged (a couple of prime-time soaps spring to mind), that is not resting as it is overly stimulating, whereas a programme on nature, for example, would be restful. I am sure you get my drift! Resting allows your body to recharge and your mind to refresh itself. Resting is so important because most Western women are expert at 'doing' and not so good at 'being'.

Getting regular quality sleep is also imperative. Sleep is not only as important to your wellbeing as eating a healthy diet and exercising frequently, but you are also so much more likely to exercise, eat healthily, feel emotionally balanced and connect with friends when you are well rested. Deep restorative sleep is absolutely essential to your health and happiness,[6] yet 40 per cent of women get less than seven hours' sleep and 70 per cent of women less than eight hours' sleep on weekdays.[7] Juggling numerous responsibilities, having a baby or young child, hormonal fluctuations, dealing with the stresses and strains of life or having a partner who snores all add to an increased risk of sleepless nights and insomnia. In fact, women are 20 per cent more likely to experience insomnia when compared with men. One investigation by the National Sleep Foundation (NSF) into the sleeping habits of more than 2,000 women aged from 18 to 64 found that almost two-thirds had between one and three disturbed nights every week.[8]

The consequences of inadequate sleep

While most people tend to associate sleep deprivation with feeling tired and cranky, in fact it's a lot more serious than that. Sleep deprivation, which is an acute or chronic lack of sufficient restorative sleep, puts you at a higher risk of developing heart disease and cancer, but it's also been shown to promote weight gain, exacerbate and trigger depression and anxiety, reduce immune function and increase the likelihood of accidents.[9] Sleep deprivation also puts you at much higher risk of making poor health choices and life decisions. For example, one study found that 80 per cent of women managed to fight through the day-time tiredness associated with sleep deprivation by drinking caffeine-rich drinks, with one-third admitting they consumed three or more such drinks every day in an attempt to escape their exhaustion. Half of the women confessed that they will sacrifice exercise and, in addition, more than one-third said they also reduce the amount of time spent with friends and family, stop eating healthily and don't participate in sexual activity when feeling tired. Sleep deprivation affects every level and aspect of your life.[10]

Why women experience insomnia

In addition to juggling responsibilities and dealing with the stresses and strains of modern-day living, one of the reasons that you might be more at risk of insomnia when compared to men is because your sleep is intimately related to hormonal fluctuations. Some women, for example, especially those with PMS, will experience bouts of insomnia just prior to their period. Women going through the perimenopause are also more likely to experience sleeplessness due to hot sweats and feeling uncomfortable. If you've noticed that your sleep has got worse after having a baby, it's probably due to the fact that women (men less so) become more acutely sensitised to the sounds that their baby makes. Unfortunately women tend to retain this heightened sensitivity to night-time noise long after their children have grown up! Studies have also shown that women who have never had children sleep better even in their fifties and sixties than women who have had children.[11]

The integrated medical approach to rest and sleep

While getting more rest and improving the quality and quantity of your sleep will help to reduce your chances of developing the health problems that I mentioned earlier on, improving your sleep increases the likelihood of you taking better care of your health quite dramatically – and that is why I place so much importance on it. If sleep is a problem for you, here are some suggestions to help you:

- **Identify and address the cause of your sleep problem.** For example, is it related to stress, your hormones, your inability to fully relax before bed or your physical environment? Wherever possible take action to address those causes, for example you might want to use blackout blinds in your room to keep it dark, try a stress reduction approach prior to bed or get your partner to sleep in a separate room if they disturb you!

- **Take a natural sleep remedy.** The ones that I use most often with my patients are valerian[12] (follow manufacturer's instructions), melatonin[13] (0.5mg to 3mg), magnesium[14] (500mg) or 5-HTP[15] (100mg to 200mg) at bedtime. Magnesium is particularly helpful if you have restless legs syndrome and 5-HTP is good if you have symptoms of depression or widespread muscular pain.

- **Get physical.** If you don't exercise, try exercising for a minimum of 40 minutes three times a week to help you discharge energy and get to sleep. Try to do this exercise early in the day, otherwise it will stimulate you when you need to be winding down.

- **Rest every day.** Write a list of all the different ways you enjoy resting and commit to taking a period of rest of at least 20 minutes every day.

- **Take a power nap.** Napping for 10 to 20 minutes in the early afternoon has been found to increase energy levels, motivation and improve mood and memory. Research also says that taking a nap of 30 minutes a day is better than sleeping 30 minutes later in the morning.

- **Avoid eating heavy meals.** If you eat just before you go to bed your body will be busy digesting and won't want to go to sleep, so leave a gap of at least two hours between a meal and bed. Avoid caffeine and nicotine late at night, too.

- **Avoid or limit alcohol.** While many insomniacs use alcohol to help them sleep, research shows that alcohol consumption prior to bed results in multiple awakenings, shallow sleep, a reduction in sleep time and a reduction in the overall quality of sleep. If you have problems with sleep my advice is to stay clear of it.

- **Take Vitamin B$_6$.** If you regularly have trouble sleeping just prior to your period, try taking vitamin B$_6$ (100mg at bedtime). This helps to make the calming brain chemical serotonin. Take this with an additional B vitamin complex.

- **Try guided imagery.** I am a big fan of guided imagery, which uses images to achieve specific objectives, and regularly encourage my patients to listen to a guided imagery sleep CD before going to bed. See Resources for details.

- **Watch the temperature of your room.** Keep a slightly cool temperature in the room, as this will help you get to sleep and achieve a deeper level of sleep: 18–21°C (65–70°F) is the ideal temperature.

- **Off-load your stress and worries.** If you have things on your mind, try off-loading them into a journal, talking about them or trying a relaxation technique (see De-stress and Relax, page 77).

- **Create a negative association to waking up.** If you are still awake after 20 minutes of attempting to sleep, get up and do something that you really don't enjoy doing, such as cleaning. This sets up a negative conditioning pattern that associates not sleeping with discomfort. By doing this you are training the brain to help you get to sleep. This method works really well for a lot of people.

- **Use the Alphastim SCS.** This portable medical device sends minute and painless electrical currents called microcurrents into your body via clips attached to the ear lobes. It is particularly effective for insomnia, and also depression and anxiety. I tend to use it with my patients when the above measures don't work. See Resources for details.

- **Use your holistic health tools.** The ones I find most helpful for insomnia are Mindfulness (see page 147), Emotional Freedom Technique (see page 151) and EmoTrance (see page 158).

- **Seek professional help.** If you have insomnia that doesn't respond to the above measures or you experience excessive daytime sleepiness, abrupt awakening during the night accompanied by shortness of breath, a morning headache, or you wake up with a dry mouth or sore throat, then I encourage you to seek the help of a sleep specialist. The latter are symptoms of a serious sleep disorder called sleep apnoea.

Healthy eating and supplements

Every aspect of you – your mood, weight, energy levels, libido, thoughts, sleep, vitality and even IQ – is influenced by the foods that you eat. Not only does eating a healthy diet reduce the likelihood of developing life-threatening diseases such as cancer and heart disease, but it can alleviate depression, reduce the symptoms of menopause and endometriosis, and even increase your level of fertility. One study found that women who consumed 30 grams of fibre a day had half the risk of developing breast cancer when compared to those who ate less than 20 grams.[16] The average woman eats only 12 grams of fibre a day! Switching to a high-fibre breakfast, using wholemeal bread and eating your five fruit and vegetables a day would take your fibre intake up to 30 grams a day. Therefore, the question is really how serious are you about your health and how willing are you to improve your diet? I'm assuming that you are committed to improving your health, otherwise you would not be reading this book, so it's up to me to convince you to adopt what I consider to be healthy eating.

The goal of a healthy eating programme is to provide you with great tasting food that sustains your energy and mood, meets the nutritional and energy requirements of your body, helps you maintain your optimum weight, supports the process of healing and recovery from illness, reduces inflammation, prevents disease and optimises your physical, emotional and psychological potential. In a nutshell, healthy eating helps you thrive and flourish as a human being.

Of course, that all sounds wonderful and straightforward but in practice it's not. While most people think of healthy eating as simply making healthy eating choices, such as eating fruits, vegetables and whole grains, in my experience there are four potential stumbling blocks or barriers to healthy eating that need to be addressed in order to increase the chances of you sticking to a healthy eating programme. They are habits, dieting, eating disorders and emotional eating.

Healthy eating barrier 1 – habit

Most of us have default eating habits. For example, Lorraine, a patient of mine, always had cereal with milk in the morning, a tuna or ham sandwich and yoghurt for lunch, and either pizza, meat and potatoes or fish, chips and vegetables for dinner, usually followed by ice cream or a chocolate bar. When I asked how long she had been eating those foods, she said 15 years! After explaining the importance of variety, not to mention the unhealthy nature of her diet, we used one of the holistic health tools – the Emotional Freedom Technique (see page 151) – to address her habit of eating the same foodstuffs. This worked well and within two weeks she had completely transformed her diet and was able to stick with it, even when under stress. If you tend to eat the same foods repetitively, here's what I suggest:

- Keep a food diary for a week, in which you record everything you eat and at what time of day you eat it. At the end of the week, look at the repeating food choices that you have made.

- Write down a list of why you stick to the same foods, for example habit, unadventurous, you like the taste of them, you're too tired to cook and so on.

- When you are under stress, what do you eat? Write this down.

- Now write down a list of all the possible benefits of eating new foods and adding variety to your diet.

- Now use the Emotional Freedom Technique (EFT) to address your food habits. You'll need to think of a statement phrase to use, so try something such as, 'Even though I always eat Cheerios in the morning, I deeply and completely accept and forgive myself without judgement.' Use EFT with your main food habits and notice how it breaks those habits. If you struggle with this you might want to consider seeing a therapist who is trained in the use of EFT.

Healthy eating barrier II – cravings

A craving is an intense, often uncontrollable desire to have a certain food. They are very common with one study finding that 91 per cent of women experience strong cravings.[17] Most people with cravings experience a degree of tension prior to eating the food, which is then followed by a wave of pleasure and relief as dopamine and other feel-good chemicals get released in response to consuming the object of craving. The key to resolving cravings for food is to address the underlying cause of your craving. In my experience the top causes, which need to be identified and addressed, are

- **Blood-Sugar Imbalance/Insulin Resistance** – see Part Five (Metabolic Syndrome – page 368)

- **Stress** – see Secret Two – De-stress and Relax (page 77)

- **Calorie Restriction** – eat no less than 1000 calories a day as less than this is known to trigger cravings.[18] Most women should eat a minimum of 1200 calories a day

- **PMS Hormonal Swings** – see Part Four (Premenstrual Syndrome – page 172)

- **Sleep Deprivation** – see Secret One – Rest and Sleep (page 45)

- **Eating Disorders** – see healthy eating barrier III (page 52)

- **Food Sensitivity/Intolerance** – see Part Five (Food Intolerances – page 344)

Healthy eating barrier III – eating disorders

In the UK alone 1.1 million people have an eating disorder and up to 20 per cent of women with an eating disorder will die as a result of it.[19] It's a serious problem. If you have any of the following signs relating to three of the most common eating disorders – anorexia nervosa, bulimia and binge eating disorder – then I encourage you to consult the eating disorders website listed in Resources, as you will need professional help.

- **Anorexia Nervosa** affects 1 to 2 per cent of women and is a serious, potentially life-threatening eating disorder characterised by self-starvation and excessive weight loss. Someone with anorexia has an intense fear of weight gain or of becoming fat, despite being underweight. They will have a distorted body image, phobias about food's ability to create fatness and also a resistance to maintaining body weight at or above a minimally normal weight for their age and height. To lose weight and maintain a low body weight the person with anorexia will starve herself, as well as possibly over-exercise and/or purge.

- **Bulimia** affects 1 to 3 per cent of women and involves the regular intake of large amounts of food, accompanied by a sense of loss of control over their eating behaviour; the regular use of inappropriate compensatory behaviours, such as self-induced vomiting, laxative or diuretic abuse, fasting and/or obsessive or compulsive exercise; and an extreme concern with body weight and shape.

- **Binge Eating Disorder** affects about 2 per cent of women and 15 per cent of women who are mildly obese. It involves episodic overeating of large amounts of foods that are perceived to be fattening, the feeling of being out of control, guilt and remorse after eating, obsessive thinking about food and weight, and then attempts to deal with the consequences of overeating by starving, dieting, exercising and weighing.

Eating disorders are whole-person illnesses that require sensitive treatment from experts experienced in the field. As with most illnesses, it's important to address eating disorders from a nutritional, emotional, psychological and spiritual level.

If you have an eating disorder, then you should seek the help of an experienced health professional or team of professionals, consisting, usually, of a nutritional therapist and psychotherapist, counsellor or addiction specialist. See Resources for more details.

Healthy eating barrier IV – emotional eating

Emotional eating refers to the repeated use of food to change the way you feel. Quite simply, emotional eating is using food to sedate and control your feelings; it's rooted in instant gratification and the desire to escape yourself. It's very common, affecting about 80 per cent of my patients. You can have the best of intentions and all the knowledge you need about a healthy diet, but if you use food to manage your stress, it will almost certainly sabotage your healthy eating programme. If you think that you could be an emotional eater, here's what I suggest:

- Starting now and for the next 24 hours, observe your eating patterns without judging yourself

- Notice how you use food to change the way you feel

- Write down a list of your favourite comfort foods, for example bread, chocolate, biscuits

- Write down a list of the events and experiences, thoughts or images that trigger you to eat your comfort foods

- Reflect on the past and work out how long you have been using food in this way

- Write a list of how emotional eating has restricted your life and health

- Read secrets three and four as they will provide you with tools to start managing your emotions more effectively

The integrated medical approach to healthy eating and supplements

What constitutes healthy eating really does depend on you. For example, your level of physical activity, rate of metabolism, lifestyle, life stage, nutrient and hormone levels, and the presence of stress all influence what an optimum diet would be for you. Things like the availability of food, your food preferences, the financial resources that you have available and also the eating habits of your family are also relevant. That said, and without over-complicating things, I find that the majority of my patients will do very well by following my healthy eating advice. If you have a serious health problem such as cancer or if you are pregnant you should consult with a nutritional therapist or integrated medical doctor.

Foods to eat

For the majority of women a diet that is high in nutrient-dense whole-foods, such as fresh fruit, vegetables and whole grains, and low in nutrient-poor processed foods, such as cakes, biscuits, pizzas and crisps, represents a healthy balanced diet. This works for about 80 per cent of my patients. However, for the remaining 20 per cent I often have to change the ratios of carbohydrate, protein and fat. Some women are genetically hardwired to eat a high-protein, high-fat and low-carbohydrate diet, whereas others need a high-carbohydrate, low-fat, low-protein diet. My suggestion is that if after four weeks of following my healthy eating programme you are not satisfied that your diet is meeting your health and energy needs, then take a look at the eating section of my other book, *The Mind–Body Bible*, which goes into this in more detail (see Resources).

Aim for

5–7   free-range, organic eggs per week – pick a brand where the chickens have been fed on flax seeds as these are rich in omega-3 essential fatty acids

3+   servings of green leafy and root vegetables a day, such as broccoli, spinach, kale, sweet potato, bok choy, celery, peppers and green beans

2+   servings of colourful fruits a day, such as apples, pears, plums and berries (fresh or frozen) – consider starting your day with a breakfast juice made from frozen berries, nut milk, whey protein powder, apples and flaxseed oil

3   servings of oily fish a week, such as wild Alaskan salmon and sardines

2–3   servings of whole grains a day, such as organic whole oats, brown rice, whole rye, buckwheat, quinoa and corn-on-the-cob

1–2   servings of beans (black soya, aduki, kidney, pinto, navy, yellow soya, black-eye), peas, chickpeas or lentils a day – these are rich in hormone-balancing phyto-oestrogens

1–2   raw cloves of garlic a day

1–2   servings of fermented foods a day, such as miso (one teaspoon a day), shoyu (3–4 teaspoons a day), umeboshi vinegar (3–4 teaspoons most days), brown rice vinegar (3–4 teaspoons most days), sauerkraut (one heaped teaspoon every other day), gherkins (1–2 most days), natto (1 packet every 1–2 weeks), tempeh (1½ packet every week) and umeboshi plums (one per week)

1+   salad (summer months) or vegetable-based soup (winter months) a day

1   serving of organic milk, and/or organic, natural live yoghurt a day

1   handful of organic nuts a day, such as organic walnuts, almonds and Brazil nuts

1   heaped teaspoon of ground seeds a day, such as sunflower, flax, sesame and hemp

1   tablespoon of organic cold-pressed flax, hempseed or extra-virgin olive oil a day

Optional extras

- Try adding sea vegetables such as agar agar, arame, dulse, hiziki, kelp, kombu, nori, turoru and wakame to your diet – they are rich in minerals and vitamins, and can add a lot of flavour to your meals.

- If you are a meat eater, I recommend you limit your consumption to no more than three times a week and, wherever possible, use wild game, organic white meat such as chicken or turkey, and meat from grass-fed animals – excessive meat consumption can trigger inflammation in the body, which is associated with an increased risk of over a hundred different diseases.[20]

Foods to limit or avoid

Trans-fatty acids – Try to avoid or limit your consumption of these

As found in crisps, biscuits, crackers, doughnuts, margarine, vegetable shortening, baked goods, French fries, fried food, snack foods and most processed foods. Trans-fatty acids are damaged fats that are linked to heart disease, insulin resistance and Alzheimer's disease.[21]

Saturated fats – Maximum of 20g (¾oz) a day

As found in meat, dairy and eggs. While there is no doubt that excessive consumption of saturated fats can increase your risk of developing heart disease, you do need some to maintain good health. As with most things, it's best to eat them in moderation.[22]

Refined carbohydrates – Maximum of three products a week

As found in white bread, white pasta, rolls, pastry, cakes, biscuits, confectionery, carbonated drinks, juice drinks and certain breakfast cereals. There is a lot of evidence linking the consumption of refined carbohydrates with obesity, heart disease, certain cancers, stroke, non-insulin dependent diabetes, atherosclerosis and a lower life expectancy.[23]

Sugar – Maximum of 10 teaspoons/40g (1½oz) a day

As found in table sugar, processed foods, soda, cereals, baked beans, sausages, beef burgers – and even cheese! The regular consumption of sugar has been associated with a considerable number of health problems, including attention deficit disorder, suppression of the immune system, obesity, tooth decay, osteoporosis, heart disease, diabetes, increased inflammation and cancer.[24]

Sweeteners – Avoid

As found in Nutrasweet, Equal and Spoonful. There is an increasing body of evidence linking the regular consumption of sweeteners to mental agitation, headaches, depression, lowered seizure threshold and even cancer.[25] Instead consider sugar substitutes such as xylitol (also shown to reduce tooth decay and risk of middle-ear infections), agave nectar, molasses (which is also rich in iron), manuka honey, date juice, amasake (from fermented rice), fruit juice, raisins and maple syrup.

Refined Soya Products – Avoid

The subject of soya and whether it is good or bad for your health tends to divide the world of nutritionists into two camps, each passionately fighting for or against it. On the one side soya is touted as nature's answer to anything from menopausal symptoms and high cholesterol to memory problems; on the other side it stands accused of blocking the absorption of key minerals, negatively interfering with thyroid function and possibly increasing the risk of breast cancer.

Having spent some considerable time reviewing the research, my concern, which is shared by many others within the field of integrated medicine, is with the processed forms of soya. I advise you to avoid any products containing any of the following: textured vegetable protein (TVP), soya protein isolate (SPI), soya oil, soya flour, hydrolysed vegetable protein or hydrolysed soya protein. I suspect that these adulterated and unnatural forms of soya, when eaten in significant quantities – as many people do – have a negative effect on our health, although this has yet to be proven conclusively. Until I see evidence to the contrary I cannot recommend them.

However, if you are not allergic to soya, traditional forms of soya can be eaten in moderation most days of the week without any detriment to your health. These include fermented forms of soya, such as miso, tempeh, tamari, natto and shoyu soy sauce, and some unfermented whole soya forms, such as organic non-genetically modified soya milk derived from whole soya, roasted soya nuts, edamame (soya beans) and organic tofu fermented with nigari (a curdling agent found in seawater). In fact, overall, the research shows that the regular consumption of traditional whole soya products does have some health benefits, but probably not of the magnitude claimed by the companies that produce them.

Salt – Maximum 6g (⅕oz) a day

As found in table salt and many processed and refined foods. Salt has been linked in some salt-sensitive people to high blood pressure, stroke, stomach cancer, heart disease and osteoporosis.[26] I also suspect that it worsens PMS and period symptoms. If you know how much sodium is in a food, you can work out roughly the amount of salt it contains by multiplying the sodium by 2.5. So if a portion of food contains 1g of sodium then it contains about 2.5g of salt. Instead try Solo salt, which is lower in sodium.

Mercury-laden fish – Limit

Coldwater fish are naturally rich in omega-3 fatty acids and excellent sources of protein. However, because most fish is now contaminated with toxins such as mercury, polychlorinated biphenyls (PCBs) and dioxins, fish really does, regrettably, need to be eaten in moderation – two to three times a week maximum. Some types of fish, such as tuna, halibut and swordfish, have such high levels of mercury they should be avoided altogether or eaten very infrequently.[27]

Soft Fizzy Drinks – Avoid

Drinks such as cola have a profound acidifying effect on the body. A healthy pH for the body is about 7.1 and the pH of cola has been calculated to be between 2.8 and 3.2. To neutralise the acidification, the body draws calcium from the bones, which leads to an increased risk of osteoporosis and bone fractures.[28]

Get saavy about glycemic index (GI) and glycemic load (GL)

Your health, mood and energy levels are intimately linked to your blood sugar. Rapid changes in blood sugar increase the risk of developing diabetes, metabolic syndrome, obesity, heart disease and stroke, as well as triggering mood swings, hyperactivity, problems with concentration and even depression. Choosing foods that raise blood sugar levels slowly, in preference to those that cause rapid changes in blood sugar, is an important goal to work towards. To help you with that researchers have developed the concept of glycemic index (GI) and glycemic load (GL). The glycemic index is a numerical value assigned to a carbohydrate-containing food. It indicates how quickly that food causes a rise in blood sugar. Glucose is 100 and a GI of 70 or more (white baguette, cornflakes, baked potato) is considered high, a GI of between 56 and 69 (wholewheat products, brown rice) is considered medium and a GI of less than 55 (quinoa, bulgur wheat, pulses and most vegetables) is considered low.

GL is even more useful than GI, because it takes into account the amount of carbohydrate in a food. A food with a GL of 20 or more is considered high, 11 to 19 medium and 10 or less low. Watermelon, for example, has a GI of 72, but because it has a low carbohydrate content (there is little of that high GI carbohydrate in it because it is mainly water) its GL is 3.6. I advise most of my patients to simply avoid or limit high-GL foods such as white breads, sugary breakfast cereals, white rice, potatoes, overcooked white pastas, sugar-containing cakes, pastries and sweets. To find out where you can get a list of the GI and GL values of different foods see Resources.

Maintain a stable blood-sugar level

In addition to eating low-GL foods, such as vegetables, beans, fruits and wholegrains, try to ensure that the three main meals and two snacks you eat every day include a protein source, as this will help to keep your blood sugar levels stable. The following are all acceptable: eggs, nut butters (such as almond, peanut butter and hazelnut), hummus, tahini (sesame seed spread), seeds (pumpkin, sesame, flax and hemp), nuts, fish, lentils, beans, meat (beef, lamb and pork), poultry (chicken and turkey) or dairy (milk, cheese, cottage cheese and yoghurt). Eating protein with carbohydrate helps prevent dips in mood and energy levels.

Eat a hearty breakfast every day

Breakfast really is the most important meal of the day. Studies show that people who eat breakfast are less likely to snack and binge, and more likely to maintain a positive mood and energy levels. As a general rule of thumb you should try to eat within 60 minutes of waking up in order to prevent your blood sugar from dropping further.

Keep an eye on your portion size

Portion size and calorie intake is an important part of healthy eating. Most women need about 2,000 calories a day. Obviously women who are smaller and less physically active will need less, while larger and/or physically active women will need more. As a general rule of thumb I encourage my patients to eat until they sense they are satisfied, to put their knives and forks down between mouthfuls, to eat off small plates and to choose smaller portion sizes, particularly when eating out at a restaurant. Another good rule of thumb is to eat no more than you can fit into your cupped hands. This works well for the majority of women.

Slow down

Most people eat unconsciously in that they are not aware of what they are tasting and experiencing as they eat. Learning how to slow down, sitting up straight, chewing your food more and bringing your attention to what you are tasting, smelling and feeling not only enhances the pleasure of eating, but it also reduces the amount of food that you eat.

Watch out for food intolerances and sensitivities

While I personally think the prevalence of food intolerances and sensitivities is exaggerated, between 10 and 20 per cent of my female patients do experience them. If you have bloating, difficulty losing weight despite exercising and eating healthy foods, skin problems and headaches, you should see the relevant section in part five. A common food sensitivity that I see amongst my patients is to sugar. This is a genetically inherited biochemical over-sensitivity to the mood-altering effects of sugar and, rather than craving sugar and carbohydrates for emotional reasons, people with a sugar sensitivity crave it for physiological reasons. Like an alcoholic who needs alcohol in order to feel normal, so the sugar addict needs sugar. It is a relatively common contributor to mood problems and should be suspected if you have two or more of the following:

- You *really* like sweet foods

- You crave sugar or carbohydrates such as cakes, biscuits, pasta, chocolate, ice cream and/or bread

- You are overweight and find it hard to lose those extra pounds

- You frequently experience tiredness and changes in your mood for no apparent reason

- You sometimes feel as though you are going crazy

- You eat a lot of sweets and/or have a strong sweet tooth

- You feel guilty about eating the sweet foods that you do

- You get cravings for alcohol

- You have a personal and/or family history of alcoholism

If you think this might apply to you go to Food Intolerances (page 344).

Use healthy cooking methods

Cooking methods have a significant impact not only on the taste of your food, but also the nutrient content. Wherever possible I recommend steaming, stir-frying, sautéing and grilling. In the winter months braise foods in the oven, using a crock pot, or roast your vegetables in the summer.

Keep hydrated

While there is no hard evidence that you need to drink eight glasses of water a day, I find, as do many other health professionals, that drinking at least 2 litres of water (preferably filtered, reverse osmosis or mineral water) and restricting your caffeine intake are key contributors to optimum health. If you drink more than one cup of coffee, two cups of tea, two cans of caffeinated drink (such as Pepsi, Coke, Diet Coke or Red Bull) or three cups of green tea or earl grey tea a day consider reducing your caffeine intake, as you might have developed a caffeine dependency and/or your caffeine intake might be contributing to blood-sugar swings, fibroids, mineral deficiencies, mood problems and low energy levels.

One study, for example, found that an intake of more than two cups of coffee a day was linked to endometriosis.[29] If you drink a lot of caffeine and do decide to stop or reduce your intake you can reduce the risk of headaches by reducing the number of caffeinated drinks you take by one a day and by taking the amino acid l-tyrosine, 500mg to 1,000mg, three times daily in between meals. For caffeine replacements try herbal teas, rooibos (redbush) tea, dandelion coffee and naturally decaffeinated coffee.

Rotate your foods

Try to rotate the foods that you eat, so you don't eat the same foods on consecutive days. This helps to reduce the likelihood of developing food intolerances and allows you to benefit from the unique nutritional content of those different foods.

Go organic

If you can afford it switch to organic. On average, organic food contains higher levels of vitamin C and essential minerals such as calcium, magnesium, iron and chromium, as well as cancer-fighting antioxidants.[30] Organic food tends to taste better and it has much lower levels of pesticides. Most people have pesticide residues in their bodies and we still don't know the health consequences of this. My advice is to play safe and go organic. If your budget is limited, spend your money on organic meat. This way you avoid eating meat laden with the hormones, steroids and antibiotics from animals that have been raised in the difficult living conditions that non-organically raised animals can endure.

Follow the 80/20 rule

If you are fairly fit and well, and you are following most of the healthy eating suggestions outlined here, you can ease up on your eating plan from time to time. As long as you eat healthily 80 per cent of the time you can enjoy less healthy options 20 per cent of the time.

Watch your alcohol intake

Most women can drink moderate amounts of alcohol (maximum of two units a day) without any detriment to their health. Indeed, there may be an overall benefit to the heart, but this needs to be balanced with an increased risk in developing breast cancer.[31] Also, the evidence is pretty strong now that if you are attempting to have a baby, you should avoid all alcohol and remain alcohol free throughout the pregnancy and breastfeeding period. While most of my patients have a healthy relationship with alcohol, some don't. It's my experience that most people who habitually use alcohol in the evening are simply using it to medicate feelings of stress and tension. Others have a dependence on alcohol. While this needs to be diagnosed by a professional trained in the assessment and treatment of addiction, one 'yes' answer to the following, indicates that you should seek the help and advice of your doctor.

1. Have you ever felt you should cut down on your drinking?

2. Have people ever annoyed you by criticising your drinking?

3. Have you ever felt bad or guilty about your drinking?

4. Have you ever had a drink first thing in the morning (an 'eye-opener') to steady your nerves or get rid of a hangover?

If you have insomnia, candida, cancer, an immune or autoimmune system problem or are simply dedicated to experiencing your full health and healing potential, you should also consider reducing your intake of alcohol or quitting it completely. I usually recommend the latter, not just because of the physical benefits, but because of the emotional benefits. Couples are much more likely to interact meaningfully when they are not drinking alcohol. Plus, having alcohol-free evenings provides the time and space to read, attend an evening course or group, or enjoy the company of your partner. While there are a couple of exceptions, the people and patients whom I consider to be enjoying the highest level of health and fulfilment tend to embrace life fully – and that usually involves giving up alcohol.

Choose your oils wisely

The oils you use both on your food and in your cooking can have a significant impact on your health, mood and risk of developing disease later on in life. The best oil to use on your vegetables and salads is organic cold-pressed extra virgin olive oil. It is rich in anti-inflammatory essential fatty acids and is regarded as being one of the main reasons why the Mediterranean diet has been shown to have so many positive benefits. Unrefined coconut oil is an excellent choice for cooking with, as it remains stable at higher temperatures, so when heated it doesn't create free radicals which damage our health. If you're not keen on cooking with coconut oil, olive oil is a good alternative. Low-salt butter is great on bread and on vegetables, but it is a saturated fat and should be eaten in moderation.

Wherever possible limit your consumption of trans fats (found in the hydrogenated and partially hydrogenated oils used in many processed foods), margarine, vegetable oils, including corn oil, hemp oil, canola oil and sunflower oil, and mayonnaise.

Supplement your diet

Most women are lacking in essential vitamins and minerals, with more than 91 per cent not getting their RNI of iron (14.8mg), more than 74 per cent not getting their RNI of magnesium (270mg) and almost 50 per cent not getting their RNI of calcium (700mg).[32] (RNI is the amount of a nutrient that is adequate to prevent deficiencies in 97.5 per cent of the population and it takes into account age and sex.)

We need vitamins and minerals in order to survive and thrive as human beings. A lack, or more accurately imbalance, of vitamins and minerals has been associated not only with deficiency diseases, but also with conditions ranging from migraine headaches and arthritis to depression and heart disease. While it would be nice to think that we can get all the nutrients we need from a so-called 'balanced diet', the reality is that only 14 per cent of the population eat five portions of fruit and vegetables a day,[33] and for those who do eat their five a day, the vegetables and fruits they are eating contain far fewer nutrients than they did 50 years ago.[34] To prevent deficiency diseases and to provide the bodymind with the nutrients it needs for optimum health, most, if not all, women need to take supplements.

Foundation supplement programme

The following are my general recommendations for supplements. They should be used in conjunction with the advice and recommendations that I make in parts four and five. For specific products see Resources.

- **Multivitamin-mineral supplement** Ideally this should contain mixed carotenoids (vitamin A) and mixed tocopherol/tocotrienols (vitamin E). It should also have at least 400IU of vitamin D, 50mg of the B vitamins except for folic acid (400mcg to 800mcg), B_{12} (50mcg to 100mcg) and biotin (50mcg to 300mcg).

- **Calcium** Because most multivitamin-minerals don't contain that much calcium or magnesium you should also take calcium in addition to your multivitamin-mineral to make up a total daily dose (including dietary sources) of 1200mg to 1500mg per day. When choosing calcium supplements go for calcium citrate, ascorbate, chelate or calcium-rich seaweed formulas, as they are absorbed much more effectively by the body.

- **Vitamin C (1000mg) with bioflavonoids** Both of these are potent antioxidants and anti-inflammatory supplements.

- **Omega-3 fish oils** Take these (1000mg to 3000mg a day) to support general health, mood, hormonal balance, heart and brain function and to reduce inflammation. It's important that the product you use is guaranteed to be free of mercury, PCBs and other pollutants.

- **Antioxidants** If you are over the age of 30, smoke or have any health problem, you should consider taking an antioxidant supplement containing any of the following: coenzyme Q10, alpha lipoic acid, n-acetyl cysteine, reduced glutathione, grape seed extract, green tea extract, astaxanthin or pycnogenol.

- **Wholefood supplements** While nothing compares to real fruits and vegetables, wholefood supplements contain concentrated wholefoods, such as tomatoes, broccoli sprouts, berries and apples. These are dried, ground up, put into powders and then drunk as a smoothie or taken in capsule form. In addition to being rich in vitamins and minerals, they also contain enzymes, coenzymes, phytonutrients, antioxidants, trace elements, activators and many other unknown or undiscovered factors. Because they are affordable for most of my patients, I recommend that they are taken every day. See Resources.

Additional supplements

- If you have blood-sugar instability, insulin resistance or diabetes you should take a total daily dose of 200mcg of chromium polynicotinate, which helps to improve insulin sensitivity and stabilise blood sugar.[35]

- If you have a high risk of breast cancer I would recommend adding in indole-3-carbinol (I-3-C), 200 to 400mg a day. This is a phytonutrient found in the cabbage family, which has been shown to reduce cancer risk.[36]

- If you get bloating after meals or feel that you aren't digesting your food properly consider adding in a digestive enzyme.

- If you need a supplement to support your immune system I recommend astralagus,[37] a mix of organic cordyceps, maitake, reishi, shiitake and trametes mushrooms taken as a tincture.[38] See Resources.

- If you have general fatigue and are addressing the underlying causes you might want to consider either Siberian ginseng[39],

Rhodiola[40] and/or Ashwagandha[41] – all three help to support adrenal gland function and help to improve stress resilience. Use products that are standardised and follow the instructions provided by the manufacturer. See Resources.

- If you are menstruating, pregnant and/or known to be iron deficient you should take an iron supplement.

- Details of other recommended supplements can be found in parts four and five, according to the health problem that you want to treat.

Physical activity and touch

Keeping active and fit, especially when balanced with rest and relaxation, is one of the keys to health, healing and happiness. To this I also add touch, which often gets forgotten.

You may find it surprising, but physical activity levels have been found to be *more* important than body weight in determining a person's risk of death.[42] For example, a study of 906 women showed that activity, or lack of it, was the biggest predictor of heart disease. The women were given angiograms to detect heart disease. They were assessed for weight and body mass index (a measure of obesity), with 76 per cent being overweight and of those 41 per cent were obese. However, those risk factors did not result in more heart disease. Instead, the least active women showed the most evidence of heart disease. Weight did not matter. They also found that moderate levels of physical activity were sufficient to lower the risk of death from all causes.[43] It is therefore better to be slightly overweight and fit, than lean and unfit! What's more, regular physical activity can reduce body fat, increase bone mass, dissolve away the symptoms of depression and stress, reduce the risk of heart disease, hip fractures and breast cancer, help stabilise hormone levels, and increase feelings of self-worth and self-confidence.[44] And if that doesn't convince you to get moving, here are a few more reasons:

- One study showed that women who exercised for about four hours a week had a 37 per cent lower risk of breast cancer than those who did no exercise.[45]

- Another study looked at the occurrence of hot flushes in post-menopausal women and found that 43.8 per cent of sedentary women experienced hot flushes, compared with 21.5 per cent of physically active women. Physical activity, particularly if amounting to more than 3.5 hours a week, produced the greatest reduction in hot flushes.[46]

I am deliberately writing about physical activity, as opposed to exercise, because the latter has negative connotations for a fair number of people, plus the word activity more accurately describes the truth that most physical activities confer health benefits. While most people tend to think of running and swimming as the best ways to get fit, there are many more, including brisk walking, rebounding (mini-trampoline), climbing stairs, yoga, pilates, cycling, gardening, weeding, mowing, raking, vacuuming, dancing, playing golf, painting, decorating and, of course, sex.

Touch is also an important physical need and its positive effects on health and wellbeing are well documented. Maybe you can recall a time when someone touched you or gave you a hug and you felt connected and lifted by the experience? In addition to feeling nice, gentle touch has been shown to help reduce stress, relieve pain and increase your ability to cope with stress. One famous study found that orphans who were given additional touch experienced fewer illnesses and gained significantly more weight.[47] Another study found that therapeutic touch reduced symptoms of Alzheimer's disease amongst residents of a nursing home.[48]

The integrated medical approach to physical activity and touch

Here are some tips to help get you into the daily habit of physical activity, although if you haven't exercised before, are aged over 50 or have a serious or debilitating medical condition always check with your GP before exercising:

- **Focus on the benefits.** Write down five reasons why you would benefit from taking daily physical activity.

- **Improve your motivation.** Score out of ten how motivated you are to take daily physical activity (0 = zero motivation, 10 = completely motivated). If you score less than seven, write down three different ways you could increase your motivation – use the Emotional Freedom Technique (see page 151) or Values-based Goal Setting (see page 166) from the holistic health tools to help you.

- **Choose your physical activities.** Make a list of all the possible physical activities that you could realistically do. Include a mix of aerobic activity (such as running, swimming), strength training (with weights, resistance bands, push-ups) and flexibility exercises (such as yoga, qi gong, pilates).

- **Honour your body and fitness level.** If you haven't exercised for a while start gradually with walking, increasing to brisk walking, then jogging and, if appropriate, running. Most gyms have personal trainers who will create a tailored programme for you. Consider this as an option, particularly if lack of motivation or inexperience is a factor for you.

- **Aim for between 30 and 45 minutes of physical activity every day.** If this is not possible start with three times a week and take it from there. It's important to set yourself a realistic target.

- **Plan the next week ahead in a diary or journal.** Write down exactly what activities you are going to do on which days. For example, Monday – brisk walk to and from work, Tuesday – swim after work, Wednesday – yoga after work, Thursday – brisk walk to and from work, Friday – weight training and push-ups before work, Saturday – gardening, Sunday – walk in countryside with family.

- **Try the talk test.** When doing aerobic exercise you should aim for moderate intensity. One way to gauge this is with the 'talk test': exercise hard enough to break into a sweat, but not so hard that you can't carry on a conversation.

- **Get your touch quota.** Each day see you receive respectful touch from another human being by asking for a hug or kiss. Making love or self-pleasuring are more intimate ways of experiencing touch. I also highly recommend that you treat yourself to a massage every so often.

- **Use a pedometer.** A useful way to monitor your activity levels and give yourself the motivation to get active is to attach a pedometer to your clothing. This measures how many steps you take. The target for most people is 10,000. If you can, do your physical activity outdoors. Not only do you benefit from being in the sunshine and fresh air, but there is good evidence to suggest that reconnecting with nature not only nourishes the soul, but helps to reduce stress and lift mood levels. If you are unsure about this, go for a walk near the ocean, in a wood or in the mountains, breathe in the fresh air and notice how good it makes you feel. Read secret five (page 127) for more information on connecting with nature.

Healthy environment and sunlight

Your environment has a major impact on your health, mood and wellbeing. That might not come as a surprise; we all know how uplifting it can be when we go on holiday or for a walk in the country. Spending 10 to 15 minutes in natural sunlight a day has been shown to have numerous health benefits. Sunlight triggers the creation of vitamin D. In fact, for most people it's the main source of vitamin D. Increasing your exposure to sunlight (without getting burnt) is associated with a reduced risk of developing cancer of the colon, breast, ovary, prostate and lymphoma. Sunlight and vitamin D are also associated with improved bone health and a lower incidence of multiple sclerosis.[49] If you become pregnant and have low levels of vitamin D, the chances of you giving birth to a son or daughter who goes on to develop type 1 diabetes are also increased.[50] So while the Cancer Research SunSmart message is to cover up and stay out of the sun in order to reduce the risk of developing the skin cancer melanoma, this needs to be balanced with the fact that the sun is a vital nutrient – and like all nutrients it just needs to be taken in the right amounts.

The flipside of our environment is that for many women it negatively impacts on their health in so many different and sometimes unexpected ways. For example, most women are unknowingly exposed to an unprecedented and vast array of toxins, including:

- **Personal care products**, such as bleaches, dyes, scents, creams, lotions, fragrances and hairsprays

- **Household chemicals**, such as household cleaners, air fresheners, disinfectants, drain cleaner, furniture polish, wax and paints

- **Heavy metals**, from amalgam fillings, vaccines, antiperspirants, cigarette smoke, paint, copper and lead pipes, and food packaging

- **Building materials and products**, including adhesives, carpeting, upholstery, manufactured wood products, copy machines, pesticides and cleaning agents, all of which may emit volatile organic compounds (VOCs) such as formaldehyde

- **Environmental toxins**, from air, food and water and including noise and light pollution

- **Electromagnetic toxins**, from PCs, lighting, TVs, freezers, wi-fi, pylons and microwaves

- **Industrial toxins**, from the outputs of large industrial plants

- **Bacteria, fungus moulds, yeasts and parasites**, from food, the water supply and body acidification

The consequences of this exposure have only come to light in the last five to ten years, for example:

- The presence of chemical toxins in the body is linked to a wide range of conditions, including autism, attention deficit hyperactive disorder, chronic fatigue syndrome, multiple chemical sensitivities, multiple sclerosis, memory loss, childhood cancers, premature puberty, low sperm counts, testicular cancer, breast cancer, undescended testicles, multiple myeloma, non-Hodgkin's lymphoma, infertility, birth defects, asthma and learning disabilities.[51]

- Light pollution is associated with sleep deprivation, headaches and increased levels of stress and anxiety. Researchers at the National Cancer Institute (NCI) and National Institute of Environmental Health Sciences have completed a study that suggests that artificial light during the night can be a factor for breast cancer.[52]

- Air pollution can be a serious contributor to ill health, particularly if you are susceptible, for example you're elderly, have a chronic disease and/or you live next to busy roads, in the city, or near power plants or chemical factories. Air pollution is composed of many environmental factors. They include carbon monoxide, nitrates, sulphur dioxide, ozone, lead, second-hand tobacco smoke and particulate matter. The latter, also known as particle pollution, is composed of solid and liquid particles within the air and is a significant contributor to inflammation and heart disease.[53]

- A report published in 1996 by the environmental think-tank World Resources Institute found a considerable amount of evidence to suggest that pesticides are suppressing the immune responses to bacteria, viruses, parasites and tumours, making millions of people significantly more vulnerable to disease.[54]

- A report based on tests of ten samples of umbilical cord blood found an average of 287 contaminants in the blood, including mercury, fire retardants, pesticides and the Teflon chemical PFOA. Of the 287 chemicals detected, 180 cause cancer in humans or animals, 217 are toxic to the brain and nervous system and 208 cause birth defects or abnormal development in animal tests. The dangers of pre- or post-natal exposure to this complex mixture of carcinogens, developmental toxins and neurotoxins have never been studied.[55]

Women are particularly susceptible to the negative effects of environmental toxicity. For example xeno-oestrogens are chemicals found in the environment (particularly in plastics and pesticides) that mimic the action of oestrogen, which in turn leads to a situation called oestrogen dominance. This occurs when your body has too much oestrogen relative to progesterone. Oestrogen dominance has been associated with a variety of symptoms and health problems, ranging from breast and womb cancer, fibroids and endometriosis to osteoporosis and infertility.[56]

The good news is that your body, and in particular the liver, can detoxify and eliminate many toxins, plus there are plenty of things you can do to reduce your exposure to toxins.

The integrated medical approach to a healthy environment and sunlight

One of the ways in which you can support your health and happiness is to ensure, to the best of your ability, that the environment within which you live and work supports and promotes your health. There are a lot of different books on the subject of non-toxic living – see Resources – and here are some tips to support you in doing this:

List your concerns about toxicity

You could also compile a list of all the potential benefits of reducing your exposure to toxins. Use this to motivate yourself to make the necessary changes to your lifestyle.

Reduce your exposure to xeno-oestrogens

You can reduce your exposure by eating organic food (pesticides and growth hormones given to animals are the two greatest sources of xeno-oestrogens), reducing your consumption of fatty foods such as full-fat dairy products and fatty meat (as xeno-oestrogens are concentrated here) and limiting the use of plastic containers, clingfilm and plastic water bottles, from which they are leached.

Drink pure water

Identify a source that is known to be free from hormone-disrupting chemicals. Plastic bottles leach these chemicals into them, but if you do drink from them make sure that the bottle has not been left out in the sun or heated – see Resources.

Limit your clingfilm use

Wherever possible use glass storage jars instead of plastic and never microwave food in a plastic bowl.

Switch to organic

While this doesn't guarantee that it is completely free from pesticides (organic farmers still use some pesticides), it will help to reduce your toxic load.

Go smoke free

Smoking not only increases the likelihood of developing lung cancer and emphysema, but in women it has been linked to premature menopause and infertility.[57] If you smoke and want to give up you are spoilt for choices as to methods and agencies that can help. Hypnotherapy, nicotine gum, cognitive behavioural therapy, neuro-linguistic programming and the NHS stop smoking services have all worked for my patients. Because nicotine addiction can mask other addictions I encourage you to read about addictions in part five as well. Second-hand smoking has also been found to have a detrimental effect on health, so avoid smoky environments wherever possible.

Use non-toxic personal care products

Deodorants, tampons, moisturisers, lipstick, hair dye, nail polish, perfumes and shower gels are made from chemicals, many of which are known carcinogens, allergens and hormone disruptors. Of particular concern is the evidence linking tampons with toxic shock syndrome, a potentially fatal infection of the blood caused by the toxin TSST-1.[58] Fortunately, there are an increasing number of companies specialising in non-toxic personal care products – see Resources.

Use non-toxic cleaning products

Because of the increasing demand for non-toxic products there is a wide range of different brands to choose from – see Resources.

Open your windows

Some research suggests indoor pollution is much more of a problem than outdoor pollution.[59] Keeping your windows open helps air to circulate.

Use a negative air ioniser

This device generates millions of negatively charged particles, which have been found to help with improved sleep, a reduction in migraines and allergies, and an improvement in mood and asthma symptoms[60] – see Resources.

Get outside

Because sunlight is the main source of vitamin D it's important to expose yourself to between five and ten minutes of sunshine on most days. I would avoid putting sunscreen and sunglasses on for this period and try to feel the warmth of the sun on your hands, face and arms. After this period it's important to cover up and use sunscreen.

Go fluoride free

It's controversial, but there is accumulating evidence that the fluoride found in our water supply increases the risk of various health problems in certain vulnerable groups, such as the elderly, children, people with magnesium and calcium deficiencies, and those with heart or kidney disease. These include increased risk of osteoporosis, dental fluorosis (damage to the enamel of the teeth), infertility, reduced IQ, increased risk of hip fractures and increased risk of osteosarcoma (bone cancer) in boys.[61] You can check whether your water supply is fluoridated by asking your water supplier. If it is, my advice would be to invest in a reverse osmosis water system – a system that removes fluoride as well as heavy metals, chlorine and other chemicals (most conventional water filters do not remove fluoride) – see Resources.

Go mercury free

Mercury is one of the most toxic metals known to man, yet it resides within the teeth, in the form of amalgam fillings, in millions of people throughout the world. To date mercury toxicity has been linked to depression, autism, lupus, memory problems, behavioural problems, birth defects, kidney disease, immune suppression, chronic fatigue syndrome, infertility and allergies.[62] Another study found high blood levels of mercury in patients with Alzheimer's disease (AD) when compared with non-AD patients.[63]

I'm not in favour of everyone having their mercury fillings removed, but if you are concerned about the potential problems associated with mercury toxicity read up on the subject before you consider having your amalgam fillings removed. Should you wish to have them removed ensure you see a dentist who follows the guidelines set out by the British Society for Mercury-Free Dentistry – see Resources. This is important, because mercury can be released during the removal process and this can make the toxicity problem worse.[64] While having your fillings removed it is also important that you take certain supplements such as selenium and chlorella to support the process.

SUMMARY

- For good health, certain physical needs need to be met.

- The foundations of good physical health are to get between seven and eight hours of sleep most nights; experience at least ten minutes of rest (not-doing) each day; consistently eat an individually tailored, nutrient-dense diet that is high in vegetables, fruits and whole grains; exercise for a minimum of 40 minutes on most days; reduce your exposure to harmful toxins in your environment; and spend 10 to15 minutes outside every day without sunscreen.

- Four of the most common barriers to healthy eating are habits, dieting, eating disorders and emotional eating. All of these should be addressed with the help of an experienced health professional.

- In addition to a nutrient-dense diet, most women need to take supplements to prevent deficiency diseases and ensure they are receiving the right vitamins and minerals for optimum health.

Secret Two
De-stress and relax

The stress factor

Of all the challenges that my patients face, the most common and potentially harmful is the failure to actively de-stress and relax on a daily basis. Most women that I see as patients are stressed, whether they are able to acknowledge it or not. Taking care of children, relationship worries, feeling isolated, managing a career, running a household, battling weight gain, debt, or low confidence ... the list is endless and all these issues contribute to an ever-increasing burden of responsibility on most women (and men).

That's not the half of it, though. Most women I see in my clinic are stressed not just because of what is happening to them, but because of the stress they place upon themselves. A perfectionist streak, a strong desire to please others and win attention, being 'nice all the time' and/or the tendency to push themselves hard – in the absence of regular healthy self-care, self-acceptance and strong social support, these pressures create an often ever-present psychic or inner tension. How that inner tension is dealt with depends on the individual. Many of my patients use food, alcohol, busyness, caretaking, TV or excessive control of others as strategies to cope – to take the edge off their feelings. Others will take their tension and stress out on others – normally their children or partners. Others will slip into depression, anxiety,

OCD or phobias. Others will experience stress-related illness or, if they repress their emotions, then they might experience an emotionally-induced illness such as tension myoneural syndrome (see page 386). Whatever the cause of stress and whatever the strategy employed to avoid the stress, the cost to your health can be considerable.

CASE STUDY

Sara, a 43-year-old mother of four, came to see me with tiredness, insomnia and vague aches and pains all over her body. Her GP had told her that it was all due to stress and that she needed a break, to take some time off. While she knew that her GP was correct, and he was, she struggled to even know how to start beginning to relax and de-stress. How do you truly relax and de-stress when your default setting is busy-busy and your life situation demands so much of you?

What is stress?

Stress is the bodymind's natural response to an event or experience, actual or imaginary, which at some level we believe we don't have the resources to deal with adequately. What determines whether something is positively or negatively stressful is mainly your perception; that is your perspective on the situation that you are in. For example, I had a situation at my clinic where I provided two consecutive patients with the same diagnosis of depression. The first was relieved, because she was worried it was more serious; the other found the diagnosis distressing, because she believed people with depression were weak-willed. Because each person attached a different meaning to the diagnosis, they responded to it very differently.

Positive stress

Stress is not inherently negative; it's a response that is built into our bodymind as a means of providing us with the fuel (energy), alertness and focused attention to take action. If I'm walking along a road and I see a car coming towards me, my stress response will kick in and I will jump out of the way. If I'm taking part in a sports event, a certain level of stress will enable me to perform more optimally. Positive stress also breeds creativity and enthusiasm, and helps us achieve our goals. A degree of stress is therefore a necessary part of being a healthy and productive human being.

Negative stress

When we suppress our stress response, experience ongoing stress or fail to deactivate and discharge the energy that arises in the bodymind in response to the stress, this can, and often will, compromise our health and vitality, and put us at risk of various diseases. Chronic stress is a contributor to many disturbances and diseases including:

- Increased deposition of fat around the abdomen (stress is a major contributor to obesity)

- Increased risk of infertility

- Reduced nutrient absorption

- Raised cholesterol and triglyceride levels

- Inhibiting the immune system

- Raised blood pressure

- Poor memory and concentration

- Suppressed thyroid function

- Reduced wound healing

- Blood sugar imbalances

- Decreased bone density

- Decrease in muscle tissue

In addition to these, stress is associated with addictions, sleep disturbances, abuse, violence, heart disease, cancer, strokes, autoimmune disease, IBS, sexual dysfunction, arthritis, diabetes, depression and anxiety![1]

Women and stress

The research on stress and sex differences is fascinating. Women experience and respond to stress quite differently from men:

- Women are physiologically primed to experience more stress than men. Women's bodies tend to produce more stress hormones than men's and it takes longer for those stress hormones to return to normal levels. This might be related to women's general tendency to worry more than men. While we all worry to a certain degree, a Gallup poll found that, on average, women worried a great deal about 7 of the 12 issues that they were surveyed on.[2]

- Women deal with stress much better than men. When under stress men tend to 'fight or flight', whereas women initially experience 'fight or flight', but are then much more likely to move on to 'tend and befriend'. When under stress women are much more likely to nurture themselves and their young ('tending') and form alliances with others ('befriending'). This reinforces the importance of women reaching out to others when under stress.[3]

- Men are less likely to talk about how they feel, less likely to admit that they are stressed (even to themselves) and less likely to seek help from a doctor or anyone else. Most men only visit their GP when medical symptoms of stress emerge, such as chest pains, headaches and stomach upsets, but some don't even bother to go then. In contrast, women will talk things over with a friend or partner and are more likely to see their GP when they feel anxious or stressed, rather than waiting for a physical problem to develop.

The integrated medical approach to de-stressing and relaxing

If you are anything like the patients who come to see me, the chances are that stress is compromising your health and you would benefit from either learning how to relax or taking regular periods of relaxation. Relaxation is an active process, the goal of which is to trigger a shift within the body's nervous system from sympathetic dominance (which is the body's accelerator) to parasympathetic dominance (the body's brakes). Over-activity of the sympathetic system is one of the most common causes of disease and the major barrier to health, healing and happiness. The body has a built-in mechanism, called the relaxation response, which switches it to the parasympathetic. When activated – for example, by taking a couple of long, slow deep breaths – your heart slows, your blood pressure drops, healing is accelerated and the immune system functions more effectively. Finding a balance between the sympathetic and parasympathetic states is one of the most important keys to good health and healing.

Step 1 • Ask yourself if you are stressed

One way to work out whether stress is compromising your health and quality of life is to honestly ask yourself, and/or a close friend or partner, 'is stress affecting my health or quality of life?' If so, fine, you can move on to step two. Unfortunately, it's not that easy for many people, usually because their awareness of themselves – their body and mind – is limited, so often they won't be aware that they are stressed. If you suspect this applies to you, look at the following list of subtle and not-so-subtle signs and symptoms of stress. If any of these are familiar, you might be experiencing stress.

Effects of stress on your body

Headache, pounding heart, shortness of breath, muscle aches, back pain, clenched jaws, tooth grinding, stomach upsets, increased sweating, tiredness, sleep problems, weight gain or loss, sex problems, skin breakouts.

Effects of stress on your thoughts and feelings

Anxiety, restlessness, worrying, irritability, depression, sadness, anger, mood swings, job dissatisfaction, burnout, forgetfulness, inability to concentrate, seeing only the negatives.

Effects of stress on your behaviour

Overeating, undereating, angry outbursts, drug abuse, excessive drinking, increased smoking, social withdrawal, relationship conflicts, decreased productivity, blaming others.

Take an adrenal test

A useful way to measure the impact of stress on your health is to measure the level of the hormones DHEA and cortisol. You can order the kit from a diagnostic laboratory (see Resources) and they will send you four specimen pots into which you place your saliva at four different times of the day. The levels and ratios of each hormone are then measured and compared with what would be expected in a healthy person. See Adrenal Fatigue (page 267) for more information.

Step 2 • Take a stress inventory

This is an important step. By being honest with yourself and facing the reality of how you do or don't manage your stress you can start to do something about it. We all have default settings to which we revert when we experience stress; these are mainly unconscious habits that kick in automatically when stress arises. More often than not we won't be aware of them.

Answer the following questions as honestly as you can (to help you, the responses given by one of my patients follows the questions):

1. What am I stressed about at the moment? Include partner, family, friends, work, money, home, health, appearance, community, world, your relationship with yourself...

2. What are my stress triggers?

3. When I get stressed I...

4. How is stress interfering with my life?

Typical patient's response

1. *I'm stressed about...*

- Partner – we seem to be getting more distant from each other and arguing a lot

- Family – my mum is always criticising me and I'm worried about my dad's health

- Friends – I've fallen out with my best friend and I don't really have any other true friendships

- Work – I'm worried I'm going to be made redundant
- Money – I'm stressed about my £2,000 credit card bill and the fact that I don't have any savings
- Home – I really don't like where I live, as it's too small and it smells of mould in the bedroom
- Health – I'm worried about getting cancer like my mother
- Appearance – I'm overweight and hate my body
- Community – I feel unsafe where I live
- World – I do worry about global warming and that we are harming our planet
- Relationship with self – I don't really know who I am or what my purpose in life is

2. *My stress triggers are...*

- My partner being critical of me
- My partner not listening
- My partner leaving the house a mess
- My girlfriend not returning my call
- My mum being critical of me
- Letters from the bank
- Having to get the kids ready for school
- Evening times with the kids – they take a long time to get to sleep
- My partner not really helping with the children

3. *When I get stressed, I...*

- Get angry and lose my temper
- Storm out of the room
- Shout at the kids

- Eat chocolate, biscuits and cakes

- Swallow my anger

- Start getting resentful and plotting how I can get even

- Drink wine

- Zone out in front of the TV

4. *How is stress interfering with my life?*

- It's making me unwell – I feel tired all of the time

- I eat a lot and because of that I am 2 stone overweight

- It makes me feel out of control

- I've lost sight of who I am and where I am going

- It interferes with my sleep

- I find it hard to really enjoy myself and have fun

The value in having done this exercise for my patient was that she was quickly able to get a real sense of the hold and limitation that stress placed on her life and health. Seeing this and really getting in touch with this was one of the first steps to making some changes to the way she managed her stress.

Step 3 • Respond proactively to stressful situations

Using the list from step one, go through each source of stress in turn and decide which one of the three options below you are going to use in order to reduce the stress that you are under.

Option 1 – Take action List in very precise and realistic terms what action you can take to change the situation. If you get stuck, imagine a friend of yours is in exactly the same circumstance as you – what advice would you give them? Write it down.

Option 2 – Change your perspective Changing the way you see the problem and the meaning you give it is a very powerful way of reducing the stress that it triggers. Again imagine you are helping a friend with the same problems to come up with three different perspectives – what advice would you give them? Write it down.

Option 3 – Accept reality If you truly can't change the situation or your perspective on it, then the way to release any stress is to stop resisting the situation and accept the reality of it as it is now. Embracing reality does not mean you are passively accepting reality; far from it, embracing reality as it is helps you access the resources and clarity to take the best possible course of action. One of the simplest and most effective ways to transform your relationship to reality, and the one I recommend to many of my patients, is The Work. Developed by the spiritual teacher Byron Katie, The Work is designed to identify and question thoughts that trigger pain, suffering and distress. Because so many of my patients have distressing thoughts about their partners and themselves, I frequently recommend it. See The Work (page 163).

Once your list is finished, for each source of stress, implement the options. Get a friend or therapist to help if you get stuck.

Step 4 • Meet your emotional needs

Emotional needs are as important to your health as your physical needs. They include the need for positive attention, respect, safety, intimacy, social connection, competency, status, meaning and purpose. Failure to get one or more of these met in a healthy and balanced way will lead to stress, even if you aren't aware of it. I ask all my patients to fill in the following emotional needs questionnaire and I invite you to do the same. (If you prefer, write it in your notebook or journal.) Read through each question slowly and spend a few moments thinking about how fulfilled you are in respect of the issue being asked about. For each emotional need, give yourself a score of between 0 and 5 (0 = emotional need completely unmet and unfulfilled, 5 = emotional need completely met and fulfilled).

Watch out for the tendency to rush this exercise or to score yourself too highly. Ask yourself once you have a score in mind, 'does this score feel accurate?' If it does, great, write it down. If it doesn't, reassess and score again.

EMOTIONAL NEEDS QUESTIONNAIRE

To what degree:

- Do you feel safe? ☐

- Do you receive enough positive attention from those around you? ☐

- Can you attain privacy when you need to? ☐

- Do you give positive attention to those around you? ☐

- Do you have a sense of autonomy and control in your life? ☐

- Do you feel emotionally connected to others? ☐

- Do you feel part of the wider community? ☐

- Are you able to experience friendship and intimacy? ☐

- Do you have a sense of competence and achievement? ☐

- Do you live your life with meaning and purpose? ☐

- Are you respected and acknowledged by your peers? ☐

- Are you respected and acknowledged by your family? ☐

- Are you respected and acknowledged by your partner? (if applicable) ☐

Having completed the questionnaire, go through it again and check whether the score you have given yourself truly reflects the facts of the situation as it currently stands. Generally, the lower the score, the greater the need for some action to be taken in order for that need to be met. Highlight those emotional needs that you have scored three or less with a marker pen and, starting with the need that you scored lowest, try using the following visualisation exercise.

EXERCISE: The miracle visualisation

Close your eyes and imagine that when you wake up tomorrow morning a miracle has occurred and you are living a life in which your unmet emotional need is fulfilled completely. Take three deep breaths and allow your imagination to create a movie of how your new life looks.

- Where are you living?

- How are you feeling and looking?

- Who is with you?

- How are they acting?

- What does your home look like?

- What work are you doing? (Give yourself plenty of time to do this.)

- What is it about this new life that confirms your emotional need is now being fulfilled?

When you start to feel as though you are really living this new life of yours, imagine the 'new you' meeting the 'old you' and tell your old self exactly what she needs to know and to do in order to make this new life a reality. Give this time, be patient and something will come. Once the insight(s) have been revealed to you, open your eyes, take a deep breath and notice how different you feel. Now write down your insights and create a plan of action that will result in that specific emotional need being met.

Step 5 • Learn some instant stress release techniques

It's very useful to have to hand a couple of tools for reducing stress at any given moment. These aren't necessarily designed to tackle the underlying causes of stress, but are more focused on increasing relaxation and shifting your state of mind. The following techniques are the ones my patients find to be most useful:

EXERCISE: 4/7 breathing

This is probably the simplest and one of the most effective stress reduction techniques.

- Next time you feel stressed, overwhelmed or tense, take a breath in to the count of four and then breathe out to the count of seven

- Repeat this at least five times and notice how much better you feel

Breathing out for a longer period of time on the out breath helps to trigger the relaxation response.

EXERCISE: Destress points

1. Lightly place the fingers of both hands on your forehead, over the points halfway between your normal hairline and your eyes (these are the frontal eminence points) and stretch your skin slightly. Now place your thumbs on your temples next to your eyes and take a deep breath.

2. Keep your fingers on these points for at least five minutes and keep breathing deeply. Notice how the emotional intensity starts to fade. Continue until you feel calm and at peace.

EXERCISE: Change the image

If there's someone you work with who winds you up or constantly annoys you, try this to change the way you react to them. Imagine that person as a small kid, wearing a big over-sized nappy. Smile at how ludicrous they look. Now next time you see that person, see them in their nappy and I guarantee that you'll feel very different about them.

Step 6 • Increase your emotional resilience

Emotional resilience is the ability to cope with pressure. It's an inbuilt psychological buffer system that enables you to withstand various potentially stressful situations. Learning how to increase your emotional resilience and your coping threshold is an important part of dealing with stress. Here are a few ideas:

Take control

Feeling that you have some degree of control in the events of your life, or controlling the way you chose to respond to those events, is a panacea for stress. Whenever you feel stressed, identify at least three ways in which you can take control of the situation. For example, if you've been in the same job for over ten years, you could be fed up of having no say in decision making and everything about the job may be starting to stress you out. Taking control could involve you 1) telling your supervisor how you feel and asking for more responsibility, control or a different role; 2) looking for a new job; 3) changing the meaning you give to the job, by seeing your job as a source of income that simply allows you to do things you enjoy.

Take the challenge

Labelling a situation as a problem creates a problem, as it implies that there's no way around it – that it's a dead end. Try and get into the habit of seeing the situations that you are in as challenges and invitations to explore different options by finding creative solutions. Taking this attitude empowers you to focus on solutions rather than problems. It also decreases your stress considerably.

Get connected

Close relationships, committed partnerships, a supportive family and involvement with the local community are powerful antidotes to stress, especially for women. The more connected we feel (and the less isolated we are) the greater our ability to cope with life's situations. Being able to share challenges with others, and draw upon other people's suggestions and support, can help prevent someone sinking into depression. I'm not suggesting that you suddenly get married, or go into the streets and find yourself a partner, but actively making the most of the people you do have in your life, getting involved in a community-based project and even volunteering can have a big positive effect on your life and health. See secret five (page 127) for more information.

Get creative

Make a commitment right now to doing something creative for at least one hour a week. Choose something unrelated to work, but make it something that allows you to 'get into the flow' – this could be anything from learning to playing an instrument, playing chess, writing or taking a dance class. Notice how good and free it makes you feel afterwards!

Start journaling

Keeping a daily diary in which you can write down your thoughts, reflect on the day's activities and put into words your worries and problems is a great stress-reliever.

Keep a pet

Pet therapy is widely used in nursing homes, prisons, hospitals and schools to reduce stress levels and improve health. Stroking a cat or dog or watching fish in an aquarium have all been found to lower blood pressure. Long term, the results are even more impressive. Owners of pets are more likely to survive a heart attack, make fewer visits to their GP, experience less loneliness and suffer less from depression.[4] However, there is a caveat with pet therapy – you have to make time to spend with your pet and you have to take care of it!

Step 7 • Take up a relaxation practice

The following are just some of the approaches that my patients use to help them de-stress and relax:

Yoga

Practised for thousands of years, this whole-body and mind form of exercise and spiritual practice can help to calm the mind, raise energy levels, increase flexibility, cultivate focus and patience, and, depending on the type of yoga you do, help you to develop emotionally and spiritually.

Massage

If you enjoy being touched, massage is a wonderful way to release tension from the muscles, relax the bodymind and encourage a good night's sleep.

Qi Gong

Qi Gong, or chi kung, refers to a variety of metaphysical practices involving movement and/or specific breathing approaches. They are designed to restore the flow of life force around the body, which in turn promotes optimum health and wellbeing.

Exercise

Physical exercise is a great way to de-stress and release pent-up emotions. If you sense things are getting on top of you, get yourself down to the gym and really go for it on the treadmill or take your anger out on the punch-bag, or go for a long run or swim. Any of these activities will make you feel a million times better.

T'ai chi

T'ai chi is an ancient moving form of meditation, involving a series of slow, controlled movements that promote strength, balance, good posture and a sense of calm. It's used to promote health and stimulate healing, and is also a martial art.

Yoga nidra

Yoga nidra, meaning yogic sleep, is a meditation practice that guides you into a deep sleep state while retaining wakefulness and awareness. It is quite a profound practice and I'm big fan of it. See Resources for details.

Meditation

There are numerous different styles of meditation designed to cultivate awareness, peace of mind and optimum health. Some of the most popular are transcendental meditation, mindfulness meditation, primordial sound meditation and heart rhythm meditation. Practised regularly, mediation can help to increase your ability to withstand stress, access states of compassion and connection, and tap into the wisdom and guidance of your heart.

Step 8 • Practise gratitude

One of the many fascinating discoveries to emerge from the field of positive psychology – the study of how human beings flourish – is that the regular and deliberate practice of gratitude can bring about significant relief from stress and significant improvements in happiness, motivation, optimism, energy levels, sleep and quality of life. It is also a powerful antidote to 'negative emotions' and depression, as well as the foundation upon which positive mental wellbeing is created.

One of the best definitions of gratitude is by the world's leading gratitude researcher, Robert Emmons, who describes gratitude as the 'felt sense of wonder, thankfulness and appreciation for life'. Summarising the findings from the studies to date, Emmons says that those who practise grateful thinking 'reap emotional, physical and interpersonal benefits'. People who regularly keep a gratitude journal report fewer illness symptoms, feel better about their lives as a whole and are more optimistic about the future.[5] If you would like to increase the level of gratitude in your life, here are four suggestions for getting started:

Keep a gratitude journal

Write in a journal some of the things you have to be grateful for. This can be anything from the beauty of the sky outside to the joy of your children – whatever works for you. Some people really enjoy doing this every day, others once a week – you will have to find out for yourself what suits you. I get my patients to start by writing down two things for which they are grateful and two things that they appreciate about themselves. For example:

Today, I am grateful for...

1. The aliveness that I'm feeling in my body, as it provides me with the inspiration and energy to do my work

2. The fingers I have as they allow me to type this message

Today I appreciate...

1. The loving respect with which I greeted my daughter this morning

2. The friendly manner with which I spoke to Susan on the phone

Write a gratitude letter

Research by Martin Seligman, the founder of positive psychology, has shown this one to be particularly effective. Write a letter to a mentor, family member or some other important person in your life whom you've never properly thanked. Deliver it in person. Read it out loud.

Savour the moment

How often do you stop and in that moment notice the beauty of what you are seeing or experiencing. Taking time to savour the moment enriches your experience and enhances your positive emotions. For more about savouring see page 147.

Have a gratitude partner

Having a partner who is also committed to your wellbeing and who is able to encourage you in your health journey can provide invaluable support and motivation. Talk to someone about your commitment to gratitude and see if they would be willing to practise gratitude with you. You might, for example, exchange gratitude lists or share gratitudes over the phone or in person. According to Robert Emmons, 'If we hang out with ungrateful people, we will "catch" one set of emotions; if we choose to associate with more grateful individuals, the influence will be in another direction. Find a grateful person and spend more time with him or her.' If you would like to discover more about gratitude see Resources.

SUMMARY

- Stress is part and parcel of life. It's how we deal with stress that really counts.

- While a certain level of stress enables us to perform optimally and access creativity and enthusiasm, chronic stress that isn't managed effectively can increase your risk of numerous health problems, including depression, anxiety, obesity, heart disease and infertility.

- Taking time out each day to de-stress and relax is an important part of creating and maintaining a high level of health and wellbeing.

- Create a stress management programme for yourself – this might include a couple of instant stress release techniques, engaging in a daily relaxation practice such as yoga or meditation, taking action to meet your physical needs and perhaps keeping a gratitude journal.

Secret Three
Face and embrace your emotions

In Western society one of the most common causes of ill health, dissatisfaction, heart ache and failed relationships is a lack of emotional body awareness. This basically means not knowing how – or not being willing – to face and embrace your emotions.

CASE STUDY

Lorraine was a highly accomplished executive who, at face value, had everything going for her. When she came to see me for advice on treating her irritable bowel syndrome symptoms she thought I would suggest some dietary changes and recommend some supplements, and that this would 'cure' the problem. While this approach is completely appropriate for some IBS sufferers, it wasn't for Lorraine. Her symptoms had started shortly after she had spilt up with her partner and although she felt she had got over him, the tension in her face and watering of her eyes suggested that she was holding on to unprocessed emotions relating to him. The body never lies.

Once I invited her to breathe into her body and the tension she was experiencing in and around her throat, she started to cry. It was at this stage that I guided her to release that emotion using a technique called EmoTrance (see page 158). Within ten minutes the emotional charge was released and she felt 'five pounds' lighter. Over two further sessions I taught her a number of different approaches for processing and managing her emotions more effectively. Within two weeks her IBS symptoms had disappeared and, just as importantly, she was experiencing a much improved level of health and wellbeing.

What are emotions?

Emotions are information. They are currents of energy that move through the bodymind in response to the internal (thoughts, beliefs, images) and external circumstances of our life. I like to think of them as messages that are trying to get our attention in order to move us in some way. If the message is acknowledged and received (for example, by embracing and feeling an emotion such as sadness), you might be moved to cry, to share your feelings with another person, or to write about those feelings in a letter or journal. You might also be moved to release that emotion using one of the processing techniques that I share later on. All of these are healthy ways of relating to emotions, because they work with, not against, the emotion. A healthy relationship with emotions arises when we allow ourselves to be present enough with our feelings in a way that allows us to be moved by them. An unhealthy relationship occurs whenever we attempt to sedate or control our feelings.

What are the different types of emotions?

There are a lot of different 'flavours' of emotions and many ways of categorising them, but the simplest system uses just four major categories. I came across it in an excellent book called *The Emotional Toolkit* by a clinical psychologist called Dr Darlene Mininni.[1] She places all the emotions under the following sub-headings:

Happiness	Anger	Sadness	Anxiety
joy	frustration	grief	panic
pleasure	resentment	shame	nervousness
gratitude	upset	inadequacy	dread
contentment	irritability	hurt	concern
love	rage	guilt	insecurity

There are far more emotions than are listed here, but it gives you a taste of how emotions can be categorised.

What do the different emotions mean?

While the specific underlying meaning of an emotion will depend on you and your circumstances in any given moment, some general rule-of-thumb conclusions can be made about different emotions.

- **Happiness**, or one of its variations, arises because we have gained something positive. The relevant question is WHAT HAVE I GAINED?

- **Anger**, or one of its variations, arises because of some threat. The relevant question is HOW AM I BEING THREATENED?

- **Sadness**, or one of its variations, arises because of some kind of loss. The relevant question is WHAT HAVE I LOST?

- **Anxiety**, or one of its variations, arises because of some threat to us, combined with a belief that at some level we can't cope. The relevant question is WHAT AM I AFRAID OF?

Think back to a moment in the past when you experienced each of these four emotions. For each one in turn ask the relevant question and find your answer. Here are some responses provided my one of my workshop attendees, Pam:

Happiness

- Situation: my husband announcing that we are going on holiday to the Maldives (I've always wanted to go there)

- Gained: sense of being appreciated and cared about

Anger

- Situation: my husband not listening to me

- Threat: watching the football is more important than me

Sadness

- Situation: finding out that the house purchase has fallen through

- Lost: my dream of living in that house

Anxiety

- Situation: one hour before having to do a presentation at work

- Afraid: of being laughed at

Women and emotions

While there is a popular stereotype of women being more emotional than men, research has found that men and women experience very similar levels of emotion, it's just that women are more likely to show that emotion. This is partly the result of social conditioning, which means that as a woman you are much more likely to be exposed to emotionally focused conversations and encouraged to express your emotions verbally, although for most women the exception is the expression of anger.

When compared with men, women[2]:

- Express their emotions more easily and are less likely to exert control over what they feel

- Are more likely to share their emotions with others

- Express their emotions with more intensity

- Use more emotive language

- Are more likely to have their behaviour affected by emotions

- Are less likely to express emotions relating to control, such as pride, anger and jealousy

- Are more likely to remember details of an emotionally charged event or experience and experience greater emotional intensity in response to those memories

- Are likely to experience mood swings because of fluctuations in their hormone levels – for example up to 60 per cent of women will experience mood swings prior to their period, mainly due to changes in hormones and levels of the brain neurotransmitters serotonin and noradrenaline

Another fascinating piece of research, using the well-known Myers-Briggs personality test, found that women and men tend to come to decisions via different pathways. Between 60 and 75 per cent of women use a 'feeling' pathway. This involves looking at a situation from the inside out, empathising with the situation and weighing it up in order to achieve the greatest harmony, consensus and fit, for example one that considers the needs of others. Between 55 and 80 per cent of men, on the other hand, prefer a more detached 'thinking' pathway, coming to what seems to them to be a logical, reasonable and consistent decision by using a set of rules. Neither of these pathways is better than the other, just different.[3]

In a nutshell, women tend to be influenced and affected by their emotions more than men, but you also have the ability to deal with this more effectively than men!

When emotions become a problem

Emotions become a problem when you sedate, control or deny them. At the heart of this is the tendency to divide emotions into two groups, positive and negative, and then further subdivide them: joy, happiness and peace (positive), and anger, rage, sadness and fear (negative). This polarisation of emotions is unfortunate, because they all contribute to being 'real' and the experience of being human. Negating any of these emotions blunts our ability to experience the full spectrum of emotions, which in turn disconnects us from a valuable source of insight and information. Emotions are therefore not inherently bad. Anger is not bad, rage is not bad, sadness is not bad; what determines whether they are healthy or unhealthy is our relationship to them. These are the five main 'relationships' we have with our emotions:

- Feeling them fully, accepting them as they are without wanting to do anything with them and allowing them to pass through and out of your awareness – healthy

- Discharging them, through physical activity or sharing your thoughts – healthy

- Allowing them to overwhelm you and acting them out – unhealthy

- Suppressing or consciously resisting them, which often involves distracting yourself or chemically changing the way you feel through behaviours such as eating, drinking alcohol or smoking – unhealthy

- Repressing them, in other words they are automatically prevented from coming up in the awareness – very unhealthy

In my own work I've found that people who suppress and repress their emotions the most are so-called 'nice' people. However, by adopting a 'nice all the time' approach in order to avoid conflict and receive positive attention from others, true feelings of anger, sadness and resentment – all of which are normal and natural – get bottled up. Doing this increases the likelihood of emotionally induced illness, such as chronic pain and irritable bowel syndrome. At another level I also believe that being inauthentic – that is, living a life that is not in accordance with the truth of your experience – is a soul sickness that can lead to a life of perpetual dissatisfaction. Getting in touch with your emotions, feeling them fully and being authentic and honest is, for me, at the heart of emotional health and wellbeing.

The integrated medical approach to facing and embracing your emotions

Learning how to face and embrace your emotions requires time, patience and commitment, but the rewards are many, including feeling more alive, being in touch with your intuition, experiencing deeper levels of intimacy and connection to others, enjoying much higher levels of emotional and psychological health, and reducing the risk of developing health problems relating to emotional repression.

Step 1 • Consider biological contributors to your emotional health

One of the mistakes that many people make is to assume that if there is a problem with emotions then the root cause must rest at the emotional or psychological level. While this is often true, it's also sometimes not. The health of your body also has a big influence on emotional wellbeing. Just think back to the last time you had a full-blown cold. Do you remember how miserable you felt? Those emotions weren't just because you weren't happy about having your cold. You felt them because your immune system released chemicals in your body that altered the way you felt, which is actually a very clever way of forcing you to rest and recuperate. All of the following biological factors can influence the way you feel.

- Diet, exercise and sleep

- Nutritional deficiencies – particularly of omega-3 and omega-6 essential fatty acids, vitamin C, B vitamins, folic acid, chromium, magnesium and zinc

- Food and chemical sensitivities – particularly to gluten (found in wheat, rye, barley and oats), casein (found in dairy products), caffeine, egg white, chocolate, aspartame (a sweetener) and moulds

- Toxicity – due to lead, mercury, cadmium and aluminium

- Blood-sugar imbalance – due to excessive consumption of refined carbohydrates and sugar

- Hormonal imbalances – thyroid, adrenal and sex hormone imbalances

- Diseases – anaemia, diabetes, chronic fatigue syndrome, chronic pain, cancer, arthritis, premenstrual syndrome, insomnia, stroke, multiple sclerosis or any chronic disease

- Prescription drugs – such as atorvastatin, amlodipine, atenolol, diltiazem, ibuprofen, propanolol, captopril, cimetidine, diazepam, levodopa, prednisolone, indomethacin and opiates

- Recreational drugs – such as caffeine, alcohol, tobacco, marijuana and cocaine

If you have any mental health problem, such as anxiety, depression or excessive anger, or if you experience mood swings, my advice is to work with an integrated medical doctor or nutritional therapist who can assess whether any of the above are influencing your mood. For example, many women with mood swings prior to having their period will experience a significant improvement in their symptoms if they take the herb agnus castus, vitamin B_6 and a high potency multivitamin-mineral.

Step 2 • Assess your emotional management style

A good starting point for exploring your relationship to emotions is to identify which of the following emotional management approaches or styles you use. While you might use a few, one tends to dominate and it's that one that you need to identify. Each style has a different philosophy, spoken or unspoken, about emotions. Read through the descriptions below and see if you can identify which group you belong to at the moment. As a clue, we tend to adopt a style similar to our parents!

Proactive approach
Someone with a proactive approach:

- Understands that emotions are information and is able to welcome them fully without needing to change, control or sedate them

- Does not label emotions good or bad, but regards them simply as movements of energy through the bodymind

- Feels comfortable with experiencing the full range of emotions, from sadness and anger to happiness and peace

- Knows how to express and use their emotions in ways that are appropriate to the situation

- Is more understanding of other people when they are experiencing emotions and will allow them to move through their emotions rather than closing them down

- Knows how to take care of themselves if they do experience strong emotions – for example by calling a friend or becoming fully present to what they are feeling

Open approach

Someone with an open approach:

- Understands that emotions are an invaluable part of being human

- Will allow themselves to experience their emotions, for instance anger or sadness, but unlike those that use a proactive approach is more likely to identify with their emotion and will just wait for the emotion to pass

- Will tolerate other people being emotional, but not necessarily be comfortable with the situation and will experience some degree of resistance

- Will lose sight of their authentic sense of self when feeling emotional

Closed approach

Someone with a closed approach:

- Keeps their so-called negative emotions, for instance anger, sadness or fear, hidden, because they are uncomfortable with them

- May or may not be aware of what they are feeling

- Will be fearful of expressing emotions, because, commonly, they have a fear of being criticised, losing control, being weak (if they believe that showing emotion is a sign of weakness) or upsetting others

- Will find it difficult to experience intimacy and connection because they struggle to reveal and share their inner experience

- Will be upset, intimidated and/or overwhelmed by those who do show their emotions

- Will tend to project their emotions onto others, for example falsely accusing someone of being angry, when the truth is that they are angry themselves

- Will probably use food, alcohol, smoking, drugs, work, sex, gambling and so on to control and sedate their emotions

- Will dismiss others who are emotional, perhaps by saying 'you really shouldn't be upset', 'it's not that bad', 'look on the bright side' and so on

Anti-emotion approach

Someone with an anti-emotion approach:

- Will either reveal very little emotion or be blown hot and cold by their emotions – there is no healthy middle ground

- Respond to other people's 'negative' emotions with hostility, for example a mother might say to her child, 'If you don't stop crying I'll give you something to cry about' or 'You can stop that now you ungrateful little so and so'

- Is constantly involved in power struggles and knows only how to 'feel in control' by putting other people down

- Is emotionally unstable and unpredictable, which can be very intimidating for people close to them

- Will probably use food, alcohol, smoking, drugs, work, sex, gambling and so on to control and sedate their emotions

Having read through these descriptions you can probably guess that the healthiest approach to emotions is a proactive one, followed by the open approach, closed approach and then the anti-emotion approach. However, these are not fixed levels. Regardless of which approach you use at the moment, everyone can move up the emotional ladder using the remaining steps.

Step 3 • Identify your beliefs about emotions

The following exercise provides a revealing and insightful way of illuminating the beliefs that you have around your emotions. It is best done with a friend or partner who can read the statements out to you and write your answers down, but if that's not possible just do it yourself. The key to this exercise is to write down your answers immediately, without thinking – it needs to be done quickly.

Anger is ....

Sadness is ....

Fear is ....

Vulnerability is ....

Happiness is ....

For example, one of my workshop attendees responded with:

- Anger is bad, anger is evil, anger is wrong, anger is dangerous, anger is awful

- Sadness is weak, sadness is not allowed, sadness is scary, sadness is threatening

- Fear is painful, fear is terrifying, fear should be hidden

- Vulnerability is terrifying, vulnerability is like death

- Happiness is bad, happiness is not OK, happiness should be controlled

What I find illuminating about this exercise is that it reveals we all make judgements about things that are completely normal and natural – our emotions. Having completed this I suggest you use either the Emotional Freedom Technique (EFT) (see page 151) or EmoTrance (see page 158) to release the beliefs that you have around your emotions. Both of these are explained in detail in part three. This is important and powerful work. EFT and EmoTrance are two self-help techniques that are very effective at bringing about deep shifts in our relationships to things, whether they are fears, situations or emotions.

Step 4 • Share your feelings

This is very important for women. One fascinating study found that women who hold back feelings of anger actually end up much more angry and irate in the long term. In the study the researchers compared different methods of regulating anger and sadness in men and women exposed to emotional film footage. The researchers instructed one group to express any feelings of anger brought about by the film clips, a second group was told to suppress their anger and a third group was told to substitute a happy memory for any feelings of anger. All three groups then watched a second film and were allowed to respond spontaneously. The results showed that the women in the study who had suppressed their anger reported feeling more angry, outraged, upset and disgusted than their male counterparts.[4] The following suggestions will help you communicate your feelings more effectively.

- The next time you feel angry about something commit to sharing it. If you are being over-run with emotions, before you say anything take three deep breaths. Breathe in for a count of four and breathe out to a count of seven. This will help to calm your mind and reduce the intensity of the emotions that you are feeling.

- If you are talking to the person that your feelings are about, use 'I' statements, as this will reduce the likelihood of them feeling criticised, blamed or attacked. For example, rather than saying, 'you never help with the kids', the 'I' approach would be, 'I'm really struggling to cope with the kids by myself and it makes me feel overwhelmed, so would you be able to help me by putting them to bed tonight?' You can see what a difference starting with 'I' makes.

- Keep a diary or journal. Expressing what you are feeling through writing is not only great for your mental health, it has been found to improve your immune system, reduce stress levels, help you get perspective on situations and help you get to know yourself better (see page 34).

- Mentally rehearse your communication skills. Close your eyes and allow an image of a confident and assertive you to appear. See yourself engaging in the types of situations that would normally make

you upset. Watch yourself keep calm, but act firmly and appropriately. Once you've got the hang of it, become one with this new
you – imagine yourself as an assertive, confident person. Get a real
experience for how it feels to be this way. What things would you
be saying that are new? If you looked in a mirror how would you
look? What would your friends and family say? Allow yourself as
much time as you need to experience and make real this new you.
Muster as much energy as you can to really allow yourself to feel
alive and confident. Experience yourself managing situations
effortlessly and enjoy the experience! Repeat this exercise as often
as you want – I suggest at least once a day for 14 days.

- Try role playing. With a trusted friend or even a practitioner, recreate a typical scenario that would lead to you becoming emotional.
  Practise different ways of asserting yourself. Remember to breathe
  deeply. Tell your friend what it is you want. Practise changing your
  voice, your posture and your body language. Work out between
  you what works and rehearse it until this becomes your new way of
  relating.

- If you are in a relationship, take a look at Secret Five: Develop and
  Deepen Your Relationships (page 127) for more suggestions on how
  to communicate more effectively.

Step 5 • Choose an emotional management tool

When I work with patients who have a significant stress or emotion-
related component to their health problem, I teach them one or more
of the three emotional management tools that I recommend. These
tools are really designed to help you process emotion. Remember
emotions are designed to flow and when, for whatever reason, they
get stuck or are ignored that leads to problems. Details of all can be
found in part three. They are:

- Mindfulness (see page 147)

- Emotional Freedom Technique (see page 151)

- EmoTrance (see page 158)

My advice is to read through all of them and start using them on various issues that you are finding challenging at the moment. You might want to use the following series of questions as a way to help you focus on what might in some way be holding your health, healing and happiness back. My advice would then be to address one issue a day. Because many issues are interconnected, you will almost certainly find that once you have successfully cleared one issue, the intensity and importance of other issues will also change, so keep reassessing whether an issue is important for you or not.

What are my five worst mistakes?

1. _____

_____

2. _____

_____

3. _____

_____

4. _____

_____

5. _____

_____

What are my five greatest fears or things holding me back?

1. _____

_____

2. _____

_____

3. _____

_____

4. _____

_____

5. _____

_____

What areas of my life am I not facing up to at the moment?

1. _____

_____

2. _____

_____

3. _____

_____

4. _____

_____

5. _____

_____

What are my five worst memories?

1. _____

_____

2. _____

_____

3. _____

_____

4. _____

_____

5. _____

_____

Which five factors or issues undermine my self-belief?

1. _____

_____

2. _____

_____

3. _____

_____

4. _____

_____

5. _____

_____

Step 6 • Deactivate any emotional trauma

I am yet to encounter someone whose health, happiness and quality of life is not, at some level, being limited and affected by trauma. Anytime we are overwhelmed by a situation we perceive as threatening it is traumatic. Most people tend to associate trauma with obvious events, such as experiencing or witnessing physical or sexual abuse, experiencing or witnessing violence, war, natural disasters, rape, accidents, major illness or the loss of a loved one. Indeed, one study interviewed women from five different countries and found that over a lifetime up to 66 per cent of women had experienced physical abuse, 37 per cent emotional abuse and 33 per cent sexual abuse.[5] However, trauma can also happen after not-so-obvious experiences, such as parental neglect, emotional, intellectual and/or spiritual abuse, minor injuries, childbirth, medical procedures, injuries and minor illness.

I have also found that many of my patients have experienced trauma within their relationships, either because of what happened during that relationship or because of the heartbreak and pain following the end of the relationship. Other patients of mine have post-traumatic stress disorder, which develops after exposure to one or more terrifying events in which grave harm occurred or was threatened, and in response to which they experienced intense fear, helplessness or horror. It causes flashbacks, nightmares, a state of hyperarousal (in which they have problems sleeping and relaxing) and has a significant impact on their life, health and relationships.

Getting to the heart of an underlying issue, such as heartbreak or abuse, and using one of the simple and safe processes in the emotional trauma techniques section can create a dramatic and immediate shift in the way you feel. If you think this might apply to you then I would recommend that you read through this section.

Are you carrying emotional trauma?

If you are reading this and feeling uneasy, anxious or nervous, or if your heart is racing, your palms are sweating or you experience a tightening in your gut, then those are clues that emotion is waiting to be deactivated and processed in your body. Another way I help my patients identify traumas that need to be processed is to ask about significant stressful events from the past, get them to breathe deeply and, as they focus on the event, to tell me what they are experiencing. A feeling of heaviness, distress, upset, anger, irritability, numbness or any negative emotional state suggests that at some level they are still being affected by that event. Try this exercise.

EXERCISE: What events from the past are still affecting you?

Make a list of five emotionally traumatic and stressful events or experiences involving people, which you would like to be free of. Once you have written them down, close your eyes, breathe deeply, think about the first one and become aware of what you are feeling. You can stop getting caught up in the emotions by commenting, silently or out loud, on what you are experiencing. For example, 'When thinking about Peter I feel heaviness in my stomach, I feel nauseous and upset.' Once you've finished, and it need only take a couple of seconds, turn your attention to the next one and repeat the exercise. The list that you create now is going to be the basis of the work that you do a little further on and if you prefer you can write this information in your private journal.

1.

2.

3.

4.

5.

How to heal trauma

Traumas should ideally be worked through with the help of an experienced professional, especially if those traumas are significant. I also find that it's not just simply a case of deactivating the emotional charge relating to the trauma, it's also about processing all the consequences of the trauma and also learning new emotion and stress management skills – see Resources for details.

There are, though, occasions when it is safe to release and process stuck emotions relating to past events by yourself. For example, I have had quite a few patients come to me who need help and support in processing the grief that they have in relation to the loss of a partner. To help them, I usually recommend EmoTrance (see page 158), which is a wonderfully simple and effective skill for releasing the blocked grief energy and it can take just 20 to 30 minutes to release completely. Minor traumas, such as arguments with others, can also be dealt with effectively with EmoTrance and/or Emotional Freedom Technique (see page 151). This tool can be used effectively by yourself, but in my experience most people prefer to seek help from a practitioner, as working with trauma can feel overwhelming at times.

SUMMARY

- Emotions are information; currents of energy that move through the bodymind in response to the internal (thoughts, beliefs, images) and external circumstances of your life. They are messages that are trying to get your attention in order to move you in some way.

- Being overwhelmed by emotion, suppressing emotion and repressing emotion are all ways of relating to emotion that represent a significant barrier to health, healing and happiness.

- Learning how to embrace and work with your emotions is not only healthy, but the key to resolving emotionally related illness and growing emotionally and spiritually.

- Taking an inventory of emotionally traumatic experiences in your life and then seeking help can result in a significant improvement in the quality of your life and help various problems, ranging from anxiety and depression to eating disorders, phobias and panic attacks.

Secret Four
Accept yourself

~

If I had to identify just one factor that had the greatest potential to create lasting health, healing and happiness it would have to be self-acceptance. This provides the foundations upon which I work with many of my patients and in my experience it is the missing ingredient in most women's health programmes.

CASE STUDY

As Lori came into my office it felt like a whirlwind had entered with her. She was chatty, energetic and, at face value, full of life and vitality. She then started to share with me her long list of 'problems' – insomnia, anxiety, excess weight around her abdomen, stress and a husband who was, according to her, 'emotionally shutdown and deliberately out to wind me up'. Many of these problems had been going on for some time and she had tried everything from Reiki, counselling and strict diets to self-help workshops, nutritional supplementation (she was taking 12 different supplements) and affirmations. None of these appeared to be working for her.

As she continued to speak, I noticed that every 60 seconds or so she would subtly, and sometimes not so subtly, berate herself. It wasn't obvious, but she used phrases like, 'I should be slimmer', 'I can't believe I let him do that', 'I just need to try harder...' Of course these are fairly common things for people to say to themselves, but what was marked about Lori was the energy and tone with which she said it. I sensed, and she later confirmed that this was true, that she didn't like herself. In fact, part of her hated herself and that part of her was trying everything in its power to change her, in order to fit an image of how she should be. The disparity between how she was and how she thought she should be was, from my perspective as an integrated medical doctor, the root source of tension and stress in her bodymind – it was this that was stopping her health from flourishing.

My first priority with Lori, therefore, was to show her how to cultivate what I refer to as self-acceptance. Within four weeks of starting the exercises and using the skills that I'm about to share with you she contacted me to say that she was feeling much calmer and being much kinder to herself. Of course, she wasn't yet achieving this all the time and it was hard, especially when she was stressed, but for the first time in her life she was really starting to get a sense of what it was like to love and accept herself. For me, showing my patients how to achieve self-acceptance is the greatest gift that I can pass on to them.

Self-acceptance and women

Many women are obsessed with the idea of improving themselves. The self-improvement industry is flourishing, increasing numbers of women are having cosmetic surgery, and millions of women are trying to lose weight and cover up the signs of ageing. What is behind this – why are so many women trying to the change the way they are?

Having worked with hundreds of women on issues relating to self-acceptance, such as depression, anxiety, emotionally induced pain, addictions and eating disorders, I have come to the conclusion that it's due to the 'I'm not good enough as I am' belief. This drives various actions and behaviours that are designed to convince the world and yourself that you *are* OK as you are. This belief is very much rooted in a competitive, consumerist society in which everyone is trying to keep up with everyone else. Of course, it's absolutely great to have goals, visions and aspirations – they provide us with momentum, hope and fuel to move forward in life. The problem comes when the decisions are rooted in fear, judgement and resistance to reality, because that perpetuates the myth that you are not OK as you are. Being stuck in this vicious cycle not only contributes to discontentment and frustration, but it is the motor behind many of the problems faced by women today, including stress-related illness, depression, anxiety and eating disorders.

What is self-acceptance?

Self-acceptance is the inner acceptance of who and what you are, just as you are. When you unconditionally accept yourself you see yourself and all the different aspects of yourself – thoughts, feelings, images, behaviours, appearance and life situation – clearly, with a welcoming attitude of non-judgement and non-attachment. What is beautiful about relating to ourselves in this way is that a freedom and joy starts to arise spontaneously and from this we begin to see new possibilities, such as taking a new job or going on a certain workshop or reading a specific book. Rather than being stimulated by fear and rejection of yourself, these thoughts come from a place of love and acceptance.

Why is self-acceptance important?

Self-acceptance is intrinsically connected to your level of fulfilment, happiness and peace of mind. People with a high level of self-acceptance:

- Are able to experience joy and freedom in most circumstances
- Feel the full spectrum of emotions without getting caught up in them
- Experience a deep connection to life, God or spirit
- Feel healthier, happier and more at peace
- Experience a deep gratitude and reverence for life

- Are present, awake and aware in the moment

- Are able to develop intimate and loving relationships with others

- Are better able to respond to life's challenges effectively and creatively

- Are much less likely to have depression or mental health problems

- Are less likely to experience addictions, take drugs or have problems with friendships and relationships

- Are more likely to treat other people with respect, care and kindness

In my experience someone with a high level of self-acceptance has an ease of being about them and an authenticity in which they accept life on life's terms. If that sounds good to you, read on!

The integrated medical approach to self-acceptance

Self-acceptance doesn't happen overnight. In fact, developing it requires a lot of patience and consistency, but I believe it is the most deeply rewarding work you can do if you are truly committed to your health, healing and happiness.

Step 1 • How much do you accept yourself?

This might appear to be a very straightforward question, but most people will answer it so quickly that they don't allow a true answer to rise within them. It's tempting to give a response that corresponds with how you would *like* to be, rather than how you actually are. Although this is a rather crude way to assess your level of self-acceptance, take a couple of deep breaths and say the following out loud:

'I deeply and completely accept myself'

How true do you feel this statement is for you? Score yourself between 100 and 0 (100 = complete and total self-acceptance and 0 = no acceptance whatsoever). If you score less than 90 continue.

Step 2 • How do you not accept yourself?

How do you not accept yourself? It's an important question to ask, because it will put you in touch with those aspects of yourself that need healing and accepting. The following exercise takes some time to do. I would recommend giving yourself at least 30 minutes to list your responses to questions one to three, and then slowly and at your own pace use the tools as instructed in part four on those responses. This can be done over days and weeks.

EXERCISE: Gaining greater acceptance

1. List the ways in which you do not accept yourself, then rank them in terms of how important they are to you, with the first your most important.

For example (these examples were given by workshop attendees):

- I hold back for fear of making a fool of myself

- I hate the way I look

- I feel embarrassed by my nose

- I don't feel confident in my abilities

- I wish I was taller and better looking

- I should be a better mother

- I don't know how to relate to people

- I should be married by now

You get the idea. It's important to be really honest with yourself and try not to hold back. One of my workshop attendees identified 55 ways in which he didn't accept himself!

2. List at least ten events and experiences from the past in which you were not accepted for who you were.

For example:

1. My mother told me that she always wanted to have a boy, rather than me

2. I was told by my parents that I was an accident

3. I was sent home from school for wearing make-up

4. My parents never listen to me

5. My husband ignores what I say

6. The other children didn't want to play with me at school

7. I was told by my parents that crying was a sign of weakness

8. I wasn't allowed to go to art school

9. I was abused by my uncle

10. My dad said he was embarrassed by me when I came last in a swimming race

3. List at least five reasons why you shouldn't accept yourself.
For example:

1. Self-acceptance will stop me from being motivated

2. It is wrong to accept myself, because I can only be accepted in the eyes of God

3. It will make me arrogant

4. I am not worthy of self-acceptance

5. I am scared of what might happen

4. Reduce the power that these statements have over you using either the Emotional Freedom Technique (see page 151) or Emo-Trance (see page 158).
Start with those at the top of your list.

As you work on the issues you have identified you will know that you have successfully released them when you tune into them and you feel at peace.

Step 3 • Watch out for the pain body

In his best-selling book *The Power of Now*, the spiritual teacher Eckhart Tolle talks about the pain body, an entity living in the bodymind which sustains itself by feeding on the negative energy created by drama. This drama includes all forms of negativity, judgements, self-criticisms, comparisons and blame. Basically any thought, image or action that is less than respectful, nurturing and loving provides the pain body with a source of sustenance. The pain body consists of all the emotional upset and trauma that we have accumulated throughout our life.

Because the pain body thrives on any negativity, one way to reduce its power and influence is to watch out for thoughts, images, feelings, sensations and stories coming from the pain body. Many patients find the idea of watching out for the pain body really useful, as it gives them a sense of the importance of being aware and alert, so that if the pain body does arise they can prevent or limit its less-than-healthy influence. This is not easy at first, but with some practise you will probably get quite proficient at it. I recommend you try the following exercise.

EXERCISE: 'I see you and I accept you'

Whenever you notice yourself getting caught up in negativity, irritation, irritability, judgements or drama, turn your attention to your body and locate where you feel the pain body is – it's often around the solar plexus, chest or throat area, although it can be anywhere. Having located it, say silently to that part of yourself, 'I see you and I accept you', breathing deeply as you do so. The pain body cannot (at this stage) feed on acceptance and love. Keep focusing on that area and on breathing deeply until whatever you are feeling and sensing passes. If it helps reduce the power it can have over you, imagine that the pain body is a harmless little gremlin.

In the early days of doing this you might get caught up in your feelings and thoughts, and that's OK. If that happens, just turn your attention back to the sensations in your body and repeat the exercise, but whatever happens, be gentle and respectful to yourself. If you criticise yourself while doing this that's the pain body speaking!

Keep a pain body journal

In addition to the 'I see you and accept you' exercise, which can be done in the moment and throughout the day, at the end of the day or whenever suits you best, write in a journal a couple of incidents in which the pain body took over your thinking. When you write, write in the third person as this helps with the process of 'dis-identifying' from the pain body. I usually get my patients to do this for about two weeks. For example you might write something like:

> 'Her pain body started to criticise her when she dropped a cup of tea on the floor. This triggered anger and sadness inside her.'

If you find it helpful, and most of my patients do, you can continue keeping a pain body journal for as long as you need to.

Pain body triggers

As a standalone exercise, write a list of all the situations and circumstances in which you experience your pain body being triggered. For example:

- When talking about money with my partner

- When watching *Eastenders*

- When reading the newspapers

- When I'm with my boss or parents

- When I'm tired or hungry

At the start of each day, briefly review your list of potential trigger events and, as best you can, watch out for the pain body during those times. There is more about healing the pain body in Resources.

Reduce the power of negative thinking

Most women suffer from negative critical thoughts about themselves and others – it's so common it's normal. In addition to the 'I see you and I accept you' exercise, I also offer my patients the following ideas to help disengage a troublesome or distressing thought. Contrary to popular belief, changing the thought to a more positive one doesn't actually work that well in the long term, because you are resisting reality, which in turn causes stress. It's much more effective to work with the reality, which is your stressful thought. Here are just a handful of useful ways to do that. Put them to the test and see which one works best for you.

Next time you get caught up in less-than-loving-and-accepting thinking, don't try and change the thought, but use one of the following strategies:

- Witness and observe your thoughts without judging them – see Mindfulness (page 147)

- Say to yourself 'oh that's my mind speaking, let's listen to what it has to say'

- Say sincerely to your thoughts 'thank you for your perspective'

- Imagine those thoughts on a karaoke screen – change the colour and font, make them small

- Sing those thoughts to yourself to the tune of 'Happy Birthday'

- Say to yourself 'my thoughts on this situation are...'

- Say those thoughts in a silly voice, such as Donald Duck's

To put this into practice, think of three thoughts about yourself, your life or health that are in some way distressing to you. Be as specific as you can. Write them down in your journal and for each one in turn get a sense of the hold, the power, it has over you. Once you have that sense use one or more of the above techniques to change the relationship that you have to that thought. Notice how different you feel about the issue now! This will hopefully give you a real sense of the power that our thinking can have over us. The real key to lasting mental wellbeing is to use these approaches every single day, until they happen automatically.

Step 4 • Take care of your inner child

While the idea of having an inner child sounds strange and challenging to some people, I find working with the inner child, alongside the pain body, to be one of the most important skills and tools for creating self-acceptance, healing the pain body and creating more joy in people's lives. The inner child is a metaphor to describe that young, vulnerable part of us that holds all our unfelt emotions, as well as our inner joy, creativity, spontaneity and source of wonder. All of us have an inner child that, like all children, simply wants to be accepted and loved for how it is. Learning how to do that is a skill that I teach to many of my patients. If you are anything less than loving and accepting of yourself then I encourage you to try the following.

EXERCISE: The inner child meditation

Once or preferably twice a day sit down in a place where you won't be disturbed, take a couple of deep breaths, close your eyes and imagine yourself as a five- or six-year-old girl. See her standing in front of you. Give that child some space and just watch her, notice how she is – is she sad, scared, angry, shy, distracted or happy? Now speak to her kindly and say that you want to take care of her, that you are sorry that you have ignored her, but that you are now committed to loving her just as she is. When she is ready, imagine picking her up and cuddling her. Tell her how much you love her and how you are going to take care of her. Do whatever feels natural. The most important thing is that she feels understood, validated, safe and loved. If you struggle to see yourself when you close your eyes you could find a photograph of yourself as a young child to look at. If you find this inner child work strange or weird, don't worry, you're not alone. Just persist with an open mind and open heart and when the time is right you will feel a connection.

EXERCISE: Inner child journal

Writing to your inner child and having a conversation is a simple and powerful way to start nurturing and communicating with her. If you are also doing the pain body journaling, try doing this afterwards.

- With your dominant hand write, 'How are you today little [your name]?'

- Then with your non-dominant hand allow her to write back to you. Don't censor the words and allow them to flow (this takes a little practice). Your inner child's response may be short.

- Then go backwards and forwards between adult and inner child until it feels right to stop.

- Finish the exercise by thanking your inner child and sharing *authentically* how you are enjoying spending the time together.

Essentially you are getting to know one another, plus it provides you with an opportunity to express how committed you are to taking care of her. The inner child needs to know this and more importantly experience it. I would recommend that you do this every day for the next 14 days.

Meeting your inner child's needs

As you go through the day check in with your inner child, especially when you are feeling out of sorts or stressed. Say to yourself silently, 'What do I need right now?' Do you need food, water, rest, sleep, to remove yourself from a situation or to pick up the phone and talk to someone? What do you need to take care of yourself? This is a very important exercise, because so many of us are out of touch with what we really need in any given moment. The pushy or perfectionist part of our personality will tend to drive us at the expense of our needs. While this is sometimes OK, done consistently it leads to stress and exhaustion. Getting in touch with your needs and taking action to meet them is just good self-care. There is more about inner child healing in Resources.

Step 5 • Love your body

This can be a real tough one for many women, as most women have a less-than-loving relationship with their body. In fact, some of the most beautiful people that I have ever worked with see and experience themselves as ugly. Other women might 'only' hate certain parts of themselves, such as their nose, thighs or breasts; others, and this is rarer, are completely accepting of themselves – stretch marks, cellulite, warts and all. In this exercise I'm going to guide you through a process that is designed to transform the relationship that you have with your body. If possible it should be done with a willing and non-judgemental partner or friend with whom you feel safe.

EXERCISE: Learning to love your body

1. Write down all of the different ways you don't accept your body. If you struggle with this ask yourself the question, 'What would I change about my body if I could?' Don't hold back with your use of language!

   For example:

   • I resent the fact that my left ear is lower than my right ear

   • I don't like my breasts, they are misshapen and ugly

   • My legs are too short

   • My bum is massive

   • I'm fat

2. Now write a list of what you do like about your body. If your instant response is, 'I don't like anything', take a couple of deep breaths and look in the mirror – you might find something.

   For example you might write:

   • I like my hazel brown eyes

   • I love my dimples

   • I like my long legs

3. Find yourself a large piece of paper and draw a picture of your body back and front – it doesn't have to be a work of art, just recognisable. Then, using different colours, shade in the areas that you don't love using a colour that feels appropriate. For each shaded area write in the thought(s) you have about that part. Once that is completed shade in the parts of you that you accept/like/love. This should be in a different colour, again one that feels appropriate.

4. Having completed your diagram, focus on each body part in turn, starting with those that you don't like first.

   • Breathe deeply and allow yourself to locate where you are feeling the unreleased emotional charge in your body. If you struggle with this, think back to an occasion when you were triggered by something and as a result started to think negatively about your body image.

- For each body part, release the emotional charge that you are feeling using either the Emotional Freedom Technique (see page 151) or EmoTrance (see page 158). Continue with each one, moving on to the body parts you do like/love.

- If you sense any block to these, release them also, until you get to the stage when you look at the diagram of your body and not only don't feel any negativity, but feel warmth towards your body.

5. Now try this powerful meditation:

EXERCISE: Loving-yourself meditation

- Sit still, close your eyes and take a couple of deep breaths in and out.

- Bring to mind someone or something that you have a deep unconditional love and appreciation for.

- If you can't think of anyone, imagine what the feelings would be like if you did have someone for whom you felt unconditional love.

- As you focus on that person or thing, notice what you are feeling in your bodymind and breathe in and out of those feelings, so that they start to expand.

- Once you can feel that loving appreciation in your body, release the image and send the loving appreciation that you are feeling down to your feet.

- Gradually move your attention up the entire length of the body, sending loving appreciation to every single cell of your body. This might take a couple of seconds or minutes – do whatever feels comfortable or natural.

- Once you reach the top of your head, take some time to enjoy the peace and stillness. If you sense any blocks anywhere use

EmoTrance (see page 158) to release it. Continue until your whole body is buzzing with warmth, expansion and self-love.

This last meditation is very powerful. I often recommend this as a standalone exercise that can be used, say, first thing in the morning or whenever you feel out of sorts.

SUMMARY

- Self-acceptance is the foundation upon which health, healing and happiness is built.

- Learning how to accept and value yourself just as you are takes time, patience and consistency.

- The intention behind the process of self-acceptance is that, no matter what, you bring a welcoming acceptance to reality – or 'what is' – because only by connecting and embracing reality can transformation and healing take place.

- The pain body is an entity that lives inside your bodymind. It thrives on negativity, so dis-identifying from it by using 'I see you and I accept you' can help to reduce the power that it has over you.

- Taking care and responding to your inner child – the vulnerable part of you that holds your unfelt emotions, as well as your joy, creativity and spontaneity – is one of the keys to self-acceptance. Doing the inner child meditation and journaling with her for a minimum of two weeks start the process of re-connection.

Secret Five
Develop and deepen your relationships

~

The quality of your relationships has a profound influence on your health, your mood, your ability to recover from disease and your level of happiness. These relationships are not just with friends, family and your partner, but with yourself, your community and even the planet.

According to Carol Gilligan, one of the world's leading authorities on gender studies, a woman's sense of worth tends to be inextricably bound up in her web of close relationships, whereas a man's sense of worth tends to be closely related to his achievements. Women therefore tend to be more diligent about maintaining and nurturing these relationships, and interpersonal details tend to be far more important to most women than they are to most men. The majority of these differences begin to emerge in early puberty: when girls talk to their friends, their conversation tends to be more emotional and to be concerned primarily with relationships, while boys tend to be more reserved and to discuss facts, statistics and achievements. Women, even more than men, need to have intimate relationships.[1]

CASE STUDY

Laura was a veteran of 12 self-help workshops and courses, a yoga devotee and someone who had travelled to many different countries, including India, Nepal, Guatemala and Peru. She had a significant amount of money, was the life and soul of the lavish parties that she threw at her country house and yet here she was sitting in my office crying. Despite her busy life and her appearance of 'togetherness', she was suffering from what I regard to be the core challenge of our time – a deeply felt sense of being isolated and alone, of being disconnected from her true self, from others and from nature.

What she yearned for, what she had spent her life searching for, was someone or something to share her beautiful, sensitive and vulnerable self with. She was not short of would-be partners, but the same pattern kept repeating itself: she would fall head-over-heels in love, open herself up to her partner and then, in her own words, would 'be stamped on and abused'. This cycle of hope–love–hurt had been repeating itself for most of her life and she was tired of it. She wanted nothing more and nothing less than an open, loving, fun and intimate relationship in which she was allowed, indeed supported, to thrive and flourish as a woman and human being. She wanted what many, if not all of us, want at the very core of our being – to experience intimacy and unconditional love.

What is emotional intimacy?

Most people agree that intimacy with others involves letting defences down, being vulnerable and sharing honestly from a place connected to feelings. When this is reciprocated it forges the experience of togetherness and connection. It feels wonderful, safe and healthy. As emotional intimacy progressively takes hold within a relationship, it provides the foundations for physical intimacy, sexual intimacy and spiritual growth.

How we learn the rules of emotional intimacy

Our capacity for intimacy is determined primarily by our parents or caregivers. We learnt how to be in relationships through the direct experience of our relationship with them and the observation of the relationship they had with one another. Our parents are our first teachers in love and intimacy. If they abused us, neglected us or were simply ignorant of or ill-equipped themselves with the skills of intimacy, it's highly unlikely that we know how to be intimate with others (and ourselves). Some experts believe that the emotional resonance of our early childhood (the first seven years) becomes imprinted in our psyche and that we, in our ignorance and innocence, come to equate this with love.[2] As adults we then seek that same resonance by drawing to us people and partners who will recreate that same resonance and dynamic. If abandonment, abuse or neglect was a theme of childhood, we tend to recreate that in adulthood until we wake up, create a new story about what love is and then learn the skills to bring that new love into being.

The healing power of intimacy

Fulfilling your basic human desire for connection and experiencing intimacy through partners, friendships, women's groups, social or sports groups, your community, animals and nature is essential for deep healing and total wellbeing. Here are just a few snapshots of some of the reasearch that has explored the influence of love and intimacy on health:

- Studies show that people who feel isolated are three to five times more likely to die prematurely and get sick than those who don't.[3]

- In one study people who had dogs had four times less sudden cardiac death that those who didn't.[4]

- Being a member of a church or bridge club can lower premature death by half or two-thirds.[5]

- In a study conducted by researchers from Yale University, 119 men and 40 women answered questions regarding their feelings of love and being supported, a factor which was independent of the effects of diet, smoking, exercise or genetics. The angiography tests that followed showed that the men and women who reported being loved and supported had significantly less blockage in their arteries.[6]

- The *American Journal of Epidemiology* reported a study that reveals the correlation between love and physical health. For a five-year period a university research project studied 8,500 men who had no previous history or symptoms of ulcers. By the end of the study 250 of the men developed ulcers. What was the variable? Men who reported a low level of love from their wives were more than twice as likely to have ulcers as the men who reported a high level of love from their wives.[7]

- A study of 7,000 residents of Alameda County, California, concluded that people who were isolated from meaningful relationships had a greater risk of premature death. Started in 1965 by Dr Berkman and her colleagues at the California Department of Health Services, the conclusion of the nine-year study was that people who lacked social and community ties – in other words those who were not married, who had little contact with family and friends, and who were not members of churches or other groups – were two to three times more likely to die prematurely than the people who had healthy relationships.[8]

What is love?

Given that most – if not all – of us are searching for it, asking the question, 'What is love?' is a vitally important part of creating more intimacy in our lives. Some of the responses I've had from my workshop participants include, love is 'feeling connected and at peace with the moment', 'the source of everything and the essence of who we are', 'it can't be described just known', 'the ecstatic feeling of being at one with someone or something' and 'what arises when we give unconditionally'. What's your definition and experience of love?

When it comes to understanding matters of the heart, and learning how to create more intimacy and love, the single most useful concept that I've discovered to date is that there are two types of love – romantic love and attachment love, and that the latter is the key to creating healthy and intimate relationships.

Romantic love

Romantic love is the passionate, head-over-heels type of love that we experience when we fall in love with someone whom we find attractive. This kind of love can last anything from days to two years. Romantic love is not to be confused with lust, the primitive 'I-need-to-gratify-my-sexual-impulses-with-you-now' experience! Romantic love can include lust, but it is so much more encompassing – it literally takes over mind, body, soul and common sense!

While studying the psychology and physiology of romantic love one of the most illuminating insights that I came across was the comparison of falling in love, or romantic love, with addictions. One interesting study found that the parts of the brain that get activated in addictions correspond exactly to the parts of the brain that get activated when we experience romantic love. This really helped to explain the experiences associated with romantic love and why it doesn't provide the foundations for lasting love.

An addiction is the compulsive continuing use of any substance or process, despite its adverse influence on a variety of areas of your life, including health, friendships, levels of awareness, spiritual growth, work, ability to stay focused and capacity for reasoning. As an addict gets pulled deeper into their addiction, whether it be to alcohol, drugs, work or sex, they will become more obsessive about their addiction, need more and more of the 'substance' to get the same high and they will become progressively powerless over the addiction. Their addiction takes them into a narrow, emotionally charged world, in which they feel disconnected from their authentic sense of self and unable to see reality as it is.

Romantic love addiction

This certainly doesn't apply to everyone, but if you do tend to lose a sense of who you are while in an intimate relationship then I encourage you to read this part on romantic love addiction. If not, great, move on to attachment love. When you fall in love your partner becomes your world; you think about them obsessively and yearn to be with them. You experience the incredible highs of being with them (and thinking about being with them), but also the lows when you can't be with them. You start to lose sight of important friendships, you find it hard to concentrate at work and you forget to take care of your physical body. You start to lose yourself in the relationship with your partner and, importantly, lose sight of yourself while doing so.

When you have fallen in love you will do anything, including deceiving yourself, in order to maintain that connection – that is until the pain, hurt and battles begin...

Why does this happen? I mentioned earlier that our definition and experience of love is based on our interaction with, and observation of, our parents and that part of us seeks to recreate that same emotional resonance, so that we might finally get the unconditional love we crave. Put simply, we are attracted to people who embody the positive and negative traits, and characteristics, of our parents in order to hopefully get the attention, acceptance, validation and love that we always wanted.

This usually isn't that obvious, but look deep (maybe with the help of a therapist) and you will find them! This is why in romance relationships each person feels as though the other is so familiar – they are! The only problem is that they, like our parents, will be unable to give us what we need or if they do give us what we need we can't receive it, because we don't know how to. As the joy of being in love wears off, your romantic partner transforms from someone who seems to bring out the best in you to someone who brings out the worst in you, by repeatedly and unconsciously (usually) poking you in your 'emotional sore spots'. You, of course, do the same to them, because romantic love is based on unfinished business from the past, not on the vitality and freshness of this moment.

Attachment love

While romantic love is a fiery, passionate, but essentially unstable kind of love, attachment love is a deep, secure connection found in committed long-term relationships. Attachment refers to the emotional bond between two people, which allows them to experience closeness and emotional intimacy, and it is more enduring than romantic love. Attachment love is actually rooted in your genes, and we have genetically programmed needs for closeness, a secure base (having someone there for you) and a safe haven (having people around you to whom you can go when you need help).

A healthy intimate adult-love relationship is based on being physically and emotionally responsive, and offering a secure base and safe haven to one another. This does not mean that you are enmeshed with one another – which is usually the first thing my male workshop attendees in particular flag up. Yes, you are dependent on your partner to give you closeness and security, but that bond provides the foundations from which you can create a life that allows you to embrace your individuality and uniqueness. It's a paradox that you need dependency in order to experience true healthy independence (which is not isolation). A securely attached love provides the firm ground upon which you live your life, but other recognised benefits include[9]:

- Higher levels of intimacy, trust and satisfaction

- Greater levels of success

- Increased likelihood of seeing oneself as loving and competent, and others as trustworthy and dependable

- Increased likelihood of resolving arguments and difficulties within a relationship

- Increased ability to deal with stress and conflict

- Greater confidence at work and more enjoyment of work

Securely attached people typically value relationships more and generally do not allow work to interfere with those relationships. They do not use work to satisfy unmet needs for love, nor do they use work to avoid social interaction.

The integrated medical approach to creating intimacy, love and connection

While the following suggestions are designed primarily for someone in a partnership, if you are single I still encourage you to read through them and to explore some of the suggestions as they will help you to prepare (as best you can) for when or if you do enter into a relationship. And if you are in an existing relationship, but are struggling or contemplating separation, I would strongly encourage you to follow the advice that I am about to share with you, while at the same time seeking professional guidance and support from a trained counsellor or relationship therapist.

Step 1 • Start facing reality and taking responsibility

For change to happen in a relationship at least one member of the partnership needs to get the ball rolling. This isn't about taking 100 per cent responsibility for the relationship, but 100 per cent responsibility for the way you are in the relationship. Commencing the process of change always starts by confronting the reality, the truth about your relationship. If you are anything less than completely secure and connected in your relationship, then for your sake acknowledge it. If you are no longer engaging one another, no longer speaking about things that truly matter, or tolerating each other's inappropriate or abusive behaviour, then take that as a warning sign. If you are simply co-existing with one another, or having the same arguments over and over again, take that as a warning sign, too.

Step 2 • Address the barriers to relationship success

While these steps will guide you in the process of creating attachment love, I find that the process of building trust, making connections and fostering intimacy is enhanced considerably when the following issues are identified and addressed in parallel with the work of relationship strengthening. If left unaddressed, each of these represents a significant barrier to a healthy and intimate relationship.

- **Addictions** This can include addictions to alcohol, drugs, prescribed medications, work, sex, love, gambling, the Internet, food and so on. See the section on addictions (page 260).

- **Trauma/abuse** A past history of trauma, abuse and neglect can have a profound effect on our ability to create intimacy. See Face and Embrace Your Emotions (page 94).

- **Codependency** While this term was once used to refer to someone who enables another person's addiction, it is now more generally used to describe someone whose emotional and psychological development has been blocked because of childhood trauma and/or neglect. See Codependency (page 307).

- **A broken heart or past relationship hurt** If you've been hurt in a relationship previously or if you still can't move on from a past love, then both of these will limit your ability to be fully present in your relationship now. Make a list of all of your ex-partners and for any that still trigger an emotional charge within you, you could try using EmoTrance (see page 158) to release it. Another way to let go of the past is to write an honest, emotionally charged letter to that person, in which you share your truth about them. Towards the end of the letter you should say something along the lines of, 'I am now moving on, I will not forget you, but I have my life to live now.' Going into the garden and having a small ritual, such as burning the letter, can provide completion. Do whatever works for you.

Of course there are many other barriers that will be personal to you. Use the space below to write down what they are or write them in your journal, followed by what needs to happen in order for you to overcome or address those barriers.

1

2

3

Step 3 • Practise respectful communication

The following exercise is something I give to patients whose communication is, shall we say, less than loving towards their partners. It's designed to create a safe way to communicate and I've found it absolutely invaluable in teaching my patients to start sharing their feelings with their partners. Because it requires a commitment to use it from both members of the couple, you should read through this with your partner and agree that when one of you announces that you would like to use the respectful communication exercise that you will do that at a mutually convenient time.

EXERCISE: Respectful communication

A = Awareness

- Become aware that you are stressed, tense or upset towards your partner.

- Say to them something along the lines of 'I need to share something important with you – is now a good time?'

- If it is, move on to the next step. If it isn't, agree exactly when would be a good time, but as a general rule of thumb it is best to do this exercise in the moment.

A = Active Listening

- Both of you should sit down opposite each other.

- The person who has asked to do this exercise should take a few deep breaths and then start talking, while the other person listens.

- The person who is listening is going to use active listening. This, as its name suggests, means actively listening to the other person without interruption. The goal of the listener is to understand what is going on for the other person, by listening to them and trying to see things from their perspective.

- The person who is speaking needs to explain what is going on for them. One very effective and relatively non-threatening way to communicate is to use 'I' statements to communicate your feelings about some aspect of your partner's behaviour. Stay clear of character assassinations. For example, 'You have absolutely no respect for all the hard work I do around the house. You just sit there and treat me like a slave. You are arrogant and selfish' would become, 'I feel taken for granted and unappreciated at the moment. I'm really tired and exhausted with doing all the housework myself. If you could help me for just 20 minutes twice a week that would make me feel so much happier. It would demonstrate to me that you really care for me.'

- Once the message has been communicated, the receiver needs to feed back the message in a way that demonstrates that they have genuinely understood the other person. At this stage you don't have to agree with what has been said, but you are validating and acknowledging what has been said.

- The receiver then asks whether he or she has correctly understood everything. The first person either says yes or communicates the areas that have been left out. The receiver once again provides feedback.

- Now you reverse roles, so that the other person shares their feelings.

A = Action

Once you have both communicated your feelings to each other, if it has been done effectively and genuinely you should notice a shift in the energy between you both.

The focus is now on what specific action, if any, needs to be taken. Using the example above, Mary and John agreed:

1. John will help with the housework for 20 minutes every Saturday morning and Wednesday evening.

2. When John gets home from work, rather than watching TV he will spend 15 minutes with Mary so they can talk about their respective days.

A = Appreciation

Once you've agreed on a plan of action, then it's time to reconnect to each other. This could be anything from hugging or going for a walk, to kissing or making love. Whatever works for you!

When arguments cross the threshold

From time to time, arguments may get out of hand. By this I mean:

- Verbally abusive

- Potentially physically abusive

- One of you feels emotionally overwhelmed

If any of these rear their head, then 'time out' can be called. Calling time out is a clear signal that this has gone too far and you can't cope.

- On calling time out, all exchanges and communication must stop instantly.

- The person who called time out says, 'I am not leaving the relationship,' and then they leave the room.

- Each person then must use whatever tools they want to calm down. I recommend Emotional Freedom Technique (see page 151), 4/7 Breathing (page 87), Journaling (see page 34) or calling a friend.

- Once the person who called time out feels calm enough, they return to the room with the other person and ask if they are ready to talk.

- If that other person is ready, then use the respectful communication exercise (see page 135).

Step 4 ● Identify your attachment style

We all have an underlying attachment style, a default way of relating that we tend to use most of the time. I have included all four here so that you can identify where you are at now and also to give you a taste of what is possible, should you do this relationship work!

Type one – securely attached

If you are securely attached in your love for your partner you trust them and you know you can count on them. Because your relationship is grounded in trust and mutual respect, you find it safe to talk about your feelings and feel able to share any problem that you might have about them with them. You are able to be present with one another and to truly listen without reacting, accusing, blaming, defending or shutting down. Your relationship no longer experiences the extremes of emotions and you walk a middle path together, secure in the freedom and joy that arises from a committed and intimate relationship. When you come together you feel safe and connected.

Type two – anxious attachment

If you really want to be in an emotionally intimate relationship, but struggle to fully trust your partner, then you are probably anxiously attached in your love for your partner. Like a small child who doesn't want to be left alone, someone with this style of attachment will either cling to their partner and/or do everything to get their attention – from waiting on their partner hand and foot, to arguing and screaming. They will do whatever they can to get close and to feel safe.

Someone with a type two attachment style is usually hypersensitive to any sign or indication that their partner is about to leave them or distance themselves. They will be sceptical about what their partner tells them and need to be reassured many times before believing them. One patient of mine would give her husband a grilling as to his whereabouts when he got back from work. She needed to know in order to make herself feel safe. Women with this type of attachment style tend to pair up with men who are type four.

Type three – fearful avoidant attachment

A person who can't trust anyone, and avoids closeness and intimacy because of an underlying fear, probably has a fearful avoidant attachment style. They learnt at some point in life that it was not safe to let down their defences and that it was safer to stay closed and protected. People with a fearful avoidant attachment style want to be in relationships, but they are fearful of being in them. They will be extremely cautious and not expect much from their partners. They almost expect things to go wrong, and when it (inevitably) does, it just confirms what they believe – that others can't be trusted. Another strong characteristic of fearful avoidants is that they tend to be plagued with worry and concerns, and are mentally battered by their own inner critic.

Type four – dismissing avoidant attachment

If you have a belief that you don't need to be close to people, and/or you prefer to avoid people and intimacy, then this type of attachment style probably relates to you. Like fearful avoidants, people with this style learnt in the past that it was not safe to be vulnerable and open within relationships. However, unlike fearful avoidants, dismissing avoidants tend to hold themselves in high regard, feel good about their 'independence' and will rarely turn to the relationship for security. For example, when faced with a potential relationship conflict they will pull down the emotional shutters, tune out of the situation or simply walk away in order to maintain their feelings of safety.

Step 5 • Increase your level of attachment love

There are many different ways to develop your emotional bond and create attachment love. The following are just some of the different strategies for achieving this.

- **Stop all blame** This is perhaps the hardest thing to do for most people, but blame only creates distance, resentment and pain. If you want to create lasting love then stopping the process of blame, and taking responsibility for reconnecting with your partner is the key to your wellbeing and the future of your relationship.

- **Know your emotions** Emotions are at the heart of attachment love. Whenever you remember, and certainly whenever you are feeling stressed or tense, try to identify what emotion you are feeling. There are a lot of different flavours of emotion, but the main ones are sadness, fear, shame, grief, disgust, anger, happiness and surprise. Then share the emotion with your partner and speak from that emotion. For example, 'I am feeling sad, it feels like we are…'

- **Resist the urge to fix** While men traditionally default to problem-solving, many women do as well. This has its place. However, more often than not women want to be heard and validated. The offer of a solution can be taken as a sign that they are a problem needing to be fixed, which is definitely not the case most of the time. Next time you experience the urge to fix your partner, swap that for listening and validating what they have just shared. Notice the impact that has.

- **Identify your dance** The dance is the default way in which you and your partner argue and interact. At the most simple level the dance usually consists of one person taking on the pursuer/controller/complainer role and the other partner the withdrawer/defender role. A typical scenario would be a husband getting home from work and sitting down to watch TV without saying hi to his wife. His lack of respect triggers her, she starts getting angry with him, this triggers him and he gets angry back, saying he's tired and that he's had a hard day, which then triggers her, and the destructive dance goes on.

The wife's anger and frustration is rooted in the distress of not feeling connected to her partner. She is simply trying to create an emotional bond, but doing so in the only way she knows how, through complaining and criticism. What she is really trying to say is this: 'I have really missed you today and when you watch TV without coming to see me first, I feel as though you don't really want to be with me, that you don't love me. I feel distant from you and I feel sad about this.' There you have it – if you can communicate the truth by getting in touch with your vulnerable emotions, nine out of ten times the other person will respond differently.

- **Listen** Of course, that's easier said than done, but one of the keys to success is to allow your partner the space to have their reality and to hear what they have to say. How do you feel when they interrupt you? Take a look at the respectful communication exercise (page 135) for some suggestions.

- **Get behind your anger and share your vulnerability** Most people experience anger, frustration and/or irritability in relationships. However, most of the time the anger is used to cover up the more subtle, vulnerable emotions such as fear, sadness and shame. It is these emotions that, once accessed and shared, can make the big difference between rekindling a connection and deepening the divide. Next time you experience anger, ask yourself, 'What other emotions am I feeling?' Then share with your partner, friend or family member what you are feeling, for example, 'I am feeling sadness or fear.'

- **Practise appreciation** Sharing genuine and sincere appreciation with the person you are with is one of the quickest and most effective ways to open the flood gates of connection. Studies consistently show that if the ratio of positive comments to negative comments is above 8:1, then the likelihood of creating and sustaining a healthy intimate relationship is increased considerably. Here are a couple of suggestions. Write down a list of all the things that you appreciate about your partner. If you get stuck, as a fair number of my patients do, recall what it was about them that first drew you to them. Having written the list, share one of those bits of appreciation with your partner each day for the next seven days. You will probably feel awkward when doing this and it might feel false, but most people relax into it very quickly. The key when sharing appreciations is to be as sincere as possible. If you feel tense about this, remember to breathe deeply.

- **Join Recovery Couples Anonymous (RCA)** Founded in the US in 1988, RCA is relatively new to the UK. It offers couples a safe environment in which they can learn how to develop the skills of healthy relating. Although it's based on the 12-step principles of Alcoholics Anonymous, you don't have to be in recovery to attend. If you and your partner are committed to transforming your relationship then I highly recommend it! See Resources.

Other pathways to intimacy and connection

In addition to developing intimacy with our partners, the following pathways to connection are also important, if not essential, to your health, healing and personal growth.

Pet connection

Keeping a pet and taking care of it can provide an invaluable source of connection. Unlike humans, pets don't tend to judge or answer us back. Keeping a pet has been found to reduce blood pressure, cholesterol levels, alleviate some of the symptoms of depression and reduce loneliness.

Friendships

Having a team of people, a network to whom you can turn to for support and enjoyment, is a critical component of mental health. It is not so much the quantity that matters, but the quality. People with a network of friends boost their chances of surviving life-threatening illness, have stronger, more resilient immune systems, improve their mental health and live longer than people without social support. Having at least one person that you can share everything with is truly life-enhancing.

Volunteering

Consider volunteering. People who commit to voluntary work are not only contributing to their community and society, but they also report a heightened sense of wellbeing, improved sleep and a stronger immune system.

Support groups

Join a social, sports or special interest club to meet like-minded people. Support groups for people going through illness or a life crisis can provide an invaluable source of support and help. There is also some good evidence that they can improve recovery and, in the case of cancer, help extend people's life. The 12-step groups, such as Alcoholics Anonymous, are absolutely invaluable to someone who has a desire to stop drinking. See Resources.

Soul connection
Following the desires of your soul is, in my opinion, one of the most important commitments you can make to yourself and to creating a deeply fulfilling life. I regard 'soul' as being your essential nature, your unique way of being that is waiting to being discovered and shared with the world. Embedded within soul are certain gifts, talents and powers that are entirely unique to you. To unearth those gifts requires a huge amount of commitment, dedication and courage. See Resources for books and events that can guide you through this process.

Spirit connection
Develop a spiritual practice. People who have a faith or belong to some kind of religious or spiritual group enjoy better health and greater support than those who don't. Meditation, prayer, mindfulness and contemplation are very effective tools for developing a deeper connection with the divine, which you could call God, Spirit or Life.

Nature connection
I believe that a significant and important contributor to the rise in distress and diseases in the developed and now developing world is our disconnection from nature. Learning how to reconnect to our own nature, through nature, is something I have a deep passion for and I invite you to explore it further. Why not consider exercising in nature? This could involve going for a walk or run, or even participating in a conservation project. 'Green exercise' as this is referred to, or simply being exposed to nature, has been found to lift mood, accelerate healing and help bring life challenges into perspective. I suggest you get into nature whenever you can and, when there, be open and receptive to nature's positive and healing influence on you.

SUMMARY

- Women, more than men, need to be in healthy relationships in order to thrive and flourish.

- Healthy relationships are rooted in honesty, respectful communication and intimacy – the ability to be vulnerable and to share your feelings.

- There are two types of love – romantic love and attachment love. The latter provides the foundations for lasting, fulfilling, intimate relationships.

- Four of the most common barriers to intimacy and relationship health are addictions, a past history of trauma, codependency and past relationship hurt.

- In addition to developing and deepening your connection to your partner, having one or more close friends, a pet, volunteering, being part of the community and having a healthy, loving relationship with soul and spirit are also important contributors to health, healing and happiness.

Part Three

Holistic health tools

In this section I outline five of the holistic health tools that I teach my patients to support them in their journey to better health, healing and happiness. These tools allow you to become an active participant in your own health and healing work, and many of my patients take some comfort from this. What this means is that whatever life situation you are in you will have a tool to hand to support you through it.

Each of the five tools has numerous applications, but to keep things simple I will provide the applications that I and my patients use most. If you have a particular health problem and will subsequently be turning to part four or part five of this book, I will also make a suggestion as to which of the tools might be most appropriate. Ultimately, however, you should trust your own intuition.

The five holistic health tools are:

1. **Mindfulness** – for pain, depression, anxiety, stress, fears and spiritual growth

2. **Emotional Freedom Technique** – for low confidence, fears, phobias, anger, self-limiting beliefs, compulsions, anxiety and psychosomatic illness

3. **EmoTrance** – for grief, anxiety, heartache, sadness, self-acceptance, love and goal fulfilment

4. **The Work** – for any stressful thought or belief and for spiritual growth

5. **Values-based Goal Setting** – for helping to get clarity around life direction, goals, meaning and purpose

While at first glance all five might seem a little overwhelming, they are actually pretty straightforward – the key is to give yourself plenty of time to try them out and to test them. Start by reading through the ones that interest you most and then try using them on any issues that you are dealing with.

Tool One
Mindfulness

To be mindful of something is to become aware of something. Mindfulness is a skill and practice that is increasingly recognised as an effective way of improving the quality of your life, reducing pain, relieving stress, decreasing addictive cravings, increasing self-awareness, reducing hot flushes and enhancing emotional intelligence.[1] One study by the University of Wales and John D Teasdale of the Medical Research Council in England found that eight weekly sessions of mindfulness halved the rate of relapse in people with three or more episodes of depression.[2]

Although mindfulness has only recently been embraced by Western psychology, it is an ancient practice rooted in the teachings of a fifth-century BC Indian prince, Siddhartha Gautama, later known as the Buddha, and it is found in a wide range of Eastern philosophies, including Buddhism, Taoism and yoga. Mindfulness involves consciously bringing awareness to your here-and-now experience with openness, interest and receptiveness. Jon Kabat-Zinn, a world authority on the use of mindfulness training in the management of clinical problems, defines it as, 'Paying attention in a particular way: on purpose, in the present moment, and non-judgmentally.' Mindfulness is about waking up, connecting with ourselves and appreciating the fullness of each moment of life.

How to develop mindfulness

Because mindfulness is a way of being, you can practise it all the time! I use the following mindfulness exercises with my own patients. Try them out and see which one of them suits you best. Here are a couple of tips to get you started with mindfulness training.

- Decide when you want to practise mindfulness. I recommend using it when brushing your teeth, washing and walking. Then, as you get better at it, use it whenever you meet someone.

- Starting tonight, when you brush your teeth, rather than brushing your teeth and thinking about something completely unrelated, become aware of the experience of brushing your teeth. Notice your thoughts, your feelings and sensations, allow yourself to become aware of the total experience without judgement or analysis. This is mindfulness – well done!

- Try this again when you have a shower or bath and when you go for a walk. Most people will be caught up in their thinking when they go for a walk, but when you walk mindfully you allow yourself to pay attention to the experience of walking. Start by paying attention to what you are feeling, then what you are thinking, then what you are seeing, then what you are hearing. Rotate around these. With time and practice you will eventually become aware of all these at the same time.

Mindfulness – observing your thoughts

If you tend to get caught up in your thinking, have mind chatter, depression or anxiety, try this:

- Sit somewhere quietly, where you won't be disturbed, and close your eyes.

- Bring your attention to your breathing. Observe the in and out breath without trying to interfere with the rate, rhythm or depth of breathing.

- Now become aware of your thoughts. Observe them without judgement or analysis, notice how they come and go. Notice the chaotic and sometimes nonsensical nature of those thoughts.

- If you catch yourself being drawn into the thoughts, just relax back once more and continue watching them as though watching a movie in the cinema.

- As you continue with this observation practice, notice how the quantity and intensity of thoughts start to settle as you start to withdraw energy from them.

- Witness how the space in between the thoughts starts to expand. This will become your focus of attention during meditative practice.

- Continue this for at least five minutes and then open your eyes.

As your awareness grows, you will start to notice how you feel uncomfortable in certain situations or that your body feels heavy after eating certain foods. Furthermore, you might start to notice patterns of predictable behaviour, in yourself and in other people. For example, you might notice that feelings of anxiety always precede the urge to eat chocolate or smoke a cigarette. Sometimes the light of awareness will result in the spontaneous changing of these behaviours and more often than not it lessens the hold they have over us. Indeed, as your awareness expands and deepens, your ability to see and acknowledge the reality of each moment deepens, and with that comes a greater connection and appreciation of life.

Mindfulness – being present with your feelings

If you feel uncomfortable with certain feelings or know that you sedate and control them, try the following:

- Sit somewhere quietly, where you won't be disturbed, close your eyes and take a couple of deep breaths in and out.

- Without getting caught up in a story or internal dialogue just notice your bodily sensations, pay attention to them and breathe into whatever you are feeling. Try not to judge your experience or attempt to do anything with it, just allow those feelings to be there and breathe.

- Next time you experience an emotion such as anxiety, anger or guilt, rather than responding by doing something with it, just simply observe it, watch it, allowing yourself to feel it deeply, completely and totally.

- By just being with the emotion you will experience it for what it is, just the movement of energy.

- Observe how that energy is constantly transforming itself, moving from one place to the next, fluctuating in intensity and changing its texture.

- Pain, suffering, stress and anxiety *all* arise when you resist the flow of energy; peace is experienced once you accept, witness and allow that energy to flow.

- As you continue observing the emotion, you will notice that it becomes focused in one particular area and that the intensity can increase before it decreases. Eventually, if you allow it unhindered expression, it will dissolve and as it does so it might present you with an insight or realisation as to what it is trying to communicate to you.

That's all there is to it. I never cease to be amazed how the simple act of allowing a feeling to be as it is, without judgement, can bring about a deep sense of peace and calm. I encourage you to experience this for yourself! For details of recommended books and CDs see Resources.

Tool Two

Emotional Freedom Technique (EFT)

Emotional Freedom Technique is a very popular self-help approach and I have successfully used it as part of my holistic health approach to helping people, mainly with issues and challenges that are emotionally focused. I find it to be especially good for helping to address low confidence, fears, phobias, anger, self-limiting beliefs, compulsions, anxiety and psychosomatic illness.

What is EFT?

The best description of EFT that I have read is one that described it as psychological acupressure. The basic procedure of EFT is to combine tapping on various parts of the body while saying specific phrases and affirmations describing the problem you wish to address and release.

How EFT works

No one really knows how EFT works, but there are plenty of theories. The most common perspective is based on the idea that in addition to having a physical body we also have a subtle energy body. This energy body provides a template for the physical body and also the medium through which our thoughts, intentions, emotions and perceptions influence matter, including the physical body. It is also believed that subtle energy, which is also known as *chi* or *prana*, moves through this subtle energy body via meridians or channels, which run the length and depth of the body.

Any time you have an emotionally charged experience that isn't fully processed and integrated, it creates a disturbance or blockage within the energy systems of the body, which in turn gives rise to self-limiting beliefs, thoughts and uncomfortable emotions. However, by tapping on certain acupuncture points (which can be thought of as gateways into this energy body), while focusing on the issue to be addressed, these disturbances can be corrected and a healthy flow of energy restored. That's one explanation. A more scientific one is that tapping induces an altered state of consciousness similar to the one you enter while dreaming and this enables the issue to be fully processed and resolved. My personal opinion is that both perspectives are valid and probably correct.

How to use EFT

Before attempting EFT you should spend some time reading through and familiarising yourself with its different steps, so that when you do start using it, you do so effortlessly and without much thought. EFT is divided into four steps.

Step One: Preparation

Step Two: The first sequence

Step Three: The second sequence

Step Four: Repetition

Step 1 • Preparation

Find somewhere quiet where you won't be disturbed. Turn your mobile phone off, unplug your phone and remove any glasses or jewellery that you're wearing.

Create your short problem statement

Identify the specific problem that you would like to resolve and create a 'short problem statement' that describes the issue you wish to work with. This should be as personalised as possible and should reflect exactly how you feel – don't hold back! Some example 'short problem statements' include:

'I have this deep anger and resentment towards Joseph'

'Sarah is driving me crazy'

'I can't stand being near Steven'

'I am over-sensitive to criticism'

'I am useless'

'I feel unlovable'

'I hate myself'

'I'm uptight about money and finances'

'I'm terrified of spiders'

'I feel scared to death about my job interview'

This short problem statement will be used with the 'tapping' part of EFT.

Create your long problem statement

Now create your long problem statement by placing your short problem statement into the template as follows:

'Even though [whatever problem it is you are working on], I deeply and completely accept and forgive myself, without judgement.'

For example, 'I have this deep anger and resentment towards Joseph' becomes, 'Even though I have this deep anger and resentment towards Joseph, I deeply and completely accept and forgive myself, without judgement.' Other examples include:

- 'Even though I hate myself, I deeply and completely accept and forgive myself, without judgement.'

- 'Even though I have this craving for cigarettes, I deeply and completely accept and forgive myself, without judgement.'

This long problem statement will be used with the 'patting the chest' part of EFT.

Rate the problem
Before you start, and to help you keep track of your progress with EFT, it's a good idea to measure the importance of the problem that you are working with, so score its importance out of ten (10 = the highest intensity level, indicating it's a major issue for you, 1 = no longer an issue for you).

Step 2 • The first sequence

Patting the chest
Place your full attention on the issue you wish to resolve and say your long problem statement slowly and out loud, while patting the upper left portion of your chest (just below your collarbone) with the flat of your hand. Repeat this three times. Keep focused on the issue, breathe deeply throughout and allow yourself to make contact with any emotions, if you can. Once you have finished, move on to the next step.

Tapping the eight points
Using all your fingertips (unless you have long nails) and with a relaxed, slightly curved hand, tap firmly on each of the following points in sequence. For each point tap about seven times and while you do so say your short problem statement. Begin with the top of the head then move on to the eyebrow, side of the eye and under eye, tapping each of these points on both sides of the face. Now tap under the nose and chin, then the collarbone and underarm. Each tap should be firm, but not painful, although some points will be more sensitive than others.

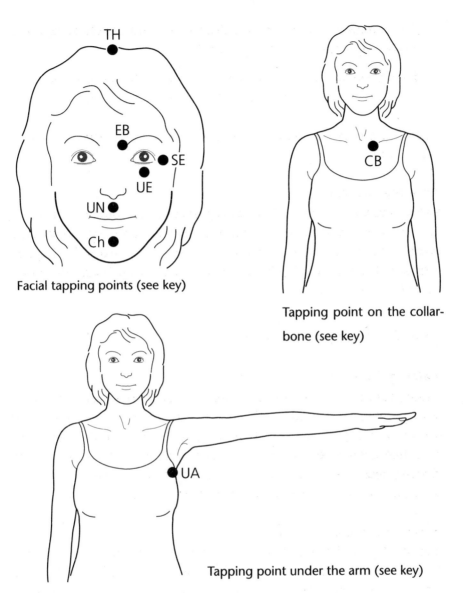

Facial tapping points (see key)

Tapping point on the collarbone (see key)

Tapping point under the arm (see key)

Key

Tapping Point	Location
Top of Head (TH)	Top of head and slightly back, to the 'soft spot'
Eyebrow (EB)	Beginning of eyebrow to the side of the nose
Side of eye (SE)	Corner of eye socket
Under the eye (UE)	Centre of bone below eye
Under the nose (UN)	Midline between mid nose and lip
Chin (Ch)	In the groove of the chin
Collarbone (CB)	Using the palm of your hand pat the area as shown above.
Underarm (UA)	On the torso under the arm, level with the seam of the bra (the nipple in men) and about 10cm below the armpit

Once you've finished, place both hands on the centre of your chest (the place you would point to if you were pointing to yourself), close your eyes and take three deep breaths. The first sequence is now complete.

Step 3 • The second sequence

Reassessment and adjustment of your statement

Take a moment to tune into the issue that you are dealing with and, using the same scoring system as before, reassess the intensity and importance of the issue. Most people will find that their score has dropped by at least a couple of points, maybe even more. Your goal is always to get the score to one. If your score is above one, make a slight adjustment to your long problem statement to reflect this. For example:

- 'Even though I *still* feel this deep anger and resentment towards Joseph, I deeply and completely accept and forgive myself, without judgement.'

- 'Even though I *still* have this loathing towards myself, I deeply and completely accept and forgive myself, without judgement.'

Now repeat step two of the EFT procedure again, but this time using your adjusted statement. So for the patting the chest part you will say something like: 'Even though I *still* feel this deep anger and resentment towards Joseph, I deeply and completely accept and forgive myself, without judgement', and for tapping the eight points, 'I *still* feel this deep anger and resentment towards Joseph.'

Once you've completed another cycle, you may get down to one, which is great, because that means you are finished. Alternatively, there may be no change in your score, and if this is the case chose a statement that more accurately reflects the issue, or you may find that a deeper issue has revealed itself. Don't be afraid to chase the issues as they come. The other possibility is that you may get your score down to two. If this is the case repeat the cycle one final time using the statement:

'I want to completely overcome this problem now and I deeply and completely accept and forgive myself, without judgement.'

Doing this will usually bring the score down to one, which indicates that you have successfully resolved the issue that you were working with!

Step 4 • Repetition

Some problems, particularly more complicated and long-standing issues, will require a number of EFT repetitions. Under these circumstances you should use EFT up to a maximum of ten times a day. If there is no obvious improvement within 48 hours, it probably means EFT is not suitable to your circumstances or that you might need some assistance from a professional EFT practitioner. For more information and recommended books see Resources.

Tool Three
EmoTrance

~

EmoTrance is a simple and highly effective tool that I use with about a third of my patients. I tend to use it most frequently for patients who are carrying unprocessed grief, anxiety, heartache and sadness, as well as for helping patients to release blocks to self-acceptance, love and goal fulfilment. If any of these are relevant to you, I encourage you to try it, particularly as the benefits are noticeable so quickly, often within a couple of minutes to an hour.

Similar to the theory of EFT, EmoTrance is based on the idea that a healthy state of mind and body arises when subtle energy (*chi*) flows without interruption through and out of the body. However, when we hold on to, suppress or repress an emotional upset this stops the energy from flowing, which in turn leads to distressing mental and sometimes physical symptoms. EmoTrance is designed to restore the flow of energy.

How to use EmoTrance

The following exercise will provide you with an experiential taste of EmoTrance. I would suggest giving yourself at least 20 minutes to do this at a time when you know you won't be disturbed.

1. Think of a statement, fact, thought or criticism that causes you to feel upset or to feel 'negative' emotions. This could be a person or a phrase that upsets you, such as 'You're fat', 'You're useless', or 'You disappoint me'.

2. Write this issue down on a piece of paper, turn it face down, take a deep breath, then turn it back over and allow yourself to feel any emotions. If you don't feel anything, choose another issue.

3. Pay close attention to where you feel it in your body. If there is more than one site, choose the one that feels strongest. What you are feeling is just trapped energy or emotion that wants to move.

4. If you can, gently place your hands on that area and get a sense of the direction in which the energy wants to go. If you don't get an immediate indication, start massaging the area with your hands, holding the intention of softening it as you do so.

5. When the energy starts to move, which it will do, get a feel for which part of your body it wants to exit through. This can be any location – top of the head, mouth, nose, hands, feet, anything goes! If it's not obvious which exit route it wants to take, just be patient and continue softening until it starts exiting your body.

6. Allow all the energy to exit your body. If it appears to get stuck, gently rub that area or trace the route you feel it wants to take with one of your hands, as that often helps.

7. More often than not, there will be residual energy in your body, so to make sure that all of the emotional charge has been deactivated, repeat the whole procedure again, starting from number 3.

8. Keep repeating until you feel no unpleasant sensation at all. On average it takes two to three cycles. If you feel lighter, more energised and much clearer around the issue, then you have successfully deactivated that emotional trauma – well done!

9. Take a moment to consider how this experience will change your behaviour and the way you feel about the issue.

Using this tool might seem complicated, but once you've tried it you'll see how straightforward it is. The key is to be patient with yourself. Part of your mind will try to rush you and convince you that it isn't working for you. If this happens to you, just slow down, breathe deeply and continue.

EmoTrance in action

To demonstrate how EmoTrance works in practice, here's a real life example of an EmoTrance session that I did with a woman called Erica, who had depression. In her own words, she told me that the greatest source of upset in her life was her relationship with her husband. This is not an uncommon situation. Here's the dialogue that took place.

Me: Tell me about your husband.

Erica: He frustrates the hell out of me. He's lazy, he won't do any work around the house and he spends more time with his mates than he does with me. He makes me feel worthless and so angry.

Me: Where do you feel that worthlessness and anger?

Erica: I feel it in the centre of my chest right here. *She points to the area.*

Me: OK, what you are feeling is energy that wants to flow out of your body. Breathe through this area, massage it gently and ask yourself, where does this energy want to go? All energy wants to flow out of the body, so where does it want to flow to?

Erica: It seems to want to go up into my throat.

Me: That's great. Gently tell that energy to soften and flow, allow it to flow, remember all energy wants to move. What are you feeling now?

Erica: It's strange. I can feel this tightness in my throat and now I feel it moving into my mouth – it wants to come out of my mouth! *Three minutes later it's all moved out.*

Me: Great, you're doing really well. How do you feel now?

Erica: I feel much better, much calmer.

Me: Fantastic. Now think about your husband again. Where do you feel him in your body? *Erica points to her stomach area. We then spend the next five minutes softening and allowing that energy to flow down and fully out of her legs.* How do you feel now?

Erica: I feel as though a heavy weight has been lifted. *There are tears in her eyes.* Wow, this is amazing. I can feel much more connected to him. I don't feel any anger, I just feel more at peace.

Me: That's great. Now breathe in deeply and spend a few moments with these new feelings that you have towards your husband. Get a real sense of how this is going to positively improve your relationship and how you will now be different towards him.

This is the beauty of EmoTrance. It requires no lengthy discussions, no interpretations and no need to talk about the problem, just the ability to feel where the problem is, soften it and allow it to flow out. The other interesting thing was that because Erica was no longer getting irritated by her husband and pressurising him to clean the house, he, of his own accord, started to do more around the house! Erica went on to use EmoTrance on a number of issues that were causing her upset. This included the beliefs 'I am not good enough' and 'I am unloveable', her grievances against two of her ex-partners and, most importantly for her, the anger she held towards her father. In addition to this she was able to start enjoying the very positive benefits that result from using EmoTrance on a daily basis, which included enhanced energy levels, improved self-acceptance, self-love and self-awareness, and the confidence that whenever she felt stuck or upset she could manage it by using EmoTrance.

In summary, when you have an emotionally charged issue to work with:

- Locate where you are feeling the energy

- Tell it to soften and flow

- Get a sense of where it wants to exit your body

- Allow it to flow and if you catch yourself trying to force it or getting frustrated by it breathe deeply and let go

- Repeat until you have gone as far as you can

For more information on EmoTrance and details of recommended books see Resources.

Tool Four

The Work

One of the most useful tools that I have come across to help individuals and couples transform their relationships, reduce stress and gain clarity is The Work. Developed by the spiritual teacher Byron Katie, The Work is designed to identify and question thoughts that trigger pain, suffering and distress. Because so many of my patients have distressing thoughts about their partners and themselves, I recommend it frequently. Byron Katie's understanding is that our most intimate relationship is with our thoughts and that the way we relate to them significantly influences the way we feel, react and behave. Because most of us believe and identify with our thoughts without questioning them, they wield considerable power over us. However, if we question them using The Work's process of inquiry, not only is it possible to reduce the negative hold they have over us, but this can also bring about a significant shift in clarity and understanding. It's not about changing your thoughts, but changing your relationship to your thoughts. At the heart of this is the realisation that most people are simply mirroring back to us dynamics that are about us, not them. You will need to try it for yourself in order to believe it. The exercise below gives you a flavour of The Work. I have modified it slightly, but I encourage you to refer to Byron Katie's original work by visiting her website or purchasing her book (see Resources).

A taste of The Work

Next time you have a self-limiting thought about yourself or your partner, such as 'he doesn't want to be with me', try the following. (for the best results write your answers down).

1. Ask yourself, 'Is this true?' Usually the immediate response is yes or no.

2. Now ask yourself, 'Am I absolutely sure it is true?' This time don't rush to answer it, breathe deeply and allow an honest answer to rise in your body. Whatever answer you get is fine. If you answer no, notice how this shifts the energy in your body.

3. Ask yourself, 'What happens when I think that thought?' How do you react? What happens? This gives you some insight into the power and limiting influence that this thought is currently having on your life.

4. Now ask yourself, 'Who would I be without this thought?' Notice the impact that this has on the way you feel and how this changes the way you would react to your partner. Give yourself plenty of time to become aware of the new feelings that arise – breathe deeply and give them plenty of space to come up. Having done this, the real key is the Turn Around.

5. In the Turn Around you are turning around the concept, idea or thought that you are working with. You turn it around in three directions – to the opposite, to the other and to the self. You then ask yourself, 'Is this as true or truer than the original statement?' For example, 'Paul should love me more' is changed to:

   • Paul should not love me (the reality in that moment, of course, is that he is not loving towards you)

   • I should love Paul (are you loving towards Paul in that moment?)

   • I should love myself (do you love yourself?)

6. Finally, write a statement in which you are willing to embrace reality, because it is fighting or resisting the reality that is at the heart of suffering. For example, your statement might be:

- I am willing to experience moments when Paul is not loving to me

Notice how freeing this is. By doing this final step, my patient was not only embracing reality – because of course there will be times when Paul is not loving to his wife – but she is learning the real so-called problem was that she wasn't loving herself. She can't control Paul, he is who he is, but she can control and influence the relationship she has to herself. As a result of doing this work my patient, Glenda, started to redirect her energy and attention from fixing Paul to taking care of and cultivating more respect for herself. This exercise took her just 15 minutes, but provided one of the most invaluable insights of her life to date.

By following these six steps you have shifted the power from the thought to your awareness. Thoughts are just perspectives and by becoming wrapped up in a particular thought it prevents us from accessing other insights and our own intuition. By going through the steps you are progressively separating yourself from the thought, so that you can decide yourself what is true for you.

Tool Five

Values-based goal setting

Helping my patients set and achieve realistic goals is a central part of the work I do and something that I really encourage you to do as well. Having goals relating to different aspects of your health and life is important. It can help you become clear about what you really want, it helps to provide focus (and reduces the likelihood of getting distracted), plus I have seen many times how committing to a goal actually helps to release the energy, enthusiasm, resources and clarity necessary to make that goal come true. Can you think of a time when this was so for you?

The key is to make sure that your goals are in alignment with your values. Values embody what is most important to you; they provide inspiration and motivation. Unlike goals, which are future-orientated, values are life directions that can be honoured now. They define what really, truly matters to you. They are the code of honour and foundations upon which you build a healthy and fulfilling life. For example, the values of one of my patients are:

- To experience *loving and respectful* relationships with the people I care about

- To live my life *authentically* and with *integrity*

- To share *honestly* when speaking with people

- To be *healthy* in body, mind and spirit

- To be more *accepting* of myself and others

The key with values is that they can be honoured every single day. While the exercise I am about to share with you is designed for medium- to long-term goals, I find it very useful to start each day by identifying a couple of 'today goals' based on my values. For example, based on the above I could ask myself:

- How can I experience *loving and respectful* relationships with the people I care about today?

- How can I live my life *authentically* and with *integrity* today?

- How can I share *honestly* when speaking with people today?

- How can I be *healthy* in body, mind and spirit today?

- How can I be more *accepting* of myself and others today?

For each of these I can then come up with one or two goals. Try it for yourself.

Setting your goals

1. Identify the values that are most important to you. Write them down in your journal.

2. Bearing in mind your values, decide on the specific goal or outcome that you would like.

3. How desirable and challenging is this goal (1 = not challenging, 10 = extremely challenging)? Your goal should score at least five.

4. Think about your goal, breathe deeply and turn your attention to your body – do you feel conflict or harmony?

Signs of conflict	Signs of harmony
Feeling contracted, uneasy or uncomfortable	Feeling expanded, light and at peace
Confusion	Clarity and alertness
Heavy, sleepy and/or tired	Uplifted, energised and/or content
Doubt	Certainty
Boredom	Enthusiasm and motivation

5. If you feel conflict, which aspect of your goal is causing the conflict? Look at each part of your goal in turn and tune into the feedback from your body. Alternatively, ask yourself, 'Am I choosing this goal because of some underlying fear, belief or worry?' If so, what is that fear, belief or worry? Create a goal around that. For example, the goal of becoming a millionaire in order to feel successful could become the goal of cultivating self-acceptance, out of which might come financial success.

6. Modify and rewrite your goal until you feel signs of harmony.

7. Now close your eyes, breathe deeply and create a movie of what your life would look like and how you would feel once this goal has been accomplished. Give yourself plenty of time to do this. It's important that you associate with the image of yourself – in other words, you should experience yourself as the person in the movie. If it helps, use the questions below to help inspire you.

   • What do you see that shows you have solved the problem or achieved the goal?

   • What are other people doing or saying that tells you that you have succeeded?

   • What does it feel like?

   • When do you realistically want to be in the position that you see in your mind's eye?

   • How will you know that you have achieved your goal?

   • Is there a measure you can use?

- How much control or influence do you have with regard to this goal?

8. Now I want you to turn your attention to the past. Try and identify a moment or experience from the past when you successfully completed a goal. Re-live it and allow yourself to become energised by it. Once you feel that energy running through you, let go of the old memory and animate your new movie with this energy. Infuse it with life and make it as real as possible.

9. Repeat this process three more times. You will know when it's complete, because when you think of your goal you will see and feel it as an energised reality. It will feel real.

10. If you get disorientated, confused or become unsure of what you are doing, just open your eyes and take a deep breath or have a glass of water and start again.

11. Once you have completed this process, the real key to achieving this goal is to reconnect with it at the start of every day. This tuning in process is important, particularly when it is preceded by a few moments of giving thanks and appreciation for what you do have in your life. Creating goals from a place of abundance, rather than poverty, appears to be another critical factor in helping goals come true.

At the beginning of each day think of at least one thing you are grateful for right now in your life – small or big, it just needs to be something that is meaningful to you. Allow that gratitude to build up within you. Breathe in and out of it until your whole body feels full of gratitude. Place your hand on your heart and now state your goal and/or intention for the day. As you say your goal, if you start to experience signs of resistance, ask yourself the question, 'What do I really need?' and rewrite your goal until it feels right in your body. Goals often change in response to shifts in circumstances and our life situation. Having said it, move on with your day.

Part Four

~

Women's health solutions

In this section I share my own integrated medicine approach to the most common women's health challenges that my female patients face. Prior to following the advice I encourage you, if you haven't done so already, to identify which of the five secrets are relevant to you, because they will provide the foundations for you. The reality is that most diseases and health problems will improve considerably just by improving your diet, getting regular physical activity, restful sleep, managing your stress and learning how to be easier on yourself.

I also highlight which holistic health tools and secrets might be most appropriate, and for all the different health conditions I suggest additional books that you might want to read. One final word of caution, though. If you are in any doubt about what your diagnosis is, are overwhelmed by your symptoms or confused as to what treatment programme you should follow, that is a clear sign that you need to work alongside an experienced health professional. In the Resources section there is a list of organisations through which you should be able to locate an integrated medicine doctor or health professional.

Premenstrual syndrome

Premenstrual syndrome (PMS) describes the presence of a variety of mental, emotional and physical symptoms that start prior to menstruation and cease with the onset – or one or two days after the onset – of menstruation. PMS is common, affecting up to 80 per cent of women, and for up to 5 per cent of those women it has a significant and detrimental impact on their quality of life.

What causes PMS?

Like so many of the hormone-related health challenges faced by women, no-one really knows what causes PMS. For example, studies have examined hormone levels in women with and without PMS and not found any differences, so while PMS is obviously related to hormonal fluctuations, because it starts after ovulation and disappears with menstruation, hormones are not directly the cause.

Another line of thinking, which I suspect might be partially correct, is that PMS is symptomatic of a general life imbalance and perhaps unresolved stress, discontentment, lack of creative expression and even undiagnosed depression. For example, some of the women who come to me with PMS have eating disorders, anxiety and addictions. One clue as to what might be happening was the discovery that for women with PMS levels of the good-mood neuro-transmitter serotonin fall quite significantly after ovulation, whereas for women without PMS they don't. One theory is that women without PMS may offset ovulation-induced susceptibility to low serotonin due to their ability to connect with other people and keep socially active. Put another way, a significant contributor to PMS might be a social one, resulting from women's increasing levels of isolation from themselves, others and possibly the natural world. The jury is still out.

What are the risk factors for PMS?

The following increase the likelihood of you experiencing PMS:

- Having a mother who had PMS

- Being in your thirties or forties

- Having two or more children

- A upheaval such as having a baby, termination of a pregnancy, mis-carriage, or coming off hormone treatment

My integrated medical prescription for PMS

The most important key to successfully treating PMS is to identify and address the underlying causes. While it's tempting to rush straight into treatment with painkillers and hormonal-based treatments, these are usually only symptomatic approaches. In my experience, most women who follow the five steps below will see a considerable improvement in their symptoms within two to three cycles.

Step 1 • Do you have PMS?

If you have any symptoms that regularly appear after the middle of your cycle (ovulation) and disappear with, or just after, the onset of menstruation then by definition these indicate you have some degree of PMS. While there are more than 150 reported PMS symptoms, the most common ones are:

- Mood swings

- Irritability

- Feeling tired

- Anxiety and tension

- Tenderness and lumpiness of the breasts

- Difficulty concentrating and making decisions

- Backache and muscle stiffness

- Crying spells

- Sugar and food cravings

- Feelings of being bloated and water retention

- Acne

- Disrupted sleep

- Weight gain

- Constipation

I encourage my patients to keep a menstrual diary, in which they record what symptoms they have over a period of at least 8 to 12 weeks. If those symptoms stop almost immediately with the onset of menstruation then a diagnosis of PMS can be made. See Resources.

Step 2 • Consider the medical options

To help relieve headaches, back pain and other aches and pains your doctor or pharmacist might recommend taking a non-steroidal anti-inflammatory medication such as ibuprofen. This can be taken as and when needed.

If you have moderate to severe PMS symptoms you might be offered a hormone-based treatment. The combined pill can certainly help some women, but for others it does not help and it can even cause a variety of side-effects, ranging from depression and headache to nausea and weight gain. While this is an option, PMS research has found that women who take inert dummy pills often experience as much relief as those who take medication. My suspicion, therefore, is that the benefit of the pill, if it has one, might be down to believing it is going to help, rather than the hormonal changes that it brings about. Other hormone options include oestrogen patches, progesterone cream and pessaries, and the following:

Danazol – this is a male hormone derivative that prevents ovulation. While it has been found to help some women experience a reduction in PMS symptoms, it is associated with side-effects such as hirsutism (increased hair growth), mood swings, rashes, acne, deepening of the voice and weight gain. I would only recommend using this if you have severe PMS symptoms that do not respond to the other suggestions I give.

Mefenamic acid – this is usually used to treat women with painful periods and heavy menstrual flow as it reduces the production of prostaglandins, which promote inflammation. It is also occasionally used to treat PMS-related symptoms such as breast pain and mood swings. The side-effects include abdominal cramps, constipation, indigestion and bloating. You might want to consider this if you have significant pain, but bear in mind that it shouldn't be taken for more than a week because of its side-effects. If pain is a problem for you, see Painful Periods (page 184).

Step 3 • Address the underlying causes

While I am going to make recommendations to treat your PMS symptoms using a variety of supplements, for lasting resolution of PMS symptoms I encourage you to fill in the questionnaires in part one, section two, to help identify possible root causes and contributors. In my experience, the ones to consider are:

- **Stress** – Solution: Secret Two – De-stress and Relax (page 77); Holistic Health Tools – Emotional Freedom Technique (page 151) and Mindfulness (page 147)

- **Poor diet** – Solution: Secret One – Nurture Your Physical Body (Healthy Eating and Supplements – page 49)

- **Environmental toxicity** – Solution: Secret One – Nurture Your Physical Body (Health Environment and Sunlight – page 70)

- **Depression** – Solution: Part Five (Depression – page 316); Holistic Health Tools – Mindfulness (page 147), Values-based Goal Setting (page 166) and The Work (page 163)

- **Food intolerances** – Solution: Part Five (Food Intolerances – page 344); Holistic Health Tools – Emotional Freedom Technique (page 151)

- **Blood-sugar imbalance** – Solution: Secret One – Nurture Your Physical Body (Healthy Eating and Supplements – page 49)

- **Nutritional deficiencies** – Solution: Secret One – Nurture Your Physical Body (Healthy Eating and Supplements – page 49)

- **Hypothyroidism** – Solution: Part Five (Hypothyroidism – page 356); Holistic Health Tools – Emotional Freedom Technique (page 151) and The Work (page 163)

- **Candida** – Solution: Part Five (Dysbiosis – page 334); Holistic Health Tools – Emotional Freedom Technique (page 151)

Step 4 • Start a PMS supplement programme

When used alongside step three, certain nutritional supplements can help to alleviate many of the symptoms of PMS. My integrated medicine prescription for PMS usually includes a combination of:

- **A multivitamin-mineral supplement**[1] plus a total daily dose of **vitamin B**$_6$[2] (100mg) and **magnesium**[3] (400mg). There is some evidence to suggest that the latter two might help to alleviate PMS symptoms.

- **Vitamin C with bioflavonoids** (1000mg) to reduce inflammation, pain and heavy bleeding.

- **Evening primrose oil** (3000mg a day) to provide the body with hormone balancing anti-inflammatory essential fatty acids.[4]

- **Magnesium citrate**[5] (500mg) and **calcium citrate**[6] (1000mg) a day if you have cramps.

- **Agnus castus**, otherwise known as vitex or chasteberry, is the most commonly used herb to support women with PMS. One study examined the effect of agnus castus in more than 1,600 women. After three months 93 per cent of the women reported an improvement in or elimination of their PMS symptoms. Four out of five women rated themselves as 'much better' or 'very much better'.[7] The dose I recommend is 40mg of dried herb or 40 drops of concentrated liquid extract once a day, or 20mg of dried herb twice a day. **Do not take this if you are on hormone treatment.**

Step 5 • Consider other complementary approaches

While there is no definitive evidence that these can help you with your PMS, some patients find the following useful in supporting their programme: acupuncture, homeopathy, massage, spiritual healing, yoga, traditional Chinese medicine and Ayurvedic medicine.

For recommended books see Resources.

Heavy menstrual bleeding

At some time during their reproductive years most women will experience a heavy period. However, if the bleeding is excessive or prolonged then it can become a problem, not only because of the inconvenience, but because it can lead to iron deficiency, anaemia and tiredness. What constitutes a normal and abnormal period is tricky because women vary so much. Generally, most women will have a period every 21 to 35 days; it will last for four to five days and produce a total blood loss equivalent to 2 to 3 tablespoons (30 to 40ml). Heavy menstrual bleeding becomes diagnosed as menorrhagia when that blood loss exceeds 80ml.

What causes heavy menstrual bleeding?

Heavy menstrual bleeding tends to be a symptom of an underlying problem, including:

- An imbalance of prostaglandins – these are the chemicals that control the muscles in your womb and can also make blood vessels wider and narrower

- Hormonal imbalances – especially an excess of oestrogen

- Fibroids – non-cancerous swellings that arise from the muscle of the uterine wall

- Polyps – non-cancerous growths in the uterus

- Pelvic inflammatory disease – sexually transmitted disease causing inflammation of the organs in the pelvis or infection

- Endometriosis or endometrial hyperplasia – overgrowth of the lining of the womb or endometrial cancer

- Problems with blood thinning and coagulation

- Contraceptive devices such as the coil or IUD (intrauterine device)

- Hypothyroidism

- Stress

- Being overweight is associated with excess bleeding

- A natural thickening of the uterine lining can occur when approaching the menopause

What are the risk factors?

While any woman may experience heavy menstrual bleeding at any time, the following increase the likelihood of you having a heavy period:

- You are within 12 to 18 months of having your first period

- You are approaching the menopause

- You have a hereditary bleeding disorder

- You are taking blood thinning medications such as warfarin

My integrated medical prescription for heavy menstrual bleeding

The most important key to successfully treating heavy periods is to identify and address the underlying causes. While it's tempting to rush straight into treatment with medications, these are only symptomatic treatments designed to reduce blood flow, not address the underlying issues. Treating heavy periods is a good example of the importance of everyone working together – including you, your GP and gynaecologist, as well as maybe a nutritional therapist and/or herbalist.

Step 1 • Do you have heavy menstrual bleeding?

The following is a list of indicators that you are experiencing heavy periods and that you need to seek professional help, support and treatment.

- You use more than nine pads or tampons (or both pads and tampons) on your heaviest days

- You have to wear both a tampon and a pad (double protection)

- Your period lasts more than six days

- You have to get up at night to change your protection

- You pass clots of blood

- You stain your bedding or clothes despite wearing tampons and pads

- You stay at home during your period because you are worried about having an 'accident'

- You feel tired, especially during your period, which could mean your body is low on iron

If you are experiencing heavy bleeding you should see your GP in order to have it investigated thoroughly and get a diagnosis. This will usually involve having some blood tests, swabs taken for infection, an ultrasound scan and possibly a hysteroscopy, in which a small camera is inserted inside the cervix in order to look inside the uterus.

Step 2 • Consider the medical options

Once you have a diagnosis or once all of the major causes have been excluded, your GP or gynaecologist might then offer you medications and/or surgery. I tend to recommend that my patients stick with the non-hormonal treatment options while the underlying causes are dealt with.

Medications

Medical options include non-hormonal treatments, such as the drug tranexamic acid (which is usually the drug of choice), and/or non-steroidal anti-inflammatory drugs (NSAIDS) such as mefanamic acid. Both of these have been shown to reduce blood loss and the latter is useful if you have pain. Hormonal treatments include the combined oral contraceptive pill, which suppresses ovulation and therefore reduces bleeding. Progestogen tablets are sometimes provided in order to cause a complete shedding of the uterus lining, after which it is hoped that the bleeding will return to normal. It doesn't usually work. Some women are offered a progestogen coil, which can help to lighten or even stop the period completely, although initially there may be spotting or prolonged periods. Finally, Danazol, a weak male hormone derivative, is sometimes used because of its ability to the stop the lining of the uterus from growing. Its ability to stop bleeding needs to be weighed up against its side-effects, which can include hirsutism (increased hair growth), mood swings, rashes, acne, deepening of the voice and weight gain.

Surgery

Surgical options for treating heavy periods include endometrial ablation, in which a thin telescope is inserted through the cervix and laser or diathermy treatment is then used to destroy most of the tissue lining of the uterus. Drugs are often used beforehand to thin the lining of the uterus. This might either stop your period or result in lighter periods. As a last resort women will be offered a hysterectomy. I only ever support the latter if all other options have been exhausted.

Step 3 • Address the underlying causes

Heavy menstrual bleeding is one of those situations where it is absolutely essential to address the root causes and contributors. That's why I insist all my patients have been thoroughly investigated prior to using supplements, lifestyle changes and so on. All the different causes of heavy menstrual bleeding should be explored as possibilities. If, for example, it turns out that you have endometriosis or fibroids then you should follow the recommendations that I make for them. If the investigations turn up blank, then my advice would be to take the questionnaires in part one, section two, and follow the secrets and imbalances that are flagged up for you. In my experience, the following factors contribute to or exacerbate heavy menstrual bleeding:

- **Stress** – Solution: Secret Two – De-stress and Relax (page 77); Holistic Health Tools – Emotional Freedom Technique (page 151) and Mindfulness (page 147)

- **Poor diet** – Solution: Secret One – Nurture Your Physical Body (Healthy Eating and Supplements – page 49)

- **Excessive weight** – Solution: Secret One – Nurture Your Physical Body (Healthy Eating and Supplements – page 49); Part Five (Weight Loss – page 401); Holistic Health Tools – Emotional Freedom Technique (page 151) and The Work (page 163)

- **Nutritional deficiencies** – Solution: Secret One – Nurture Your Physical Body (Healthy Eating and Supplements – page 49)

- **Hypothyroidism** – Solution: Part Five (Hypothyroidism – page 356); Holistic Health Tools – Emotional Freedom Technique (page 151) and The Work (page 163)

- **Candida** – Solution: Part Five (Dysbiosis – page 334); Holistic Health Tools – Emotional Freedom Technique (page 151)

Step 4 • Start a heavy menstrual bleeding supplement programme

As long as the underlying causes and contributors are being addressed, my typical heavy menstrual bleeding prescription would consist of:

- **A multivitamin-mineral supplement**, although in addition to this you might want to consider taking 25,000IU of **vitamin A** twice a day for 15 days, as in one study this reduced menstrual flow in more than 90 per cent of women.[1] You should only do this under the supervision of a nutritional therapist or integrated medical doctor and do not take if you are at risk of becoming pregnant.

- **Vitamin C with bioflavonoids** (1000mg) to reduce inflammation, pain and heavy bleeding. One study showed that taking 600mg of vitamin C and 600mg of bioflavanoids a day helped to reduce the symptoms of a heavy period.[2] Vitamin C also helps you to absorb iron from your diet and supplements.

- **Omega-3, 6 and 9** (taken in capsule or liquid form in a 2:1:1 ratio) to provide the body with hormone-balancing anti-inflammatory essential fatty acids.

- If iron deficiency anaemia is a problem I usually also add an **iron** supplement – see Resources.

- **Agnus castus** is a herb that's commonly used to reduce heavy menstrual bleeding.[3] The dose I recommend is 40mg of dried herb or 40 drops of concentrated liquid extract once a day, or 20mg of dried herb twice a day. **Do not take this if you are on hormone treatment.** My advice, however, is to only take it under the guidance of a herbalist, as they will be able to provide you with a more personalised combination of herbs. For example, the short-tem herbs shepherd's purse, yarrow, cranesbill and goldenseal are all used to control bleeding. Longer-term herbs might include ladies' mantle and dong quai.

Step 5 • Consider other complementary approaches

While there is no definitive evidence that these can help you with your heavy menstrual bleeding, some patients find the following useful in supporting their programme: acupuncture, homeopathy, Western herbal medicine, traditional Chinese medicine, Ayurvedic medicine and Tibetan medicine.

For recommended books see Resources.

Painful periods

~

Most women have experienced dull or throbbing lower abdominal pain or cramps just before or during their periods. For most it's not that much of a problem. However, for about 10 per cent of women it's painful enough to cause significant distress and disruption to their life.

What causes painful periods?

Doctors talk about two types of dysmenorrhoea (the medical term for painful periods): primary and secondary. Primary dysmenorrhoea usually applies to women whose periods have always been painful and it tends to begin 6 to 12 months after the first period. It is thought to result from an excessive production of prostaglandins (inflammation-causing chemicals), which causes the muscles of the uterus to contract during the period. Secondary dysmenorrhoea starts later in life and is due to a specific underlying cause, such as:

- Endometriosis – in this painful condition the type of tissue that lines your uterus becomes implanted outside your uterus, most commonly on your fallopian tubes, ovaries or the tissue lining your pelvis.

- Adenomyosis – in this condition the tissue that lines your uterus begins to grow within the muscular walls of the uterus.

- Pelvic inflammatory disease (PID) – this infection of the female reproductive organs is usually caused by sexually transmitted bacteria.

- An intrauterine device (IUD) – these small, plastic, T-shaped birth control devices are inserted into your uterus. They may cause increased cramping, particularly during the first few months after insertion.

- Uterine fibroids and uterine polyps – these non-cancerous tumours and growths protrude from the lining of your uterus.

What are the risk factors?

The risk factors associated with developing painful periods are:

- Age younger than 20
- Early onset of puberty (age 11 or younger)
- Heavy bleeding during periods
- Depression or anxiety
- Attempts to lose weight (in women aged 14 to 20)
- Never having delivered a baby
- Smoking

My integrated medical prescription for painful periods

The most important key to successfully treating painful periods is to identify and address the underlying causes. While it's tempting to rush straight into treatment with medications, these are only symptomatic treatments designed to reduce pain, not to address the underlying issues. Once the main causes have been identified and excluded, then I focus on reducing inflammation in the body, as there is good evidence to suggest that an excess of pro-inflammatory prostaglandin chemicals, in particular PGE2, which increases womb contractions and inflammation, is involved in painful periods.

Step 1 • Do you have painful periods?

Symptoms of painful periods include:

- Cramping, lower abdominal pain that might radiate to the legs and lower back

- A dragging sensation in the pelvis

- Symptoms relating to the underlying cause, such as fibroids (heavy periods) or endometriosis

Other signs and symptoms that can occur along with painful periods include nausea and vomiting, loose stools, sweating and dizziness.

If you have painful periods you should see your GP in order to have it investigated thoroughly and get a diagnosis. This will usually involve having some blood tests, swabs taken for signs of infection, an ultrasound scan and possibly a hysteroscopy, in which a small camera is inserted inside the cervix in order to look inside the uterus.

Step 2 • Consider the medical options

Once you have a diagnosis or once all the major causes have been excluded, your GP or gynaecologist might then offer you medications and/or surgery.

Medications

Medical options include non-hormonal treatments such as the drug tranexamic acid, which is usually the drug of choice, and/or non-steroidal anti-inflammatory drugs (NSAIDS) such as mefanamic acid. Lots of studies have also shown that NSAIDS reduce pain and help women to function on a day-to-day basis.[1] Most of these medications are thought to work equally well. You can purchase ibuprofen (Nurofen) and naproxen (Feminax Ultra) over the counter. These can be taken in combination with paracetamol for extra pain relief.

An alternative approach is the use of the combined oral contraceptive pill, which might help make periods shorter and lighter. However, there is a lack of evidence to say that they help with period pain. If you need to take painkillers every month, my advice is to follow the remaining steps, so that the underlying cause of pain can be resolved.

Surgery

Only as a last resort, and if your life and pain are unbearable, should you consider having a hysterectomy (removal of the uterus).

Step 3 • Address the underlying causes

Like heavy menstrual bleeding, the presence of painful periods is one of those situations where it is absolutely essential to address the root causes and contributors. That's why I insist all of my patients have been thoroughly investigated prior to using supplements, lifestyle changes and so on. All the different causes of period pain should be explored as possibilities. If, for example, it turns out that you have endometriosis or fibroids, then you should follow the recommendations that I make for them. If the investigations turn up blank then my advice is to take the questionnaires in part one, section two, and to follow the secrets and imbalances that are flagged up for you. In my experience, the following factors contribute to or exacerbate period pain:

- **Stress** – Solution: Secret Two – De-stress and Relax (page 77); Holistic Health Tools – Emotional Freedom Technique (page 151) and Mindfulness (page 147)

- **Poor diet** – Solution: Secret One – Nurture Your Physical Body (Healthy Eating and Supplements – page 49)

- **Excessive weight** – Solution: Secret One – Nurture Your Physical Body (Healthy Eating and Supplements – page 49), Part Five (Weight Loss – page 401); Holistic Health Tools – Emotional Freedom Technique (page 151) and The Work (page 163)

- **Nutritional deficiencies** – Solution: Secret One – Nurture Your Physical Body (Healthy Eating and Supplements – page 49)

- **Hypothyroidism** – Solution: Part Five (Hypothyroidism – page 356); Holistic Health Tools – Emotional Freedom Technique (page 151) and The Work (page 163)

- **Candida** – Solution: Part Five (Dysbiosis – page 334); Holistic Health Tools – Emotional Freedom Technique (page 151)

- **Environmental toxicity** – Solution: Secret One – Nurture Your Physical Body (Healthy Environment and Sunlight – page 70)

- **Depression** – Solution: Part Five (Depression – page 316); Holistic Health Tools – Mindfulness (page 147), Values-based Goal Setting (page 166) and The Work (page 163)

- **Food intolerances** – Solution: Part Five (Food Intolerances – page 344); Holistic Health Tools – Emotional Freedom Technique (page 151)

- **Blood-sugar imbalance** – Solution: Secret One – Nurture Your Physical Body (Healthy Eating and Supplements – page 49)

Step 4 • Start a period pain supplement programme

As long as the underlying causes and contributors are being addressed, my typical period pain prescription would consist of:

- **A multivitamin-mineral supplement.** The B-vitamin components of these, particularly B_1, B_6 and B_{12}, have all been found to help relieve period pain.[2] In addition to this you might want to consider taking extra **magnesium**[3] to make a total daily intake of 300mg. You should also make sure that you are taking 300IU of **vitamin E**[4] a day as this can help to relieve period pain. In a study, nearly seven in ten women taking vitamin E felt better.

- **Vitamin C with bioflavonoids** (1000mg to 3000mg) to reduce inflammation, pain and heavy bleeding.[5]

- **Omega-3, 6 and 9** (taken in capsule or liquid form in a 2:1:1 ratio) to provide the body with hormone-balancing anti-inflammatory essential fatty acids.[6]

- As an alternative to painkillers I recommend **bromelain** (standardised to 2000 mcu) at a dose of 200mg three times daily on an empty stomach.

Step 5 • Consider complementary approaches

I find there are quite a few different approaches that can help to relieve period pain; in no particular order they include:

- **Heat**, either in the form of a hot water bottle or a self-heating or microwave pack, can work as well as ibuprofen to relieve pain. See Resources.

- **Menastil** consists of a diluted calendula oil mixture which is applied directly over the area in which you are experiencing pain. See Resources.

- **MagnoPulse MN8** is a magnet therapy device designed to alleviate period pain. See Resources.

- **Pain Ease** patches can be worn under clothing and send minute electrical currents into the painful area. This helps to trigger healing and in some women can help to reduce pain. See Resources.

While there is no definitive evidence that these can help you with your period pain, some patients find the following useful in supporting their period pain programme: aromatherapy, acupuncture, acupressure, spiritual healing, massage, guided imagery, yoga, meditation, homeopathy, Western herbal medicine and traditional Chinese medicine.

For recommended books see Resources.

Fibroids

Fibroids are non-cancerous growths of muscle and connective tissue found in or on the muscular wall of the uterus. They are very common, affecting 25 to 40 per cent of women of reproductive age, although less than half will have any symptoms.

The size of a fibroid may vary from as small as a pinhead to as large as a watermelon. The average number of fibroids in a woman is six, with the average size being around 2cm. Fibroids are classified according to where they grow:

- Submucosal (or submucous) fibroid – this type is located beneath the lining of the uterus. The fibroid can develop a thin stalk or even enter the vagina.

- Intramural fibroid – this type is mostly located in the wall of the uterus.

- Subserosal fibroid – this type grows towards the outside of the uterus and can press on the organs surrounding it, such as the bladder or rectum.

- Pedunculated fibroid – this type of fibroid can develop when a fibroid grows on a stalk. It can be a subserosal fibroid growing out into the abdomen or a submucosal fibroid growing into the endometrial cavity. The stalk can get twisted, which can cause severe pain, although this is extremely rare.

What causes fibroids?

No-one really knows what causes fibroids, but what we do know is that fibroids are sensitive to oestrogen and will grow when levels of oestrogen are high, for example when a woman is on an oestrogen-only pill. Interestingly, during pregnancy, when levels of oestrogen are high, they don't tend to grow, which might suggest that the high levels of progesterone that also accompany pregnancy might have some protective effect on fibroids. Another factor that might explain the increased prevalence of fibroids is xeno-oestrogens – chemical contaminants that have oestrogen-like effects on the body.

Other possible contributors include stress and emotional problems. Fibroids can be a problem, because they can be painful and lead to excessive bleeding (and anaemia), but they can also contribute to infertility in many different ways. These include preventing the sperm or egg from reaching the uterus by blocking the cervix and fallopian tubes respectively. They can distort the uterus so the fertilised egg can't attach itself properly and they can also increase the risk of miscarriage.

What are the risk factors for fibroids?

The following are associated with an increased risk of developing fibroids:

- You are of childbearing age (you're most likely to get fibroids in your thirties or forties)

- You started having your periods early (before about 12)

- You don't have any children

- You had your last child at a young age

- You're very overweight

- Someone in your family has fibroids

- You are Afro-Caribbean – black women are three times more likely than white women to have fibroids

My integrated medical prescription for fibroids

The majority of women with fibroids don't have any symptoms or experience only minor problems, such as slightly heavy menstrual bleeding. If you know you have fibroids – because they were found accidentally – and they aren't bothering you, my advice would be either to do nothing or, preferably, follow the five secrets of health, healing and happiness, to prevent them from becoming a problem. It's also worth bearing in mind that if you are approaching the menopause, your fibroids and any symptoms they are causing will reduce considerably – so if you were considering medications and surgery it might be worthwhile putting them on hold. Most women, however, come to me with symptoms resulting from fibroids that haven't been diagnosed yet. For them my focus is on getting an accurate diagnosis and then using an integrated holistic approach to reducing the size of the fibroids (although this can be difficult), addressing any underlying causes and managing the symptoms.

Step 1 • Do you have fibroids?

If you have any abnormal menstrual bleeding (often heavy and/or irregular periods), and/or a feeling of fullness/pressure in the pelvic area there's a strong possibility you might have fibroids. Other symptoms associated with fibroids include:

- A swelling of the lower abdomen and/or pressure on the bowels (leading to constipation) and bladder (leading to an increased desire to pass urine)

- Painful periods

- Infertility or miscarriage (rarely)

- Problems with childbirth because of the fibroid obstructing the birth canal

- A constant chronic ache in the back or pelvis

- An urge to urinate when lying down

- Pain during sexual intercourse

- If the fibroids are severe enough to cause bleeding, then symptoms might also include tiredness, shortness of breath, pale skin and headaches

If you have any of these symptoms you should see your doctor. He or she will want to know about your periods, sex life, general health and lifestyle. If there is any possibility you are pregnant, they will do a pregnancy test, and probably arrange a blood test to check for anaemia and infection. They might do an internal (vaginal) examination and attempt to feel the fibroids themselves.

It is, of course, easy to miss fibroids this way and there other conditions, such as ovarian cysts and adenomyosis (where the lining of the uterus infiltrates the wall of the uterus, causing a thickening), that might cause some confusion. For this reason you will probably be referred for a transvaginal ultrasound scan or MRI scan. In the former a probe is placed inside your vagina. It emits sound waves which bounce off the organs in your pelvis to create a picture. The latter provides a very detailed picture and the doctor looking at it will be able to distinguish between fibroids and adenomyosis. If you are perimenopausal or post-menopausal your doctor will want to rule out a malignancy as a potential cause of any bleeding.

Step 2 • Consider the medical options

Most women who come to me are looking for a non-medical approach to their fibroids, because of their concern about the side-effects of conventional treatment. However, if the fibroids are bleeding excessively or if they are particularly large I almost always suggest that they get a referral from their GP to see a gynaecologist for treatment as in my experience natural approaches rarely work sufficiently well.

Medications

Your doctor will probably talk you through the following different types of medications. If you have heavy periods and your fibroids are relatively small, you will probably be offered one or more of the following:

Tranexamic acid – this is taken three to four times a day, for three to four days during each period. It works by reducing the breakdown of blood clots in the uterus.

Anti-inflammatory medicines – these include ibuprofen and mefanamic acid and they also help to ease period pain. They are taken for a few days each period. They work by reducing the high level of prostaglandin in the uterus lining, which seems to contribute to heavy periods.

The contraceptive pill – this may help and often helps with period pain, too.

Levonorgestrel intrauterine system (LNG-IUS) – this is similar to an intrauterine device (IUD) used for contraception. It is inserted into the uterus and slowly releases a regular small amount of a progestogen hormone called levonorgestrel. It works by making the lining of the uterus very thin (atrophied), so bleeding is lighter.

Gonadotropin-releasing hormone analogues (GnRHas) – these include goserelin, leuprorelin, nafarelin, buserelin and triptorelin and they may be offered to you if you are close to the menopause or are going to have surgery. They are synthetic hormones that stop your brain making two hormones: follicle-stimulating hormone (FSH) and luteinising hormone (LH). As their levels decrease, the ovaries produce less oestrogen and this causes your fibroids to shrink. Side-effects of these medications include menopausal symptoms, such as hot flushes, dry vagina, sweats and insomnia, and also bone loss (osteoporosis). Treatment is usually limited to between three and six months. GnRHas might be effective in reducing the size and symptoms caused by fibroids for the duration they are taken, but I believe their side-effects outweigh their benefits. If you are absolutely convinced that you want to go this route, you could consider taking low dose HRT with progestogen or the drug Tibolone at the same time in order to limit the menopausal side-effects.

Surgery

If your symptoms are severe, or there's been no improvement with medications, your doctor will probably refer you for surgery. Surgery is the most common conventional treatment for fibroids and fibroids are the number one reason for women having a hysterectomy. The three main options available to you are:

Myomectomy – this is an operation in which the fibroids are removed from the womb. The type of surgery you have will depend on the size, number and position of the fibroids. Most myomectomies are done through a cut (incision) in the abdomen. Others are done with keyhole surgery (laporoscopically through small cuts to your abdomen). Some fibroids near the lining of the uterus can be removed through the vagina without an abdominal cut. Recurrence of the fibroid may occur after myomectomy.

The advantage of a myomectomy over a hysterectomy is that you will still be able to become pregnant. If your fibroids are small, it is generally better to go with a laparoscopic myomectomy as you will generally bleed less, have less pain afterwards and will probably recover quicker than you would from an open myomectomy. If you have large fibroids and many fibroids, open myomectomy is generally the approach of choice. A vaginal myomectomy can be used if the fibroids are small, plus it doesn't require a general anaesthetic like the other two. However, understandably many women don't like the idea of having an operation involving the vagina. Fibroids might grow back after having a myomectomy and the more fibroids you have removed the higher the chance of that happening. One study found that one in four women get fibroids again in the three years after a myomectomy.[1]

Uterine artery embolization – this is a newer technique used to treat large fibroids. It involves putting a catheter (a thin flexible tube) into an artery (blood vessel) in the groin. It is guided using x-ray pictures to the arteries of the uterus. Once there, a chemical is injected along the catheter to the uterine arteries. This causes a blockage in the arteries. The fibroid then loses its blood supply and shrinks. As this treatment is quite new, its long-term safety and effectiveness are not yet clear. However, early reports are encouraging. It may only be available in certain hospitals, but is likely to become more widely available in the future. Unlike the other forms of surgery this procedure is performed by an interventional radiologist.

Hysterectomy – this is the most common treatment for fibroids which cause symptoms. This is the removal of the uterus (womb). It is a fairly major operation. I would only ever recommend a hysterectomy if all other avenues have been exhausted first and the woman has completed her family.

Step 3 • Address the underlying causes

While I am going to make recommendations to treat your fibroids, if they are big and causing significant problems you might have to go down the surgical route. Either way, I highly recommend that you fill in the questionnaires in part one, section two, in order to identify possible root causes or contributors to fibroids. In my experience, the ones to consider are:

- **Environmental toxicity** – Solution: Secret One – Nurture Your Physical Body (Healthy Environment and Sunlight – page 70)

- **Excessive weight** – Solution: Secret One – Nurture Your Physical Body (Healthy Eating and Supplements – page 49); Part Five (Weight Loss – page 401); Holistic Health Tools – Emotional Freedom Technique (page 151) and The Work (page 163)

- **Poor diet** – Solution: Secret One – Nurture Your Physical Body (Healthy Eating and Supplements – page 49)

- **Hypothyroidism** – Solution: Part Five (Hypothyroidism – page 356); Holistic Health Tools – Emotional Freedom Technique (page 151) and The Work (page 163)

Step 4 • Start a fibroid supplement programme

When used alongside step three, certain nutritional supplements can help to reduce the size of your fibroids and the associated symptoms. My integrated medicine prescription for fibroids usually includes a combination of:

- **A multivitamin-mineral formula**

- **Vitamin C with bioflavonoids** (1000mg to 3000mg) to reduce inflammation, pain and heavy bleeding.[2]

- **Omega-3, 6 and 9** (taken in capsule or liquid form in a 2:1:1 ratio) to provide the body with hormone-balancing anti-inflammatory essential fatty acids.

- **Indole-3-Carbinol** (300mg daily), which can help the liver to detoxify excess oestrogen.[3]

- **Acidophilus probiotic** to ensure that there are sufficient numbers of 'friendly' bacteria in the gut to help prevent deactivated oestrogen that has been excreted in the gut being activated again by certain 'unfriendly' bacteria.

- **Milk thistle and dandelion** are herbs that work well in combination, helping to support optimum liver function and reduce circulating levels of oestrogen.

- **Agnus castus**, otherwise known as vitex or chasteberry, is often used if there is a high ratio of oestrogen to progesterone.[4] A nutritional therapist or integrated medicine doctor can arrange testing to see if this is relevant for you – see Resources. The dose I recommend is 40mg of dried herb or 40 drops of concentrated liquid extract once a day, or 20mg of dried herb twice a day. **Do not take this if you are on hormone treatment.**

- **Natural progesterone cream** is used by some integrated medicine doctors to reduce the size of fibroids. This should only be used under medical supervision – see Resources.

- If anaemia is present (and as long as it is being medically monitored) you should consider taking an **iron** supplement – see Resources.

- If you have excessive bleeding please refer to the advice on heavy menstrual bleeding (page 178) and if you have associated pain, to my advice on painful periods (page 184).

Step 5 • Consider other complementary approaches

While there is no definitive evidence that these can help you with your fibroids, some patients find the following useful in supporting their fibroids programme: acupuncture, homeopathy, yoga, Western herbal medicine and traditional Chinese medicine.

For recommended books see Resources.

Endometriosis

Endometriosis is believed to affect 10 to 15 per cent of menstruating women between the ages of 25 and 40. The National Endometriosis Society estimates that between 1.5 and 2 million women in Britain have endometriosis.[1]

Endometriosis is a condition in which cells that normally line the inside of your uterus (the endometrium) are found elsewhere in the body. This endometrial-like tissue is most commonly found in the pelvis, ovaries, fallopian tubes and the ligaments supporting the womb, but also, and much more rarely, in the bowels, bladder, lung, heart, kidneys, joints and even the eye. These patches of endometrial tissue look and function like the cells that line the womb. They respond to the hormonal fluctuations in your body in the same way your womb does and at the time of your period the cells will start bleeding, but unlike in the womb, where blood escapes through the vagina, this blood has nowhere to go. This leads to pain, inflammation, damage to the surrounding tissues, scar tissue and adhesions (fibres that connect parts of the body that aren't normally connected).

What causes endometriosis?

There are a lot of different theories as to what causes endometriosis. They include:

- Genetic predisposition – the likelihood of you developing endometriosis may depend on your genes. Women with a first-degree relative who has endometriosis have a tenfold increased risk of developing the disease.

- Retrograde menstruation – this happens to most women and involves small amounts of blood flowing along the fallopian tubes and out into the pelvis. Most women will not, however, develop endometriosis because of this and this process doesn't explain how deposits can be found elsewhere in the body.

- Cells spread via the lymphatic or circulatory system – this theory proposes that endometrial cells are carried to different parts of the body by the blood and lymph system.

- Immune imbalance – interestingly, many women with endometriosis often have an immune system that is not working efficiently and effectively. In some women with endometriosis the macrophages and natural killer cells that are designed to mop up rogue endometrial cells don't work very well, so those cells are left to bleed and cause symptoms. The autoimmune theory of endometriosis is supported by the frequent finding of auto-antibodies in women with endometriosis and by the high incidence of other autoimmune conditions among women with endometriosis, including rheumatoid arthritis, multiple sclerosis and systemic lupus erythematosus.

- Metaplasia – this theory suggests that normal cells exposed to certain influences, such as chemicals, toxins, hormones and infection, can transform into endometrial cells. This can explain why, following hormonal treatment, some men have been found to have patches of endometriosis.

- Excessive oestrogen stimulation – endometrial cells are oestrogen responsive and oestrogen dominance is the norm in developed societies. Many researchers believe that oestrogens and their close relative xeno-oestrogens (environmental oestrogens) play a significant causative role in this disease.

While I don't know this for sure, my suspicion is that endometriosis arises from a combination of genetic inheritance, excessive oestrogen stimulation and immune system imbalance.

What are the risk factors?

The following are associated with an increased risk of developing endometriosis:

- Family history of endometriosis, especially mother or sister

- Late childbearing (after age 30)

- History of long menstrual cycles with a shorter than normal time between cycles

- Abnormal uterus structure

- Diet high in hydrogenated fats (trans fats) as found in processed foods

- Stress

In addition to the distressing symptoms associated with endometriosis, half of women with endometriosis will be infertile. It used to be thought that endometriosis caused infertility by producing scarring on the ovaries and the fallopian tubes (which connect the ovaries to the uterus), but there is some research that infertility, such as unruptured follicles, might, in fact, cause endometriosis. The jury is still out.

My integrated medical prescription for endometriosis

One of the first things I tell my patients is that many women do not actually require treatment. One study showed that over a 6- to 12-month period, endometrial deposits resolved spontaneously in up to a third of women, deteriorated in nearly half, and were unchanged in the remainder.[2] Also, because endometriosis is oestrogen-sensitive, you might find that if you are approaching the menopause your symptoms will naturally improve. That said, there are many women who do suffer considerably from endometriosis and I find that an integrated medical approach can help reduce the symptoms considerably, primarily by reducing inflammation in the body. Many of the approaches that I mention can be used alongside medication-based treatment, but check with your GP before doing so.

Step 1 • Do you have endometriosis?

Endometriosis is notoriously under-diagnosed and difficult to diagnose. It is not uncommon for a delay of up to 12 years between the onset of symptoms and a definitive diagnosis. About half of women with painful periods will have endometriosis. Other symptoms include:

- Pain in the pelvic area – between the hips and the top of the legs – which can be present all the time or just some of the time

- Painful menstrual cramps, starting a couple of days before the period starts and worsening with the onset of bleeding

- Pain during or after sex

- Heavy and/or irregular periods

- Difficulty getting pregnant – about one-third of women with endometriosis will need medical help in getting pregnant

- Painful ovulation

- Premenstrual vaginal spotting of blood

- Back pain, especially during menstruation

- Nausea and/or vomiting, usually just before menstruation

- Fatigue, insomnia and/or mood swings

- Diarrhoea, painful defecation and/or constipation

- Blood in the stool or urine

If you have some of these symptoms, and certainly if you have the tell-tale endometriosis symptom of pain during and/or after sexual intercourse, you should see your GP, who will want to exclude other possible problems that may mimic endometriosis, such as adenomyosis, interstitial cystitis, pelvic floor muscle spasm, irritable bowel syndrome, pelvic inflammatory disease and pelvic congestion syndrome (in which blood backs up in the veins inside a woman's pelvis).

To make a diagnosis they will arrange a referral for a laparoscopy. A laparoscopy is a routine surgical key-hole procedure in which a small fibre-optic tube with a light on the end is inserted into the pelvis via a small incision just under the belly button. It is usually done under general anaesthetic. Carbon dioxide is then pumped into the abdomen, so that the surgeon can see the organs more clearly. Prior to the procedure you could discuss the possibility with your surgeon of cutting out or lasering any endometrial patches found. However, most women opt for treatment to take place at a different time. If you have endometriosis, the surgeon will look carefully to see how much you have, where it is, and whether there's any damage to your organs. Laparoscopy shouldn't be performed during or within three months of hormonal treatment as this will increase the chances of failing to make a correct diagnosis.

Step 2 • Consider the medical options

Conventional medical treatment focuses on pain management, reduction of oestrogen stimulation and preservation of fertility. Often treatment begins at diagnosis when visible lesions are removed or destroyed during a laparoscopy. I encourage most of my patients to try my integrated medicine approach for three months before turning to hormone-based treatment or surgery. Of course, if the symptoms are severe then they should be considered.

Medications
Painkillers – most doctors will recommend that you take non-steroidal anti-inflammatory painkillers before and during the period of pain. Recognised side-effects include gastric irritation and ulceration. Some women benefit from these painkillers, but in my experience many more don't. The evidence as to their effectiveness is inconclusive.

The contraceptive pill – when used in high doses, the hormones within the pill can prevent ovulation and the bleeding associated with menstruation. Side-effects are common and include nausea, vomiting, headache, increased risk of blood clots, depression and breast tenderness. The pill is usually used for women with mild symptoms. Alternatives to the oestrogen-contraceptive pill are progestogen-only pills or coils, which work by putting the body into a pseudo-pregnant state. Side-effects can include nausea, bloating, tender breasts and irritability.

Danazol – this drug used to be a popular treatment, but is now falling out of favour due to its side-effects. Danazol is a weak synthetic male hormone, which works by preventing ovulation and the subsequent hormonal changes that lead to the womb lining growing and then shedding. Its side-effects include deepening of the voice, mood swings, sensitivity to sunlight, nausea, acne, facial hair, dizziness and weight gain. Danazol can be administered as a vaginal ring and this has been found to significantly reduce its side-effects.

Gonadotrophin-releasing hormone analogues (GnRHas) – these are synthetic hormones that can be given as a nasal spray, injection or implant. These work by preventing the pituitary gland from producing FSH (follicle stimulating hormone) and LH (luteinsing hormone), which in turn stops the ovaries from producing their hormones and, in particular, oestrogen. This puts the body into a temporary menopause, causing the endometrial patches to shrink by essentially starving them of oestrogen. Side-effects include hot flushes, mood swings, vaginal dryness and insomnia. The length of time you can be treated using GnRHas is between three and six months. One of the most significant side-effects is a possible 6 per cent loss in bone mineral density in the first six months, which might not be reversible.

According to a review of clinical evidence published by the *British Medical Journal*, all the hormonal drug treatments reduced severe and moderate pain at six months compared with a placebo, and all were similarly effective, although all also had side-effects.[3] Although combined oral contraceptives may be less effective than GnRHas, they have fewer side-effects and are generally recommended to be used (if it is safe to do so).

Danazol and GnRHas can only be used for a maximum of six

months, so the advantage of taking the contraceptive pill is that it can be used for longer periods of time and, of course, can be used as contraception as well. This should, though, be offset against the known side-effects. However, some women do not respond at all to hormonal treatment and of those that do some will experience a return of their symptoms, usually within six months following the end of their hormonal treatment programme.

Surgery

Diathermy/laser – when used in combination with laparoscopy, the surgeon can treat the patches of endometriosis by burning them with intense heat (diathermy) or a laser. The surgeon can also separate any adhesions that might be present, although the chances of those adhesions reforming is high. Some surgeons will offer to ablate a nerve called the uterine nerve, but this has not been shown to help. One study found that surgery to remove endometriosis helped reduce pain for about three-quarters of women, but the pain may come back.[4]

Hysterectomy – the removal of the uterus, usually along with the ovaries, is the most radical of all the treatments and should generally be used as a last resort.

Step 3 • Address the underlying causes

While I am going to make recommendations to treat your symptoms relating to endometriosis using a variety of supplements, for lasting resolution of endometriosis I encourage you to fill in the questionnaires in part one, section two, in order to identify possible root causes and contributors. In my experience, the ones to consider are:

- **Environmental toxicity** – Solution: Secret One – Nurture Your Physical Body (Healthy Environment and Sunlight – page 70)

- **Candida** – Solution: Part Five (Dysbiosis – page 334); Holistic Health Tools – Emotional Freedom Technique (page 151)

- **Poor diet** – Solution: Secret One – Nurture Your Physical Body (Healthy Eating and Supplements – page 49)

- **Stress** – Solution: Secret Two – De-stress and Relax (page 77); Holistic Health Tools – Emotional Freedon Technique (page 151) and Mindfulness (page 147)

- **Nutritional deficiencies** – Solution: Secret One – Nurture Your Physical Body (Healthy Eating and Supplements – page 49)

Step 4 • Start an endometriosis supplement programme

When used alongside step three, certain nutritional supplements can help to alleviate many of the symptoms of endometriosis. My integrated medicine prescription for endometriosis usually includes a combination of:

- **A multivitamin-mineral supplement**

- **Vitamin C with bioflavonoids** (1000mg) to reduce inflammation, pain and heavy bleeding.[5]

- **Omega-3, 6 and 9** (taken in capsule or liquid form in a 2:1:1 ratio) to provide the body with hormone-balancing anti-inflammatory essential fatty acids.[6]

- **Indole-3-Carbinol** (300mg daily), which can help the liver to detoxify excess oestrogen.[7]

- **Acidophilus probiotic** to ensure that there are sufficient numbers of 'friendly' bacteria in the gut to help prevent deactivated oestrogen that has been excreted in the gut being activated again by certain 'unfriendly' bacteria.

- **Milk thistle and dandelion** are herbs that work well in combination, helping to support optimum liver function and reduce circulating levels of oestrogen.

- **Agnus castus**, otherwise known as vitex or chasteberry, is often used if there is a high ratio of oestrogen to progesterone.[8] A nutritional therapist or integrated medicine doctor can arrange testing to see if this is relevant for you – see Resources. The dose I recommend is 40mg of dried herb or 40 drops of concentrated liquid extract once a day, or 20mg of dried herb twice a day. **Do not take this if you are on hormone treatment.**

- **Natural progesterone cream** is used by some integrated medicine doctors to treat the symptoms of endometriosis. This should only be used under medical supervision – see Resources.

- If you have excessive bleeding please refer to the heavy menstrual bleeding advice (page 178) and if you have associated pain to my advice on painful periods (page 184).

Step 5 • Consider other complementary approaches

The pain associated with endometriosis varies from nothing or slight to absolutely crippling. The last two steps will help reduce pain, but in addition to that you might want to consider any combination of the following:

- There is some evidence that using a TENS machine (which uses strong electrical currents) will help reduce period pain. However, I find that microcurrent therapy, which uses minute, painless electrical currents, works much better for my patients – see Resources.

- Try this visualisation technique. Take a couple of long, slow and deep breaths and imagine the area of pain as a ball of red fire. Now see or sense a constant stream of ice cold water pouring into the ball. Keep doing this until the fire is completely extinguished and repeat as often as you need to.

While there is no definitive evidence that these can help you with endometriosis, some patients find the following useful in supporting their endometriosis programme: acupuncture, homeopathy, massage, spiritual healing, yoga, traditional Chinese medicine and Ayurvedic medicine.

For recommended books and websites see Resources.

Polycystic ovary syndrome

Polycystic ovary syndrome (PCOS) is a condition that affects up to 20 per cent of women, 90 per cent of women with infrequent periods and 30 per cent of women whose periods have ceased permanently. In PCOS, there are multiple fluid-filled cysts on the ovaries and also a number of sex hormone imbalances, including raised testosterone. If the cysts are present, but hormone imbalances absent, the term polycystic ovaries is used instead. According to research, a woman with untreated PCOS is more likely to develop diabetes[1] and put on weight (about half of women with PCOS will be obese),[2] and three-quarters of women with PCOS will have difficulty getting pregnant.[3] Fortunately there is plenty that you can do to help yourself.

What causes PCOS?

It's unclear what actually causes PCOS, but it appears to be a number of factors, including:

- A genetically inherited vulnerability to PCOS – about two in ten women with PCOS have a mother with the condition.

- Insulin resistance – in which cells of the body become progressively resistant to the effects of the blood-sugar-lowering hormone insulin. To compensate the pancreas produces extra insulin, which increases the production of the male hormone testosterone, which in turn disrupts the normal functioning of the ovaries.

- Failure of the ovaries to communicate effectively with the pituitary gland – this results in high luteinising hormone (LH) levels.

- Obesity – this appears to be associated with PCOS, as does binge-eating disorder.

- Low quantities of sex hormone-binding globulin (SHBG) – this is a protein produced by the liver, which controls levels of hormones in the blood by binding to them.

My personal opinion is that PCOS is probably due to a combination of a genetically inherited vulnerability and insulin resistance.

My integrated medical prescription for PCOS

PCOS responds very well to an integrated medical programme that focuses on helping you achieve your ideal weight, stabilising your blood-sugar and providing your body with a healthy diet and various nutritional supplements. If you are considering hormonal or surgical treatment I encourage you to give my programme a try first for a minimum of three months, although obviously if your symptoms are severe then you may want to consider medications or surgery.

Step 1 • Do you have PCOS?

One of the difficulties in diagnosing PCOS is that sometimes the symptoms are so mild or absent that most women and their GPs might not even consider there is a problem. Add to that the fact that more than 50 per cent of women with PCOS don't have the classic signs of weight gain and hirsutism (facial hair growth) and it's no wonder the majority of women with PCOS don't know they have it. The following symptoms may suggest the presence of PCOS:

- Heavy bleeding during menstruation
- Abdominal pain similar to menstrual cramps

- The urge to urinate when lying down

- Pain during sexual intercourse

- Constipation

- Palpable lumps in the lower abdomen

- If the PCOS is severe enough to cause bleeding then symptoms might also include tiredness, shortness of breath, pale skin and headaches

If you have any of these you should go and see your doctor, who can arrange hormonal testing and an ultrasound scan. If PCOS is present, the blood tests will usually show high levels of luteinising hormone (LH), high levels of testosterone and low levels of progesterone. The ultrasound scan will probably show a 'necklace' around the periphery of the ovary consisting of at least ten cysts. These are usually very small, measuring 2mm to 8mm in diameter.

Step 2 • Consider the medical options

Medications

In addition to recommending that you lose weight (if appropriate), your doctor will probably offer you some form of medication, including:

The contraceptive pill – the two brands most commonly prescribed for women with PCOS in the UK are Dianette and Yasmin. The research shows that they can help you have regular periods (although they won't make the ovaries release eggs) and they can help with spots and acne.[4] This needs to be balanced with the slightly increased risk of breast cancer and deep vein thrombosis. While the contraceptive pill will probably be the first treatment that you are offered by your GP, my advice is to follow steps three and four for three months before turning to it, as PCOS responds very positively to more natural approaches.

Metformin – this is a drug traditionally used to lower blood-sugar, but it is increasingly being used to treat women with PCOS. This is probably due to its ability to make the cells of the body more sensitive to the effects of insulin, as well as possibly encouraging the liver to make less glucose. It has been found to increase the likelihood of you having a period, make your periods more regular and reduce the amount of unwanted hair that you have.[5] Side-effects may include nausea, indigestion and possibly diarrhoea. Because of its side-effects and lack of good research on its usefulness to women with PCOS, before taking it I usually recommend that my patients follow my integrated medical prescription first. The exception to this is if you have type 2 diabetes, in which case I would recommend taking it for six months and then reviewing your need for it with your doctor.

Clomiphene – this is usually recommended for women who are trying to conceive. It works by reducing the body's supply of oestrogen, which in turn stimulates the pituitary glands to produce follicle stimulating hormone (FSH), which then stimulates the ovaries to produce an egg. Clomiphene is then stopped and doing so results in a surge of LH, which stimulates the release of the egg. That's the theory anyway. Clomiphene is normally taken for a maximum of six months, after which another type of medication called gonadotrophins might be tried. The side-effects of clomiphene include multiple pregnancies and increased risk of miscarriage.

Surgery
If none of these work then you will probably be offered surgery:

Laparoscopic ovarian diathermy – this surgical procedure, also known as ovarian drilling, involves making small holes in the ovary during a laparoscopy (in which a viewing instrument is introduced through a small incision in the abdominal wall). These small holes, which are made using diathermy (heat), are believed to increase the sensitivity of the ovary to FSH and to the drug clomiphene.

Step 3 • Address the underlying causes

For most women, losing weight is probably the most important step you can take, because one study found that as women lost weight their PCOS symptoms improved, their testosterone levels fell, their insulin levels went down and their sex hormone-binding globulin (SHBG) went up. Because SHBG binds to testosterone this helps to reduce testosterone-related symptoms such as facial hair.

While I am going to make recommendations to treat your PCOS symptoms using a variety of supplements, for lasting resolution I encourage you to fill in the questionnaires in part one, section two, in order to identify possible root causes or contributors to PCOS. In my experience, the ones to consider are:

- **Excessive weight** – Solution: Secret One – Nurture Your Physical Body (Healthy Eating and Supplements – page 49); Part Five (Weight Loss – page 401); Holistic Health Tools – Emotional Freedom Technique (page 151) and The Work (page 163)

- **Blood-sugar imbalance** – Solution: Secret One – Nurture Your Physical Body (Healthy Eating and Supplements – page 49)

- **Stress** – Solution: Secret Two – De-stress and Relax (page 77); Holistic Health Tools – Emotional Freedom Technique (page 151) and Mindfulness (page 147)

- **Poor diet** – Solution: Secret One – Nurture Your Physical Body (Healthy Eating and Supplements – page 49)

- **Nutritional deficiencies** – Solution: Secret One – Nurture Your Physical Body (Healthy Eating and Supplements – page 49)

Step 4 • Start a PCOS supplement programme

When used alongside step three, certain nutritional supplements can help to alleviate many of the symptoms of PCOS. My integrated medicine prescription for PCOS usually includes a combination of:

- **A multivitamin-mineral supplement**, plus a total daily dose of **magnesium**[6] (300mg). The latter might help to reverse the insulin resistance that is associated with PCOS.

- **Vitamin C with bioflavonoids** (1000mg) to reduce inflammation and improve skin.

- **Omega-3, 6 and 9** (taken in capsule or liquid form in a 2:1:1 ratio) to provide the body with hormone-balancing anti-inflammatory essential fatty acids.

- **Chromium**[7] (200mcg) to help stabilise blood-sugar and improve insulin sensitivity.

- **Milk thistle and dandelion** are herbs that work well in combination, helping to support optimum liver function and reduce circulating levels of oestrogen.

- **Agnus castus**, otherwise known as vitex or chasteberry, is probably the most commonly used herb among women with PCOS and works by normalising hormone levels in the body. It is also used for irregular menstruation, amenorrhea and PMS.[8] **Do not take this if you are on hormone treatment.**

- **Saw palmetto**[9] (320mg of a standardised extract) is better known for its use in treating benign enlargement of the prostate gland, but its anti-androgen properties make it useful for reducing testosterone levels and treating excess hair growth and acne in PCOS sufferers.

Step 5 • Consider other complementary approaches

While there is no definitive evidence that these can help you with your PCOS, some patients find the following useful in supporting their PCOS programme: acupuncture, homeopathy, massage, yoga, traditional Chinese medicine and Ayurvedic medicine.

For recommended books see Resources.

Cystitis

~

Cystitis is the medical term to describe inflammation of the bladder wall. Cystitis occurs most often when bacteria grow in your bladder and in doing so cause inflammation and irritation of the bladder wall. This leads to painful, frequent urination. About one-third of all women will get cystitis at some time in their life and one in five will get repeated episodes of cystitis.[1] Women are more likely to get cystitis than men because their urethra (the tube connecting the bladder to the outside world) is shorter and nearer to the anus.

What causes cystitis?

The majority of cases of cystitis are caused by the bacteria Escherichia coli (E. coli), a species of bacteria commonly found in the genital area. Non-infectious causes include:

- Chemical cystitis – some women may be hypersensitive to chemicals contained in certain products, such as bubble bath, feminine hygiene sprays or spermicidal jellies, and may develop an allergic-type reaction within the bladder, causing inflammation.

- Interstitial cystitis – no-one yet knows the cause of this distressing chronic bladder inflammation, but an immune attack against the bladder wall and a failure to prevent irritants from entering the bladder wall have all been suggested.

- Drug-induced cystitis – certain medications, particularly chemotherapy drugs, can cause inflammation of the bladder.

- Cystitis associated with other conditions – cystitis may sometimes occur in association with other problems, such as cancer, endometriosis, Crohn's disease, diverticulitis and lupus.

What are the risk factors?

The risk factors for women developing cystitis are:

- Wiping from back to front, especially after a bowel movement
- Using a contraceptive cream (vaginal spermicide)
- Candida overgrowth
- Having diabetes
- Having a tube to drain urine from your bladder (catheter)
- Being elderly – you might get infections if your bladder doesn't empty completely because of medical problems or if you have a hard time getting to a toilet
- Reaching the menopause – your defence against infection can become weaker because of changes to the lining of your vagina and urethra
- Being pregnant – the baby can press down on your bladder and other parts of your urinary tract, so your bladder can't empty completely and flush out any bacteria

My integrated medical prescription for cystitis

It's important to differentiate between a bacterial and non-bacterial cause of cystitis as that will determine the most appropriate treatment approach, so you should always see your GP to receive a diagnosis.

Because bacterial causes are the most common cause, that's what I will deal with here.

Step 1 • Do you have cystitis?

Any of the following symptoms may indicate the presence of cystitis:

- Burning pain when urinating

- Frequent and urgent need to pass urine

- The passing of only small amounts of urine

- Cloudy urine with or without blood

- Smelly urine

- Painful sexual intercourse

- Feeling that the bladder has not emptied properly

- Pain in the lower abdomen

If the pain spreads to the kidneys (which is serious) you may also have:

- High temperature

- Pain in your side

- Nausea and vomiting

If you have symptoms of cystitis you should see your GP or practice nurse who will do a simple urine test to determine whether you have an infection. They might also send the urine sample away to find out which bacteria is causing the infection.

Step 2 • Consider the medical options

If the diagnosis of cystitis is confirmed then you will probably be offered medication.

Medications

Antibiotics – as long as you are not allergic to them, you may be pre-scribed a three-day course of an antibiotic such as trimethoprim (Trimopan), nitrofurantoin (Furadantin, Macrobid, Macrodantin), cefalexin (Ceporex, Keflex) or amoxicillin. Side-effects include nausea, headaches, dysbiosis (see page 334) and possible subsequent bacterial resistance. I am really not a fan of the repeated use of antibi-otics. This is not only because of the potential of bacterial resistance, but because natural approaches can work so well, especially if the underlying causes are also dealt with.

Alkalising powders – your doctor or pharmacist might recommend potassium citrate or sodium citrate to alkalise your urine. This will help to reduce irritation.

If you have recurrent cystitis, you might be offered:

- Low dose of antibiotics every day for 2 to 12 months to prevent more infections.[2]

- If you tend to get cystitis a day or so after having sex, taking anti-biotics within two hours of having sex can help prevent infection.[3]

- Having antibiotics to take as soon as your symptoms start might help clear your infection fast, but we need more research to know this for certain.

If you choose to go for the antibiotic option, you should also take an acidophilus probiotic during and after treatment to offset the nega-tive effects of the antibiotics on the balance of gut bacteria.

Step 3 • Address the underlying causes

While I am going to make recommendations to treat your cystitis symptoms using a variety of supplements, for lasting resolution of cystitis I encourage you to fill in the questionnaires in part one, section two, in order to identify possible root causes or contributors to cystitis. In my experience, the ones to consider are:

- **Candida** – Solution: Part Five (Dysbiosis – page 334); Holistic Health Tools – Emotional Freedom Technique (page 151)

- **Stress** – Solution: Secret Two – De-stress and Relax (page 77); Holistic Health Tools – Emotional Freedom Technique (page 151) and Mindfulness (page 147)

- **Poor diet** – Solution: Secret One – Nurture Your Physical Body (Healthy Eating and Supplements – page 49)

- **Food intolerances** – Solution: Part Five (Food Intolerances – page 344); Holistic Health Tools – Emotional Freedom Technique (page 151)

- **Constipation** – Solution: Part Five (Constipation – page 312)

- **Environmental toxicity** – Solution: Secret One – Nurture Your Physical Body (Healthy Environment and Sunlight – page 70)

- **Nutritional deficiencies** – Solution: Secret One – Nurture Your Physical Body (Healthy Eating and Supplements – page 49)

Step 4 • Start a cystitis supplement programme

When used alongside step three, certain nutritional supplements can help to alleviate and prevent cystitis. My integrated medicine prescription for treating cystitis usually includes a combination of:

- **D-mannose** (dose as advised by manufacturers), which is a sugar supplement that works by preventing the bacteria that are causing the cystitis from attaching to the bladder wall.[4] This enables them to be flushed out of the bladder. See Resources.

- **Alkaline mineral salts** (dose as advised by manufacturers), which create an inhospitable environment for bacteria. If started immediately they can very quickly reduce irritation and other symptoms.

- **Bromelain** (200mg three times a day) is a natural anti-inflammatory that helps to reduce inflammation in the bladder and also has been found to increase the effectiveness of antibiotics.[5]

- **Vitamin C with bioflavonoids** (3000mg daily) is appropriate, because studies have found that vitamin C can help increase the acidity of urine. Increasing the dose to 500mg every two hours if you have cystitis may actually inhibit the growth of E. coli, the most common cause of cystitis. Vitamin C at these levels stimulates the immune system and is antibacterial. The bioflavanoid component prevents the release of chemicals that promote inflammation.[6]

To prevent cystitis I recommend to my patients:

- **Cranberry juice extract**, because two good studies found that women who drank cranberry juice or took cranberry capsules were less likely to get cystitis over a 12-month period than women who took a placebo. Out of the women who took cranberry juice or capsules, two in ten got cystitis during the 12-month period. Among those who took a placebo, four in ten got cystitis.[7]

- **Acidophilus probiotic**, because probiotics are supplements that contain 'friendly' bacteria, whose job, amongst many, is to crowd out disease-causing bacteria. They also help to make the urine acidic, which helps to prevent the growth of unwanted bacteria. If you have or are taking antibiotics you should take probiotics for at least six months, as antibiotics wipe out health-promoting bacteria from the body.

In addition to the supplements that I recommend, it is also important to:

- Avoid or restrict sugar, refined products, alcohol and caffeine, all of which lower the immune system

- Always wipe from front to back after a bowel movement

- Empty your bladder frequently and completely

- Urinate after intercourse

- Take showers rather than using baths

- Do not douche

- Drink at least 2 to 3 litres of water and herbal teas a day

- Avoid perfumed toiletries or bubble baths

Step 5 • Consider other complementary approaches

While there is no definitive evidence that these can help you with cystitis, you might want to consider supporting your programme with: Western herbal medicine (especially uva ursi and echinacea), homeopathy, acupuncture, aromatherapy, reflexology, Ayurvedic medicine, spiritual healing, yoga and traditional Chinese medicine.

For recommended books see Resources.

Fibrocystic breast disease

The term fibrocystic breast disease is a rather inaccurate medical term used to describe the presence of lumpy and/or tender breasts. Rather than thinking of it as a disease, I regard these signs as a reflection of a woman's hormone fluctuations, diet and even stress levels. More often than not if all three of these are addressed the tenderness and lumps will subside. While it is, of course, important not to miss breast cancer, most lumps and tenderness are benign. It's also a very common issue, with over 70 per cent of women reporting breast changes such as tenderness, swelling and/or lumps in relation to their menstrual cycle. The main types of problems that occur under the label fibrocystic breast disease are:

Cyclical pain and swelling – if you notice that your breasts are sensitive or painful just prior to menstruation, but then are fine with menstruation, then you are probably experiencing a normal physiological response to the hormonal changes that are taking place. Most women just need to be reassured that this is the case.

Mastalgia – if your breast pain interferes with your quality of life you have a condition called mastalgia. This can be due to a more severe form of physiological pain or hormonal changes, infections or trauma.

Breast lumpiness – this is the number one concern for most women. Breast lumpiness is either cyclical or non-cyclical, painful or not painful. While breast tissue is irregularly textured, if the lumpiness is the same on the other breast, this is highly indicative of a normal condition.

Lumps that merge with the breast tissue – if you find a lump in one breast that merges in one or more places with the surrounding breast tissue, then you have what is called a non-dominant breast lump. However, 95 per cent of these lumps are non-cancerous, and your GP will probably recommend that they be observed over a couple of months and then reassessed.

Lumps that separate from the surrounding tissue – a solid lump occurring in one breast, which doesn't fluctuate with your menstrual cycle and is clearly distinct from the surrounding breast tissue, does need to be investigated. The most common diagnosis is a fibroadenoma. They are round, smooth, benign growths that feel rubbery. Because they can be moved easily under the skin they are sometimes referred to as breast mice. Most fibroadenomas are between 1cm and 3cm in size and will not usually grow, the exception being in pregnancy and while breastfeeding.

What causes fibrocystic breast disease?

Because it is so common, it's almost fair to describe it as a normal part of being a woman. However, it is less common in women who take the oestrogen contraceptive pill, so a high ratio of oestrogen to progesterone might be a possible cause. This is usually due to a combination of poor diet, being exposed to xeno-oestrogens (chemicals that mimic oestrogen) and possibly stress.

What are the risk factors?

The risk factors for fibrocystic disease (although some of these are controversial) include:

- Family history

- Excessive consumption of saturated fat

- Caffeine – consumption of between 30mg and 250mg a day of caffeine increases the risk of developing fibrocystic breast disease 1.5-fold, and consuming more than 500mg a day by 2.3-fold (five cups of instant coffee is equivalent to about 500mg).[1]

My integrated medical prescription for fibrocystic breast disease

The majority of breast lumps are absolutely harmless and with some simple adjustments to diet and lifestyle, and with a few targeted nutritional supplement products, you should find that they improve and at least become less uncomfortable within one to three months.

Step 1 • Do you have fibrocystic breast disease?

To assess whether you have lumps in your breast, you should get into the routine of examining your breasts regularly. The best time to do this is just after your period. The basic principles of breast awareness are:

- Know what is normal for you

- Know what changes to look and feel for

- Look and feel

- Report any changes to your GP without delay

- Attend for routine breast screening if you are aged 50 or over

The basic approach to breast self-examination is a visual and manual check:

Visual check

- Remove your bra and have a careful look at your breasts in a mirror.

- With your hands clasped together behind your head, straighten and lower the arms a few times to see if the nipples on both breasts move in the same way.

- Look at your breasts in profile.

- Bend forward and look at your breasts in profile and straight on.

Manual check

- Always use the flat of your hand for this part, with your fingers straight and together. Make circular movements with your hands to check the tissue in and around your breasts for irregularities.

- If you start with the right breast, raise the right arm above your head, and use the left hand to feel the top and outer part of your breast, then the underarm.

- To make sure you check the whole breast thoroughly, move the left hand in a complete circle round the outside of the breast, then move a couple of centimetres in towards the nipple and repeat. Continue until you reach the nipple.

- Squeeze the nipple gently to check for any discharge.

- Repeat the same moves on the left breast using the right hand.

Some women like using a Liv Aid, a soft, polyurethrane self-examination pad, as it provides increased sensitivity. For more information see Resources.

Changes to be aware of:

- Size – if one breast becomes larger or lower

- Nipples – if a nipple becomes inverted (pulled in) or changes position or shape

- Rashes – on or around the nipple

- Discharge – from one or both nipples

- Skin changes – puckering or dimpling

- Swelling – under the armpit or around the collarbone

- Pain – continuous, in one part of the breast or armpit

- Lump or thickening – different to the rest of the breast tissue

If you have any of the changes above, or if you are at all concerned, you should see your GP or breast health professional. Your GP will do a breast examination and, if appropriate, arrange a referral to a breast clinic. Most patients will then be offered a triple assessment consisting of:

- Breast examination

- Mammogram or ultrasound scan

- Core biopsy and/or fine needle aspiration

An alternative option to mammograms is Digital Infra-Red Thermal Imaging (DITI). This is a technique that uses a specialised infra red camera to create a heat map of the body. Because cancer has an increased blood supply and higher rate of metabolic activity than the surrounding breast tissue it will show up on the heat map. The advantage of DITI is that it is 100 per cent safe and risk free and it is able to pick up cancerous lumps before they can be detected by self-examination and mammography. This can lead to a much earlier diagnosis and treatment. For more information see Resources.

Step 2 • Consider the medical options

If you have been given a diagnosis of fibrocystic breast disease you might be encouraged to do nothing, wait and observe or start some medications.

Medications

I encourage you to try my suggestions in steps three and four before resorting to hormone-based treatments. The most common hormone-based treatments that you may be offered are:

The contraceptive pill – because fibrocystic breast disease is related to hormonal fluctuations, the theory behind prescribing the pill is that this will stop the pain and tenderness. While this does work for some women, it can actually make it worse for others. Other side-effects include nausea, headache, increased risk of thrombosis (blood clot), breast tenderness and a slightly increased risk of breast cancer.

Bromocriptine – this drug reduces levels of the hormone prolactin, which for some women can help reduce breast discomfort. Side-effects include nausea, dizziness, leg cramps, dry mouth and hallucinations.

Danazol – this is a male hormone derivative that prevents ovulation. While it has been found to help some women experience a reduction in breast pain, it is associated with side-effects such as hirsutism (increased hair growth), mood swings, rashes, acne, deepening of the voice and weight gain.

Step 3 • Address the underlying causes

While I am going to make recommendations to treat symptoms such as breast tenderness using a variety of supplements, for lasting resolution of fibrocystic breast disease, I encourage you to fill in the questionnaires in part one, section two, in order to identify possible root causes or contributors. In my experience, the ones to consider are:

- **Constipation** – Solution: Part Five (Constipation – page 312), (one study found that women who have less than three bowel movements a week have a risk of fibrocystic breast disease four to five times greater than women who have at least one bowel movement a day)

- **Excessive weight** – Solution: Secret One – Nurture Your Physical Body (Healthy Eating and Supplements – page 49); Part Five (Weight Loss – page 401); Holistic Health Tools – Emotional Freedom Technique (page 151) and The Work (page 163)

- **Food intolerances** – Solution: Part Five (Food Intolerances – page 344); Holistic Health Tools – Emotional Freedom Technique (page 151)

- **Environmental toxicity** – Solution: Secret One – Nurture Your Physical Body (Healthy Environment and Sunlight – page 70)

- **Poor diet** – Solution: Secret One – Nurture Your Physical Body (Healthy Eating and Supplements – page 49)

- **Nutritional deficiencies** – Solution: Secret One – Nurture Your Physical Body (Healthy Eating and Supplements – page 49)

- **Candida** – Solution: Part Five (Dysbiosis – page 334); Holistic Health Tools – Emotional Freedom Technique (page 151)

- **Hypothyroidism** – Solution: Part Five (Hypothyroidism – page 356); Holistic Health Tools – Emotional Freedom Technique (page 151) and The Work (page 163)

Step 4 • Start a fibrocystic breast disease supplement programme

When used alongside step three, certain nutritional supplements can help to alleviate many of the symptoms associated with fibrocystic breast disease. My integrated medicine prescription for fibrocystic breast disease usually includes a combination of:

- **A multivitamin-mineral supplement**, although you should also make sure that you are taking a total daily dose of 400IU to 800IU of vitamin E a day as this has been shown to reduce pain and tenderness in some women.[2]

- **Vitamin C with bioflavonoids** (1000mg) to reduce inflammation and tenderness.

- **Omega-3, 6 and 9** (taken in capsule or liquid form in a 2:1:1 ratio) to provide the body with hormone-balancing anti-inflammatory essential fatty acids.

- **Indole-3-Carbinol** (300mg daily), which can help the liver to detoxify excess oestrogen.[3]

- **Acidophilus probiotic** to ensure that there are sufficient numbers of 'friendly' bacteria in the gut to help prevent deactivated oestrogen that has been excreted in the gut being activated again by certain 'unfriendly' bacteria.

- **Milk thistle and dandelion** are herbs that work well in combination, helping to support optimum liver function and reduce circulating levels of oestrogen.

- **Agnus castus**, otherwise known as vitex or chasteberry, is often used if there is a high ratio of oestrogen to progesterone.[4] A nutritional therapist or integrated medicine doctor can arrange testing to see if this is relevant for you – see Resources. The dose I recommend is 40mg of dried herb or 40 drops of concentrated liquid extract once a day, or 20mg of dried herb twice a day. **Do not take this if you are on hormone treatment.**

- **Natural progesterone cream** is used by some integrated medicine doctors to treat fibrocystic breast disease. This should only be used under medical supervision.

Step 5 • Consider other complementary approaches

While there is no definitive evidence that these can help you with your symptoms, some patients find the following useful in supporting their programme: acupuncture, homeopathy, Western herbal medicine, yoga and traditional Chinese medicine.

For recommended books see Resources.

Infertility

Trying and failing to have a baby is one of the most incredibly stressful, traumatic and expensive experiences you can go through, and it is affecting more and more couples. About one in six couples will have a problem getting pregnant.[1]

Doctors will generally make the diagnosis of infertility if you and your partner have not conceived after two years of trying. This is based on the statistics that 85 per cent of couples will naturally conceive within one year of having unprotected sex. That figure increases to 95 per cent within two years.

However, two years is a very long time! From an integrated medical perspective, the real key is not just to use lifestyle and natural approaches to increasing the likelihood of having a baby, but to increase the likelihood of the new baby and mother being as healthy as possible. I am all for a proactive approach to childbirth, in which mum and dad do everything they can to prepare and then nurture the baby in utero. If after one year of doing this you haven't conceived, then that would be an indication that further testing and investigation is needed. If you have a history of infertility or are over the age of 35, you might want to do this even earlier.

What causes infertility?

There are many different factors that can delay getting pregnant or cause infertility:

- In two out of ten infertile couples, the man has a problem

- In about four out of ten couples, the woman does

- In a further three or four out of ten couples, both partners have a problem

The most common causes in women are ovulation problems and damaged or blocked tubes, and in men low sperm count and poor-quality sperm. In up to one-third of infertile couples, doctors can't find a reason for the infertility.

What are the risk factors for infertility?

The following risk factors are associated with female infertility:

- Age – after the age of 30, the quantity and the quality of your eggs start to decline. This process accelerates considerably after the age of 35, by which time you are at a higher risk of miscarriage and having a baby with chromosomal abnormalities.

- Weight – being overweight or significantly underweight may inhibit normal ovulation and reduce the likelihood of pregnancy.

- Smoking – this is associated with an increased risk of miscarriage and is thought to deplete your eggs prematurely, reducing your ability to get pregnant.

- Sexually transmitted diseases – chlamydia and gonorrhoea can cause fallopian tube damage and reduce the chances of you becoming pregnant naturally.

- Caffeine – consuming more than the equivalent of six cups of coffee a day may decrease your fertility.

- Alcohol – heavy drinking is associated with an increased risk of ovulation problems and endometriosis.

My integrated medical prescription for infertility

Most infertility experts would encourage mothers and fathers to prepare for pregnancy by making dietary and lifestyle changes at least four months before beginning to try for a baby. If you have been diagnosed as having infertility, you might want to consider implementing the lifestyle changes and taking the supplements that I am going to recommend while stopping trying to conceive for a couple of months. This may sound counter-intuitive, but it actually gives your body time to respond to the changes and to provide you with the best possible chances of conceiving, and then giving birth to, a healthy baby.

Step 1 • Are you infertile?

If you have yet to conceive after one year of unprotected intercourse or if you are over 35 years of age and/or have a history of infertility and have been trying for six months or more, you should see your GP. They will take a full history, check your weight and examine your pelvic area for vaginal infection or tenderness, which could be an indication of endometriosis or pelvic inflammatory disease (PID). After this they will probably refer you for some tests, which may include:

- Pelvic ultrasound – this uses high-frequency sound waves to create an image of an organ in your body, in this case an image of your womb and ovaries.

- Progesterone test – this blood test checks to see if you are ovulating and should be taken seven days before you expect a period.

- Chlamydia test – chlamydia can affect fertility and if you have it your GP will be able to prescribe antibiotics to treat it.

- Thyroid function test – it is estimated that between 1.3 and 5.1 per cent of infertile women have an abnormal thyroid.

- Hysterosalpingogram – this is a type of x-ray that checks your fallopian tubes.

- Laparoscopy – a small cut is made in your lower abdomen and a thin, tubular microscope, called a laparoscope, is used to look more closely at your womb, fallopian tubes and ovaries, with dye sometimes being injected into the fallopian tubes through the cervix (entrance to the womb) to highlight any blockages.

Step 2 • Consider the medical options

Your medical treatment programme will depend on your age, the clinic and the underlying cause. For example, if you have an infection antibiotics might be prescribed, or large fibroids might be treated with a combination of drugs and surgery. In addition to addressing the underlying causes, you might also be offered one of the following medical treatment options to support fertility. With the exception of metformin for women with PCOS or diabetes, I encourage all my patients to follow my integrated medical prescription for at least six months before moving on to these.

Medications

Clomifene (clomid) – this is used early in the menstrual cycle in order to encourage ovulation in women who do not ovulate regularly or who cannot ovulate at all. If your doctor has confirmed you have an ovulation problem, taking this increases the possibility of getting pregnant three-fold.[2] The side-effects, which are usually mild, include feeling bloated, weight gain and hot flushes. You are also more likely to give birth to twins or triplets. If you are overweight, I would recommend taking metformin with it.

Metformin – this is a drug used for people with diabetes, but if you have polycystic ovary syndrome (PCOS) you might be offered this in conjunction with clomifene. Over a six-month period you have about a one in three chance of getting pregnant taking the combination, compared to about a one in ten chance if you take just clomifene.[3] Side-effects include an upset stomach and sometimes diarrhoea. If you have PCOS or diabetes I would recommend taking metformin.

Gonadotrophins – medicines containing gonadotrophins can help to stimulate ovulation. These are usually used if clomifene doesn't work.

The side-effects include putting on weight, feeling bloated, swelling in your legs and arms, nausea, breathlessness and possibly problems with your kidneys and liver. Because of the side-effects and limited evidence to support their use, gonadatrophins should be low down on your list of priorties.

Surgery
Fallopian tube surgery – if your fallopian tubes have become blocked or scarred no amount of supplements will change this and you may require surgery to help repair the tubes and make it easier for eggs to pass along them.

Laparoscopic surgery – a laparoscopy involves having a small cut (incision) made in your abdomen. A thin, flexible microscope with a light on the end, called a laparoscope, is then passed through the incision. This type of procedure can be used to look at internal organs, take samples and perform small operations. It is often used for women who have endometriosis.

Assisted conception
While all the following assisted conception techniques can support you in becoming pregnant, the likelihood of them being successful is still low. I therefore recommend that you follow my integrated medical prescription either prior to trying them (give yourself at least one year) or alternatively alongside them. For example, giving up smoking and caffeine, switching to a healthy diet, taking supplements and managing your stress will help to increase the likelihood of success.

Intrauterine insemination (IUI) – this procedure involves sperm being placed into the womb through a fine plastic tube. The tube is passed through the cervix and into the womb. Sperm is collected from the man and then washed in a fluid, after which the best quality specimens are selected. The sperm is then passed through the tube. This procedure is performed to coincide with ovulation and increase the chance of conception. You may also be given a low dose of ovary-stimulating hormones to again increase to chance of conception. IUI tends to be used when infertility cannot be explained or when a man has a low sperm count or decreased sperm mobility. It is also helpful for men who experience severe impotence. Provided that the man's sperm and the woman's tubes are healthy, the success rate for IUI is around 15 per cent per cycle of treatment.

In vitro fertilisation (IVF) – if you have blocked or damaged tubes, then IVF might provide an option for you, although success rates do vary between clinics, and the treatment is physically and emotionally demanding. In IVF the woman takes medication to stimulate the ovaries to produce more mature eggs than normal. These are then removed from her ovaries and fertilised with sperm in a laboratory dish. One or two fertilised embryos are then placed into the womb using a fine tube that is put up the vagina and through the cervix. National statistics show that infertile couples who have IVF have about a one in five chance of having a baby after one attempt, but that IVF works best for women under the age of 35.[4]

Intracytoplasmic sperm injection (ICSI) – if standard IVF hasn't worked, or if the male has a low sperm count, then you might be offered ICSI. This technique involves an individual sperm being injected directly into an egg. The egg containing the sperm is then placed in the uterus in the same way as with IVF.

Gamete intrafallopian transfer (GIFT) – in this so-called more 'natural' approach, eggs and sperm are collected as per the IVF protocol, but the eggs and sperm are then placed inside the woman's fallopian tube or uterus (by surgery). For this to work, the woman's fallopian tube needs to be healthy.

Egg donation – if IVF has failed, or if the woman is unable to produce eggs, then egg donation might be considered. This involves stimulating the ovaries of a female donor with medications, collecting the eggs which form and fertilising them with the sperm of the recipient's partner (similar to IVF). After two to three days embryos are placed in the uterus of the recipient via the cervix.

The provision of these fertility treatments on the NHS varies between different health authorities. If the waiting time is extremely long, you might want to consider going private with a clinic that is registered with the Human Fertilisation and Embryology Authority (HFEA) – see Resources.

Step 3 • Address the underlying causes

While I am going to make supplement recommendations to support the likelihood of you conceiving, I encourage you to fill in the questionnaires in part one, section two, in order to identify possible root causes or contributors to infertility. In my experience, the ones to consider are:

- **Excessive weight** – Solution: Secret One – Nurture Your Physical Body (Healthy Eating and Supplements – page 49); Part Five (Weight Loss – page 401); Holistic Health Tools – Emotional Freedom Technique (page 151) and The Work (page 163)

- **Smoking** – Solution: Secret One – Nurture Your Physical Body (Healthy Environment and Sunlight – page 70); Holistic Health Tools – Emotional Freedom Technique (page 151) and The Work (page 163)

- **Alcohol and caffeine** – Solution: these should be stopped completely

- **Stress** – Solution: Secret Two – De-stress and Relax (page 77); Holistic Health Tools – Emotional Freedom Technique (page 151) and Mindfulness (page 147)

- **Poor diet** – Solution: Secret One – Nurture Your Physical Body (Healthy Eating and Supplements – page 49)

- **Environmental toxicity** – Solution: Secret One – Nurture Your Physical Body (Healthy Environment and Sunlight – page 70)

- **Hypothyroidism** – Solution: Part Five (Hypothyroidism – page 356); Holistic Health Tools – Emotional Freedom Technique (page 151) and The Work (page 163)

- **Eating disorders** – Solution: Secret One – Nurture Your Physical Body (Healthy Eating and Supplements – page 49); Secret Four – Accept Yourself (page 113); Holistic Health Tool – Emotional Freedom Technique (page 151) and Mindfulness (page 147)

- **Nutritional deficiencies** – Solution: Secret One – Nurture Your Physical Body (Healthy Eating and Supplements – page 49)

Step 4 • Start a fertility support supplement programme

When used alongside step three, certain nutritional supplements can help to support your own health, and increase the possibility of you conceiving and then giving birth to a healthy baby. I have also included suggestions for men as well. My integrated medicine pre-scription for infertility usually includes a combination of:

- **A multivitamin-mineral formula** containing at least 400mcg of **folic acid** (to prevent spina bifida).[5]

- **Fish oil** (3000mg a day) for healthy hormone functioning (for you) and supporting healthy sperm (for men).[6]

- **Vitamin C with bioflavonoids** (1000mg) might support conception (for you), enhance the effect of clomifene and also support sperm function (for men)

- **L-arginine** 2000mg,[7] **L-carnitine** 1500mg[8] and **zinc** 30mg[9] twice daily to support sperm motility and health (for men).

- **Agnus castus** is usually the herb of choice if there is hormonal imbalance.[10] It is particularly useful if there is a luteal phase defect (shortened second half of the cycle) or high levels of prolactin. The dose is 160mg to 240mg of a 0.6 per cent aucubin extract each morning. **Do not take this if you are on hormone treatment.** In one study 48 women aged 23 to 39 who were diagnosed with infer-tility took agnus castus once daily for three months – seven of them became pregnant and another 25 regained normal progesterone levels.

Step 5 • Consider other complementary approaches

While there is no definitive evidence that these can help you with infertility, some patients find the following useful in supporting their programme: acupuncture, homeopathy, Western herbal medicine, massage, guided imagery, yoga and traditional Chinese medicine.

Also bear in mind that the optimum frequency to have sex when trying to conceive is two to three times a week, and the most fertile time is between four days before ovulation to a couple of hours afterwards.

For recommended books, websites and clinics see Resources.

Menopause

The menopause has been treated by Western medicine as a disease
or a problem that needs to be fixed ever since oestrogen derived
from horse urine and synthetic progestin were prescribed en masse to
women in their forties to help alleviate menopausal symptoms. Fortunately, more women and some doctors are starting to embrace the
changes associated with menopause not as a disease, but as the
normal and natural cessation of menstruation following the down-
regulation of ovarian activity. This marks the end of the reproductive
period and the entrance into a new stage. In many cultures the
menopause is viewed as a rite of passage, a natural process and an
invitation to women to reshape and reprioritise how they live their
lives.

Before exploring the diagnosis and treatment of the menopause I
want to familiarise you with the definitions peri-menopause,
menopause and post-menopause:

- Peri-menopause is the period from when your ovaries start to fail
  (you still have periods, but they become heavier, lighter and/or
  erratic, and you can start experiencing symptoms such as hot
  flushes and mood changes) to 12 months after your final menstrual
  period. On average, the onset of peri-menopause occurs around age
  47, with the average duration being four to five years.

- Menopause is the point in time when you had your final menstrual period. However, one year without a single period must pass before the menopause can be officially declared. It is still theoretically possible to become pregnant until this has happened. In the Western world the menopause occurs, on average, at age 51, but it can occur normally within a range of 40 to 58 years of age.[1] Smoking is known to bring the menopause date forward by an average of two years.

- Post-menopause is the period following cessation of menstruation. You can only be certain that you are post-menopausal when you have not had any periods for 12 months. It is estimated that by the age of 54, 80 per cent of women are post-menopausal.

The definitions of menopause and post-menopause are somewhat confusing because they suggest that you are menopausal and post-menopausal at the same time! In fact the menopause is a particular date – officially 12 months after your last menstrual period. The post-menopausal phase begins after that date.

What causes menopause?

From the late thirties onwards your ovaries start to produce less oestrogen and progesterone, the two hormones that prepare your body for ovulation and menstruation. A clue that this might be happening is that you start to experience changes in your periods, for example they might become lighter or heavier, shorter or longer, more frequent or less frequent. This is the peri-menopause phase I mentioned earlier. With the continuing decline in hormones your periods eventually taper off, until ovulation ceases completely.

What are the risk factors for menopause?

The menopause is a natural process so all women will pass through it. However, there are a number of factors that increase the risk of a premature menopause. Premature menopause affects one in 100 women and occurs when the menopause occurs before the age of 40. This most often occurs in women who have undergone chemotherapy and radiation treatment or those who have had their ovaries surgically removed. Other causes include eating disorders, adrenal fatigue, excessive amounts of exercise and diseased ovaries. The majority of women, however, will not have an obvious medical reason for their premature menopause.

My integrated medical prescription for the menopause

For many women the symptoms and changes associated with the menopause are mild and of a short duration. A healthy diet, regular exercise, plenty of rest and sleep, avoiding smoking and caffeine, limiting alcohol and sugar, effective stress management and loving support will make for a safe, relatively symptom-free passage through this period of transition. For women who do find their symptoms to be distressing, then a personalised integrated medicine programme is necessary. In addition to restoring a natural hormonal balance, alleviating distressing symptoms and preventing some of the diseases that are more common during this period of a woman's life, such as osteoporosis, heart disease, stroke and cancer, an optimum programme should be designed to lift your mood, increase your energy and improve your quality of life.

Step 1 • Are you peri-menopausal or menopausal?

The majority of women (about 84 per cent) who are peri- and post-menopausal will experience menopausal symptoms and about half of these will find them distressing.[2] The most common symptoms associated with the menopause include:

- Menstrual cycle may shorten or lengthen in duration

- Amount of menstrual blood may increase (most commonly) or decrease

- Hot flushes and sweats, including night sweats

- Urinary and vaginal symptoms such as vaginal dryness, discomfort during intercourse, recurrent urinary tract infections and urinary incontinence

- Sleep disturbances and insomnia

- Mood swings, including anxiety, nervousness, depression, forget-fulness and difficulty concentrating (of the women who do experi-ence these symptoms, most will already have a history of similar symptoms)

- Other symptoms include loss of libido, thinning of bones (osteo-porosis), headaches, hair loss, brittle nails, dizziness, palpitations, cold hands and feet, loss of muscle tone and skin elasticity, skin rashes and lethargy

- In addition to this the risk of developing a number of health chal-lenges also increases, including osteoporosis, heart disease, stroke and a redistribution of body fat to the abdomen

In addition to the presence of those symptoms above, the simplest and most immediate way to work out whether you have entered the menopause is to get your doctor to do a blood test or to purchase a home menopause test – see Resources. Both test for a hormone called FSH which is raised in the menopause. Two positive tests done within a month of each other, combined with the presence of menopausal symptoms, suggest that you have entered the menopause.[3] FSH levels of greater than 30IU/L are generally considered to be in the post-menopausal range.

One caveat with this test, though, is that FSH levels can fluctuate quite considerably, so it is possible to have normal FSH levels and still be peri-menopausal. Another caveat is that if you are on the oral con-traceptive pill you will need to stop it for a couple of months prior to the test, as women on the pill will always have a low FHS level. I rec-ommend that you see your GP for hormone testing as he or she will also be able to make an assessment of risk factors for heart disease, osteoporosis and breast cancer.

Step 2 • Consider the medical options

While I don't personally prescribe Hormone Replacement Therapy (HRT), because there are so many safer, more natural approaches to resolving menopausal symptoms, it's important to know about it and also how to safely come off it if you choose to do so (see page 252). In the UK HRT is currently licensed for helping to relieve some of the symptoms that accompany the menopause, including hot flushes, night sweats and vaginal dryness. It can also be used as a second-line option for women at high risk of fractures who cannot take other medicines that are licensed for this purpose. HRT works by providing your body with low-dose oestrogen, with or without progestogen, to replace the hormones that your body can no longer make in sufficient quantities. HRT is available as patches, tablets, implants, vaginal rings, gels and as a nasal spray.

What are the HRT options?

If you do not have a uterus (in other words you have had a hysterectomy) you will be offered an oestrogen-only HRT, consisting of either oestradiol or conjugated oestrogen. This is taken every day (continuously).

If you still have your uterus you will be offered combined HRT, containing oestrogen and progestogen. The progestogen component is included in order to reduce the risk of endometrial cancer. The two types of progestogen most commonly in use in combined HRT tablets are the 17-hydroxyprogesterone derivatives (medroxyprogesterone or dydrogesterone) and the 19-nortestosterone derivaties (norethisterone or levonorgestrel). The latter increase levels of testosterone. Combined HRT patches use the latter and combined HRT is available as a continuous or cyclical regime.

If you are peri-menopausal you will probably be offered a cyclical regime, in which you take oestrogen every day and the progestogen at the end of the cycle. This will cause a withdrawal bleed every month in response to the drop in your progesterone level. Continuous regimes aren't usually recommended in this group because they cause unpredictable bleeding. The only way to have a 'no-bleed regime' is have an intrauterine device containing progestogen (levonorgestrol) inserted, while also taking oestrogen in the form of a patch, tablet, implant or nasal spray.

If you are post-menopausal you will probably be offered the choice of taking a cyclical regime, which will result in a withdrawal bleed, or a continuous regime, which does not produce a withdrawal bleed. Some women, however, do experience spotting or irregular bleeding for the first four to six months after starting this regime.

An alternative to combined HRT is Tibolone, a synthetic oral steroid with mixed oestrogenic, progestogenic and androgenic actions.

What dosage?
There are numerous factors influencing the optimum dose for a particular individual, but as a general rule of thumb the lowest dose that controls symptoms should be used.

Oestrogen – if you have decided to go on HRT (and I encourage you to read about the side-effects first) then you should start with a low dose of oestrogen, equivalent to 1mg of oral oestradiol or 25mcg to 50mcg of transdermal oestradiol per day.

Progestogens – generally these should be taken for the last 12 to 14 days of a 28-day cycle or continuously. For a cyclical dosing regime 10mg of oral medroxyprogesterone acetate or 10mg to 20mg of oral dydrogesterone is recommended for the last 14 days and 1mg of norethisterone.

Tibolone – the standard dose of Tibolone is 2.5mg daily.

What about contraception?
It is generally accepted that contraception should be continued for one year after the last menstrual period for women over 50 years old or for two years after the last menstrual period for women under the age of 50. Women taking HRT should use barrier methods, an intra-uterine device, or the levonorgestrel-releasing intrauterine system (IUS).

The benefits of HRT
In the short term HRT will help to stop hot flushes and night sweats within a couple of weeks, as well as helping to reverse vaginal dryness and related vaginal symptoms within a couple of months. Indeed, a meta-analysis of 24 trials involving 3,000 women taking HRT for symptom relief found that HRT reduced hot flushes and night sweats

by 74 per cent.[4] If your sleep disturbance is related to the hot flushes you should also find your sleep pattern improving,[5] which in turn will help improve your mood.

Long-term use of HRT, for several years or more, has been found to offer women a small benefit in helping to prevent osteoporosis and bowel cancer. Studies have shown that if 1,000 healthy women who take HRT are compared to 1,000 healthy women who do not take HRT, in those who take HRT, over a ten-year period there will be approximately:[6]

- Five fewer women who develop a hip fracture – this is because you are less likely to develop osteoporosis and therefore less likely to fracture a bone

- Six fewer women who develop cancer of the bowel (colon), although it is not clear how HRT reduces the risk of developing this cancer

That's the positive side of HRT, now for the flip-side.

The side-effects of HRT

The most common short-term side-effects of HRT include nausea (particularly with the tablets), skin irritation (with the patches), leg cramps, breast tenderness, irregular and heavy bleeding, dry eyes and fluid retention. What's more, research studies dating back to the 1970s have raised numerous concerns about the safety of HRT[7] and when taken long term, compared to women of the same age who do not take HRT, you have an increased risk of developing the following:

Breast cancer – a number of studies, including the UK's Million Women Study, set up to investigate the influences on women's health in over one million UK women aged 50 or over, have found that HRT users are more likely to develop breast cancer than those who are not using HRT.[8] The Million Women Study was also able to show that this effect is greater for combined (oestrogen-progestogen) HRT than for oestrogen-only HRT and that the effects are similar for all specific types and doses of oestrogen and progestogen, for oral, transdermal and implanted HRT, and for continuous and cyclical patterns of use. It found:

On average, the number of new cases of breast cancer per 1,000 women over a five-year period is:

- 14 in those who have never taken HRT

- 18 in those taking the oestrogen-only HRT

- 20 in those taking Tibolone

- Between 28 and 38 in those taking combined HRT

In addition to this the Million Women Study also found that:

- The duration for which you take HRT has a direct impact on your risk of developing breast cancer. In women taking HRT for between one and three years, the oestrogen-only HRT and Tibolone have a very small risk and for combined HRT that risk is slightly higher.

- With all types of HRT, the risk of breast cancer begins to decline when HRT is stopped and by five years it reaches the same level as in women who have never taken HRT.

Endometrial cancer – it is well known that post-menopausal women who have not had a hysterectomy are at increased risk of cancer of the endometrium (the lining of the womb) if they take oestrogen-only HRT. The unopposed oestrogen causes the cells of the uterus lining to proliferate, which in turn increases the risk of cell mutation. A follow up of over 700,000 women in the Million Women Study has confirmed this and shown that the risk of endometrial cancer is also increased in women who take Tibolone, but is not altered, or may even be reduced, in women taking combined HRT.[9]

On average, the number of new cases of endometrial cancer per 1,000 women over a five-year period is:

- 3 in those who have never taken HRT

- 6 in those taking Tibolone

- 5 in those taking oestrogen-only HRT

- Between 2 and 3 in those taking combined HRT

These effects also depend on a woman's body mass index (BMI, a measure of obesity) in that adverse effects of Tibolone and oestrogen-only HRT are greatest in thinner women, and the beneficial effects of combined HRT are greatest in fatter women.

Because breast cancer is more common than endometrial cancer, researchers believe that when considering the overall effect of HRT it is important to look at both breast and endometrial cancer. When rates for breast and endometrial cancer are taken together, the overall risk is highest in women taking combined HRT. The study shows that around three out of every hundred women on combined HRT will develop either breast or endometrial cancer over a period of five years. This compares with about two and a half per hundred who take oestrogen-only HRT or Tibolone, and around one and a half per hundred who have not taken HRT.

Dementia – the Women's Health Initiative Memory Study sought to evaluate the influence of combined HRT on the risk of dementia and cognitive impairment on women aged 65 and over. The study found that HRT doubled the risk of dementia within one year of commencing HRT and did not prevent mild cognitive impairment. However, the increased risk of dementia was only significant for women over the age of 75 and then it was relatively small – of 500 women being treated with HRT, one will develop dementia because of taking HRT.[10]

Blood clots – blood clots forming within a blood vessel in the leg can cause a deep vein thrombosis (DVT), which might then break off and travel to the lungs causing a pulmonary embolism. In women in their fifties, over a five-year period:[11]

- About 3 in 1,000 women who do not use HRT are likely to have a serious blood clot

- About 7 in 1,000 women who do use HRT are likely to have a serious blood clot

The increased risk of having a blood clot is mainly within the first year or so of starting HRT. See a doctor urgently if you develop a red, swollen or painful leg, or have sharp pains in your chest.

Heart disease – an American study, called the Women's Health Initiative Study, was set up to examine the long-term benefits and risks of combined, continuous HRT, particularly in relation to the development of heart disease, in asymptomatic women aged 50 to 79. While it was originally designed to go on for longer, it was prematurely stopped after five years, due to the findings that the overall level of risk outweighed the level of benefit. The results implied that during one year, for every 10,000 women treated with combined HRT, an extra:[12]

- 7 women would develop heart disease

They also found that:

- 8 women would develop breast cancer

- 8 women would have a stroke

- 18 women would develop a serious blood clot

HRT summary

Given the conflicting stories and research findings it's easy to understand why so many people are confused about HRT. HRT should only be considered after a full discussion of the relative risks and benefits for the individual women. This should take into account age, history, risk factors and personal preferences. So to help my patients come to a decision about HRT, I offer them, and you, the following guidelines:

- If you have no menopausal-related symptoms do not take HRT.

- If you have any of the following contra-indications to HRT you should not take it: a history of thrombosis (blood clots); breast cancer or hormone-dependent cancer; active, recent arterial thromboembolic disease (for example, angina or myocardial infarction); venous thromboembolic disease; pulmonary embolism; current pregnancy; severe active liver disease; undiagnosed breast mass; or uninvestigated abnormal vaginal bleeding.

- HRT should be used with caution if you have fibroids, endometriosis, raised blood pressure, migraine or benign breast disease.

- If you are currently on the combined contraceptive pill, you should not use HRT.

- If you have osteoporosis or are at risk of osteoporosis, do not take HRT to prevent it; use a combination of dietary and lifestyle changes instead.

- If you suffer from very severe menopausal symptoms that do not respond to more natural approaches, or if you have had your ovaries removed, you should consider taking HRT, or preferably bio-identical hormones (see Step 4), for a couple of years.

- If you do decide to take HRT, be clear about why you are taking it, have your health, risk and therapy reviewed annually, review your decision every year and do not remain on it for more than one to three years, as most menopausal symptoms will have resolved by this time, plus you reduce the increased risk of developing breast cancer that is associated with HRT. Most menopausal symptoms will resolve naturally within two to five years.

- Use the lowest dose that controls your symptoms for the shortest period of time.

- Continuous combined HRT should only be used by non-hysterectomised women who are at least 12 months menopausal.

- Peri-menopausal women are best treated with either sequential or cyclical combined HRT.

- Only women who have had a hysterectomy should receive oestrogen-only HRT.

Step 3 ● Address the underlying causes

While I am going to make recommendations to support your health and reduce your menopausal symptoms, I encourage you to fill in the questionnaires in part one, section two, in order to identify possible root causes or contributors to menopausal symptoms. In my experience, the ones to consider are:

- **Adrenal fatigue** – Solution: Part Five (Adrenal Fatigue – page 267), (in my experience adrenal fatigue is common in menopausal women and addressing it can bring about a significant reduction in menopausal symptoms); Secret Two – De-stress and Relax (page 77); Holistic Health Tools – Values-based Goal Setting (page 166) and Mindfulness (page 147)

- **Hormonal imbalance** – Solution: Secret One – Nurture Your Physical Body (Healthy Eating and Supplements – page 49), (while it's assumed that post-menopausal women are deficient in oestrogen, some research suggests that this simply is not true in up to two-thirds of women up the age of 80 as these women get all the oestrogen they need from an aromatase enzyme in body fat and breasts that converts an adrenal hormone, androstenedione, into oestrone, so I measure my patients' hormone levels and encourage you to do the same – see Resources)

- **Excessive weight** – Solution: Secret One – Nurture Your Physical Body (Healthy Eating and Supplements – page 49); Part Five (Weight Loss – page 401); Holistic Health Tools – Emotional Freedom Technique (page 151) and The Work (page 163)

- **Blood-sugar imbalance** – Solution: Secret One – Nurture Your Physical Body (Healthy Eating and Supplements – page 49)

- **Stress** – Solution: Secret Two – De-stress and Relax (page 77); Holistic Health Tools – Emotional Freedom Technique (page 151) and Mindfulness (page 147)

- **Poor diet** – Solution: Secret One – Nurture Your Physical Body (Healthy Eating and Supplements – page 49)

- **Food intolerances** – Solution: Part Five (Food Intolerances – page 344); Holistic Health Tools – Emotional Freedom Technique (page 151)

- **Nutritional deficiencies** – Solution: Secret One – Nurture Your Physical Body (Healthy Eating and Supplements – page 49)

- **Hypothyroidism** – Solution: Part Five (Hypothyroidism – page 356); Holistic Health Tools – Emotional Freedom Technique (page 151) and The Work (page 163)

Step 4 • Start a menopause support supplement programme

When used alongside step three, certain nutritional supplements can help to alleviate many of the symptoms of menopause. My integrated medicine prescription for menopause usually includes a combination of:

- **A multivitamin-mineral supplement** and in addition to this you should take a daily dose of 400IU of vitamin E as this might help to alleviate hot flushes.[13]

- **Vitamin C with bioflavonoids** (1000mg) helps to build collagen, keep skin smooth and elastic, and reduce heavy bleeding, plus bioflavanoids have also been shown in clinical studies to reduce hot flushes.[14]

- **Omega-3, 6 and 9** (taken in capsule or liquid form in a 2:1:1 ratio) to provide the body with hormone-balancing anti-inflammatory essential fatty acids.

- **Calcium** (at least 1000mg to 1500mg), either as calcium citrate, malate or hydroxyapatite, **magnesium** (citrate) (300mg to 600mg), **vitamin D** (400IU), **vitamin K** (2mg to 10mg), **zinc** (30mg) and **boron** (3mg) – use a formula that ensures that you get this from your diet and supplements in order to protect your bones and prevent osteoporosis. Increase the vitamin D to 800IU to 1200IU for the treatment of osteoporosis.

- **Black cohosh** is a North American herb that has been found in several randomised, double-blind, placebo-controlled (the gold standard) trials to reduce the severity, duration and incidence of hot flushes and night sweats. Women taking black cohosh also report improved sleep and energy levels, and a reduction in palpitations and headaches.[15] Another published study compared the efficacy and safety of black cohosh extract to a standard hormone replacement regime (low-dose oestradiol administered by skin patch). The researchers concluded that the two treatments were equally effective in reducing hot flushes, both patient groups experienced improvements in anxiety and depression, and both significantly lowered LDL cholesterol, but only black cohosh raised beneficial HDL cholesterol.[16] The recommended dose is 40mg to 80mg of standardised extract twice daily. Please note that black cohosh is recommended for use for six months and shouldn't be used while on HRT.

- **Fermented soya products** (dose as advised by manufacturers) containing the equivalent amount of active isoflavones found in the average Japanese diet – about 40mg are good for alleviating hot flushes.[17] I tend to use them alongside black cohosh – see Resources.

- **Natural progesterone cream** is used by some integrated medicine doctors to treat the symptoms of menopause. One study found that 83 per cent of women using bio-identical progesterone reported that their menopausal symptoms were either significantly or totally relieved, compared to 19 per cent taking a placebo.[18] Other positive benefits include improving skin health and appearance, reversing osteoporosis, reducing mood swings and improving sleep. This should only be used under medical supervision – see Resources.

Step 5 • Consider other complementary approaches

Many of the women who come to me for advice and support on how to treat menopausal symptoms are also very interested in their own emotional and spiritual growth. Our emotions and spirituality have a very powerful influence on our health and indeed there is good evidence to suggest that hormones (along with the body's nervous system) provide the interface between mind and body. Creating a rich and meaningful spiritual life, while also healing the emotional upsets and traumas from the past, helps to dissolve the blocks within the bodymind that are preventing it from experiencing vitality and well-being. As well as being enlightening, doing this 'inner work' can support your passage into mature womanhood significantly. While there are thousands of books available to you that will help nurture your emotional and spiritual growth, I have provided a list in the Resources section of those that my patients feed back to me as being the most helpful.

Coming off HRT

If you have taken the decision to come off HRT, my advice is to do it slowly. Over a period of two to three months is about right for most people. Stopping HRT suddenly can cause some of the original and new menopausal symptoms to come back with a vengeance. The longer you have been on HRT, the higher the dose and the more severe the original symptoms you were experiencing, the greater the likelihood that this will happen. There are, of course, a lucky few who can stop HRT without any problems.

If you have decided to come off HRT, there are a couple of things you can do to ease the transition:

- Restore optimum function and health of the body by following the advice in Secret One – Nurture Your Physical Body (page 41). If you are thinking of stopping HRT, read through this secret and start implementing those changes. The sooner you do this the better.

- If you do start experiencing any symptoms such as hot flushes, you should avoid known triggers, such as sugar, caffeine, alcohol and hot places, and consider taking black cohosh or a fermented soya product (see pages 250–51). For sleep disturbance you could try valerian – see Resources.

- If you still experience vaginal dryness, you could consider chang-ing the soap and personal hygiene products you use to more gentle ones, using a natural lubricant, taking black cohosh or a fermented soya product, and, if that fails using low dose bio-identical vaginal oestrogen cream or a pessary.

If you are concerned about the possible withdrawal effects of HRT and want to reduce your dose gradually, you should do so under the super-vision of your doctor.

While there is no definitive evidence that these can help you with menopausal symptoms, some patients find the following useful in supporting their programme: acupuncture, homeopathy, massage, spiritual healing, yoga, traditional Chinese medicine and Ayurvedic medicine.

For recommended books see Resources.

Part Five

Integrated medical solutions

In this section I share my own integrated medicine approach to 25 of the most common health challenges that women experience (in addition to those that I have already covered in part four).

Prior to following my advice, if you haven't done so already I encourage you to identify which of the five secrets are relevant to you, because they will provide the foundations for you. As I've said before, most diseases and health problems will improve considerably if you improve your diet, get regular physical activity and restful sleep, manage your stress and learn how to be more self-accepting.

One final word of caution, though: if you are in any doubt about what your diagnosis is, are overwhelmed by your symptoms or confused as to what treatment programme you should follow, that is a clear sign that you need to work alongside an experienced health professional. There is a list of organisations which should be able to help you locate an integrated medicine doctor or health professional in the Resources.

Acne

~

While I don't tend to see many women in clinic with acne, when someone does come in for advice I am very mindful of the amount of distress that they are usually experiencing. Acne can be a very distressing condition to have; it is not only physically uncomfortable and painful, but psychologically it can undermine self-esteem, reduce confidence, and even trigger anxiety and depression.

Acne is basically an inflammatory skin condition, which causes skin eruptions, such as whiteheads and blackheads on the face, back, shoulders and chest. It is, of course, more common in the teenage years (approximately 80 per cent to 95 per cent of adolescents develop some degree of acne),[1] but despite its decline in prevalence with ageing, about 12 per cent of women, compared with 3 per cent of men, will experience acne in middle age.

What causes acne?

As is often the case with skin-related conditions, acne shouldn't be viewed entirely as an external and localised problem of the skin, but as a symptom of a problem that has its origins within the body. In the case of acne, this problem tends to be a combination of a genetically inherited vulnerability to acne, hormonal imbalance (particularly in women) and a reduced ability of the liver to detoxify toxins and deactivate hormones.

One of the reasons that acne is so prevalent in adolescents and can be quite common in premenstrual and peri-menopausal women is because of hormonal imbalances. Acne sufferers show a greater activity of an enzyme called 5-alpha reductase, which converts testosterone into a more potent form, dihydrotestosterone (DHT). The conversion into DHT appears to be responsible (along with testosterone) for stimulating the cells in the hair follicle to produce more keratin (a hard protein that forms hair, skin and nails). What's more, male hormones such as testosterone cause the oil glands to enlarge, produce more oil and cause a blockage of the sebaceous glands. In addition to hormonal imbalances, in adults, acne tends to arise primarily from a combination of intestinal toxicity (usually because of constipation and/or candida) and sub-optimal liver function. Drugs such as the oral contraceptive pill, progesterones and steroids can also cause acne.

What are the risk factors?

The following are risk factors for developing acne:

- Hormonal changes associated with puberty, pregnancy and two to seven days prior to a menstrual period

- Medications such as steroids

- Family history of acne

- Exposure to greasy substances or certain cosmetics

- Excessive sweating

- Friction or pressure on the skin

My integrated medical prescription for acne

In my experience acne responds very well to an integrated medical approach, because it deals with the underlying imbalances that are responsible for acne. Here are my recommendations:

Step 1 • Do you have acne?

Acne is pretty straightforward to diagnose. The most superficial form of acne, acne vulgaris, causes blackheads (dilated skin follicles, with a small dark central plug), whiteheads (red, swollen follicles with or without pustules) and red inflammation around the eruptions. Acne conglobata, a more severe form, is characterised by pustules (tender nodules of pus that discharge to the surface) and cysts (deep, firm, non-discharging nodules).

Step 2 • Consider the medical options

The most common medical treatment for mild to moderate acne are products containing benzoyl peroxide (Brevoxyl and PanOxyl). They are effective at reducing inflammation and can be applied as a gel, cream or face-wash. Benzoyl peroxide works by killing bacteria, unblocking pores and making your skin less oily. About one-third of women using it will experience side-effects such as burning, a tingling feeling and/or dry, red skin.[2]

For moderate severity acne your GP might offer you antibiotics as a cream and/or medication. There's good research to show that both are effective at getting rid of red or inflamed spots, but not great at helping with whiteheads and blackheads.[3] They often have to be used for weeks and months, and in addition to causing nausea and diarrhoea, increase your chance of developing candida (see Dysbiosis, page 334). If you decide to take an antibiotic preparation you should take an acidophilus probiotic before and after completing the antibiotic course.

For very severe acne with cysts, your GP might refer you to a dermatologist (skin specialist) who may prescribe a drug called isotretinoin (Accutane). It's very effective, but it has a lot of severe side-effects, such as headaches, hair loss, very dry skin and severe mood disturbances. I would urge you to use this as an absolute last resort. I have had at least three patients who have suffered terrible side-effects from it. I do not recommend it.

Step 3 • Address the underlying causes

While I am going to make recommendations to treat your acne using a variety of supplements, for lasting resolution of acne I encourage you to fill in the questionnaires in part one, section two, in order to identify possible root causes or contributors. In my experience, the ones to consider are:

- **Poor diet** – Solution: Secret One – Nurture Your Physical Body (Healthy Eating and Supplements – page 49)

- **Constipation** – Solution: Secret One – Nurture Your Physical Body (Healthy Eating and Supplements – page 49); Part Five (Constipation – page 312)

- **Stress** – Solution: Secret Two – De-stress and Relax (page 77); Secret Three – Face and Embrace Your Emotions (page 94); Secret Four – Accept Yourself (page 113); Holistic Health Tools – Emotional Freedom Technique (page 151) and Mindfulness (page 147)

- **Dysbiosis/candida** – Solution: Part Five (Dysbiosis – page 334); Holistic Health Tools – Emotional Freedom Technique (page 151)

- **Food intolerances** – Solution: Part Five (Food Intolerances – page 344); Holistic Health Tools – Emotional Freedom Technique (page 151)

- **Nutritional deficiencies** – Solution: Secret One – Nurture Your Physical Body (Healthy Eating and Supplements – page 49)

- **Polycystic Ovary Syndrome (PCOS)** – Solution: Part Four (PCOS – page 208)

Step 4 • Start an acne supplement programme

When used alongside step three, certain nutritional supplements can help to alleviate many of the symptoms associated with acne. My integrated medicine prescription for acne usually includes a combination of:

- **A multivitamin-mineral supplement**, plus a total daily dose of **vitamin B$_6$**[4] (100mg) if your acne appears to be related to your menstrual cycle, for example your acne flares up prior to your period starting.

- **Vitamin C with bioflavanoids** (1000mg) to reduce inflammation and pain.

- **Fish oil** (3000mg a day) is an anti-inflammatory and can help to soothe inflamed skin.

- **Zinc gluconate**[5] (50mg to 100mg daily for up to two months) has an important role in hormonal balance, tissue regeneration and immune system activity and has been found to be extremely effective for treating acne.

- **MSM** (1000mg three times a day) is a supplement containing sulphur that helps to nourish the skin.

- **Milk thistle and dandelion** (dose as advised by manufacturers) help to support liver detoxification and deactivation of hormones.

- **Agnus castus**, otherwise known as vitex or chasteberry, is the herb most commonly used to support women with acne related to their menstrual cycle.[6] The dose I recommend is 40mg of dried herb or 40 drops of concentrated liquid extract once a day, or 20mg of dried herb twice a day. **Do not take this if you are on hormone treatment.**

- **Colloidal silver** is a natural anti-bacterial agent can be used as an effective alternative to the benzoyl peroxide products that I mentioned earlier. Another alternative is **tea tree oil**,[7] which has been shown to lower the bacteria and inflammation associated with acne as effectively as benzoyl peroxide. When using tea tree oil, make sure it is diluted – adding a few drops to aloe vera gel works well.

- **Acidophilus probiotic** to ensure that there are sufficient numbers of 'friendly' bacteria in the gut is important as this helps to prevent deactivated oestrogen that has been excreted in the gut to be activated again by certain 'unfriendly' bacteria.

Step 5 • Consider other complementary approaches

While there is no definitive evidence that these can help you with acne, some patients find the following useful in supporting their programme: colon hydrotherapy, reflexology, homeopathy, spiritual healing, traditional Chinese medicine and Ayurvedic medicine.

For recommended books see Resources.

Addictions

An addiction is the compulsive, continuing use of any substance, activity or behaviour that is beyond your control and affects your life for the worse. Any behaviour that removes one from reality, responsibility or relationships places you at risk of addictions. While most people tend to think of addictions relating to alcohol and drugs, addictions can be to pretty much anything, including shopping, compulsive spending, alcohol, food, gambling, drugs, prescription medication, sex, work and even love and relationships.

What causes addictions?

There are many different perspectives on why addictions come about and how best to treat them. One camp believes that addictions, such as alcoholism, are progressive, genetically based diseases, which are rooted in painful emotional and psychological problems, which, over time, through therapy, abstinence and support groups, need to be identified and addressed. The focus is then on learning to live a healthy and fulfilling life with the disease of addiction. Another camp takes the nutritional approach and believes that addictions are brain- and body-based diseases with their roots in your genetic make-up, and that full and sustained recovery can be brought about through nutritional rehabilitation and biochemical repair. Another camp again says that addictions are the consequence of not living a healthy and fulfilling life, and not having the skills and tools to regulate emotions, manage stress and build on innate strengths and talents. My own take on it is that addictions are influenced by all of these different factors. I view addictions as a desperate, but resourceful way of attempting to control, escape and sedate the emotional pain relating to childhood stresses and a genetically-inherited imbalance of the brain's neurotransmission system.

What are the risk factors?

A past history of trauma, abuse, mental illness, ongoing stress, low self-acceptance, being brought up in a less-than-nurturing environment and codependency all increase the likelihood of that vulnerability triggering an addiction.

My integrated medical prescription for addictions

Recovering from addictions can be very challenging work. In my experience the real key to successful recovery is to build a team of people – friends and professionals – who are supportive of you. While there are many different approaches to addiction treatment, I find that an integrated approach – one that addresses the psychological, emotional, social, spiritual and biological and nutritional elements of addiction – to be the key. In the Resources section I have provided details of addiction treatment centres and also where to find health professionals who specialise in helping people with addictions.

Step 1 • Do you have addictions?

One of the challenges of addiction is the fact that denial is built into the disease, so more often than not the person with the addiction will be the last person in the world to see and acknowledge that they have an addiction. If you haven't already I encourage you to fill in the addictions questionnaire in part one, chapter two.

Addictions might be a possibility if any of the following apply to you:

- You keep certain activities and experiences a secret

- You feel that a certain substance or activity has a strong hold over you

- People are afraid of you or tip-toe around you

- When you stop a certain activity, you start to get withdrawal effects, you get irritable or you switch to another means of managing your emotions

- You have a degree of shame around certain things you do

- People around you tell you that they are concerned that you have an addiction and you react with anger

- You start covering up, lying or being deceitful around certain activities

- You are gradually withdrawing from life and certain experiences – your life is becoming increasingly imbalanced

- You need more and more of a substance – food, sex, alcohol, drugs, gambling – in order to prevent yourself feeling low

- You experience mood swings, switching between Jekyll and Hyde

- You are experiencing increasing unmanageability in your life – arguments, financial problems, broken relationships, ill health

- You are becoming more detached and self-centred

Another way to work out whether you have addictive tendencies is to fill in an in-depth questionnaire that was developed by the UK-based PROMIS Recovery Centre – see Resources for details. I find it a very useful way of screening my patients for addictive tendencies. If you do have addictive tendencies, I encourage you to work with a practitioner who has experience in treating addictions.

Step 2 • Consider the medical options

Admitting to yourself and others that you have an addiction, and that you need help, is a significant step forward in your recovery programme. As to what you do next, it really depends on what addictive tendencies are present, the severity of the situation, your existing physical, emotional and psychological level of health, the financial resources you have available, your life circumstances, the impact on your family and the immediate risk of your problems.

For example, the needs of a woman addicted to relationships, who is living a fully functional life, is very different to someone with a severe eating disorder and addiction to exercise and work. Some people will need to go into a residential treatment programme for intensive specialist care. This is usually for a minimum of one month, but it can be up to 12 months in some cases. Most addiction treatment programmes offer a service in which they will assess your suitability. They might, for example, advise you to take part in an outpatient treatment programme. See Resources for recommended addiction treatment programmes and books.

Step 3 • Address the underlying causes

In my experience, addressing the biochemical, nutritional, emotional and psychological factors that led to and are maintaining the addiction process is the key to recovery, but the order in which you address them, how you address them and when you address them really does depend on you. It is for this reason that I strongly encourage you to work with a team of health professionals. In addition to this, I encourage you to fill in the questionnaires in part one, section two, so as to help identify possible root causes or contributors to your addiction. In my experience, the ones to consider are:

- **Codependency** – Solution: Secret Three – Face and Embrace Your Emotions (page 94); Secret Four – Accept Yourself (page 113); Secret Five – Develop and Deepen Your Relationships (page 127); Part Five (Codependency – page 307)

- **Trauma** – Solution: Secret Three – Face and Embrace Your Emotions (page 94); Holistic Health Tools – Emotional Freedom Technique (page 151), EmoTrance (page 158) and Mindfulness (page 147)

- **Blood-sugar imbalance** – Solution: Secret One – Nurture Your Physical Body (Healthy Eating and Supplements – page 49)

- **Stress** – Solution: Secret Two – De-stress and Relax (page 77); Holistic Health Tools – Emotional Freedom Technique (page 151) and Mindfulness (page 147)

- **Poor diet** – Solution: Secret One – Nurture Your Physical Body (Healthy Eating and Supplements – page 49)

- **Nutritional deficiencies** – Solution: Secret One – Nurture Your Physical Body (Healthy Eating and Supplements – page 49)

- **Sleep deprivation** – Solution: Secret One – Nurture Your Physical Body (Rest and Sleep – page 45); Holistic Health Tools – Emotional Freedom Technique (page 151) and Mindfulness (page 147)

- **Adrenal fatigue** – Solution: Part Five (Adrenal Fatigue – page 267); Secret Two – De-stress and Relax (page 77); Holistic Health Tools – Values-based Goal Setting (page 166) and Mindfulness (page 147)

- **Depression** – Solution: Part Five (Depression – page 316); Holistic Health Tools – Mindfulness (page 147), Values-based Goal Setting (page 166) and The Work (page 163)

- **Food intolerances** – Solution: Part Five (Food Intolerances – page 344); Holistic Health Tools – Emotional Freedom Technique (page 151)

- **Low self-acceptance** – Solution: Secret Four – Accept Yourself (page 113); Secret Three – Face and Embrace Your Emotions (page 94); Secret Five – Develop and Deepen Your Relationships (page 127); Holistic Health Tools – Mindfulness (page 147), Emotional Freedom Technique (page 151) and Values-based Goal Setting (page 166)

Step 4 • Start an addiction recovery supplement programme

When used alongside step three, certain nutritional supplements can help to support you in your recovery. My integrated medicine prescription for addictions usually includes a combination of:

- **A multivitamin-mineral supplement** – taking this will help treat any nutritional deficiencies that are present, plus when combined with a healthy diet may help you to stay off alcohol.[1]

- **Vitamin C with bioflavanoids** (1000mg) to reduce inflammation and support the healing and repair of the body.

- **GLA** (360mg a day), which can be found in evening primrose oil or starflower oil, was found to significantly improve the liver function of people recovering from alcohol addiction.[2]

- **Chromium polynicotinate**[3] (800mcg) and **L-glutamine**[4] (5g daily) powder may help to alleviate sugar and carbohydrate cravings.

- **L-tyrosine** (500mg to 1000mg three times daily between meals) is an amino acid that, if you are addicted to coffee, may help to ease the process of coming off it.

- **Taurine** (3g a day) is an amino acid that can help to reduce alcohol cravings.

- **Zinc**[5] (50mg a day) helps with anorexia and bulimia.

- **5-HTP**[6] (100mg twice daily) can help alleviate low mood and depression that occurs in many addictions.

- **Calcium citrate** (1000mg) and **magnesium citrate** (500mg) can help alleviate the cramps associated with opiate withdrawal.

- **L-theanine**[7] (100mg to 200mg a day), a green tea extract, can help to alleviate underlying anxiety and worry.

- **Alkalising minerals** my help to alkalise the body, thus enabling it to recover more quickly from withdrawal.

- **Milk thistle and dandelion**[8] are herbs which work well in combination to help support optimum liver function, which is often compromised in substance addictions.

Step 5 • Consider other complementary approaches

Support groups such as Alcoholics Anonymous, Narcotics Anonymous, Overeaters Anonymous, Marijuana Anonymous, Codependents Anonymous and Emotions Anonymous are based on the famous 12-step programme. The 12 steps provide a set of guiding principles for recovery from addictive, compulsive, or other behavioral problems. These principles include admitting that one cannot control one's addiction or compulsion; recognising a greater power that can give strength; examining past errors with the help of a sponsor (experienced member); making amends for these errors; learning to live a new life with a new code of behaviour; and helping others who suffer from the same addictions or compulsions. Many people who attend these groups find them to be an important source of support, learning, insight and inspiration. They are, however, not treatment-based programmes and are therefore best used alongside the other steps that I share with you here.

In addition to support groups, you might also want to consider supporting your programme with: hypnotherapy, breathwork, core energetics, ear acupuncture, homeopathy, spiritual healing, yoga, traditional Chinese medicine and Ayurvedic medicine. If you are a smoker I recommend a specialised approach to hypnotherapy called CBT hypnotherapy. Researchers at the University of Minnesota found that women who gave up smoking before ovulation (about day 14 of your menstrual cycle) were half as likely to remain smoke-free as those who gave up after ovulation, but before the start of the next period.[9]

For recommended books and websites see Resources.

Adrenal fatigue

~

If you are tired on waking up in the morning, chronically stressed out or suffer from any long-standing health problem, then you might be experiencing adrenal fatigue. The adrenals are two small pyramid-shaped glands sitting on top of your kidneys. Despite their small size, they are vitally important to your health and wellbeing – they help your body respond to stress, maintain the body's energy, regulate the immune system and keep your blood-sugar, fluid levels and blood pressure within a healthy range. Healthy adrenal glands secrete very precise amounts of steroid hormones. However, too much ongoing physical, emotional, environmental and/or psychological stress can cause an imbalance in the function of the adrenals, and the result is adrenal fatigue, also known as adrenal burnout syndrome. This is a common condition that arises when the adrenal glands are no longer able to meet the demands placed upon them.

What causes adrenal fatigue?

Essentially, anything that causes prolonged physical, emotional and/or psychological stress can cause adrenal fatigue. This includes:

- Nutritional deficiencies

- Work pressure

- Relationship difficulties

- Chronic repressed emotions

- Emotional trauma

- Chronic illness, infection, surgery, inflammation or pain

- Grief, loss, financial difficulties

- Depression and anxiety

- Allergies and intolerances

- Toxicity

- Lack of quality sleep

- Noise pollution

- Electromagnetic pollution

My integrated medical prescription for adrenal fatigue

Adrenal fatigue isn't a medically recognised phenomenon, so it's highly unlikely that your doctor will know of it or be able to guide you in addressing it. Whenever a patient shares a life history that includes prolonged periods of stress, I always have the possibility of adrenal fatigue in the back of my mind, because it represents a significant barrier to physical health and emotional wellbeing. The key to recovery is to address the underlying sources of stress, learn stress reduction techniques and provide the body with what it needs so that it can recuperate and regenerate. Also bear in mind that recovering from adrenal fatigue does not, regrettably, happen overnight, and depending on your health and degree of adrenal fatigue it can take anywhere from six months to two years – it requires a real commitment!

Step 1 • Do you have adrenal fatigue?

If you haven't already, I encourage you to fill in the adrenal fatigue questionnaire in part one, section two. In addition to this, and particularly if you score more than ten, I encourage you to arrange an adrenal stress index (ASI) saliva test. This measures levels of two adrenal hormones – DHEA and cortisol – and it will give a pretty accurate indicator of the severity of your adrenal fatigue. See Resources for details.

Step 2 • Consider the medical options

Unfortunately Western medicine doesn't recognise adrenal fatigue as a problem, so your GP is unlikely to know what you are talking about if you go to discuss it with them.

Step 3 • Address the underlying causes

While I am going to make recommendations to increase your energy levels using nutritional supplementation, for lasting resolution of adrenal fatigue symptoms, I encourage you to fill in the questionnaires in part one, section two, in order to identify possible root causes or contributors. In my experience, the ones to consider are:

- **Stress** – Solution: Secret Two – De-stress and Relax (page 77); Holistic Health Tools – Emotional Freedom Technique (page 151) and Mindfulness (page 147)

- **Blood-sugar imbalance** – Solution: Secret One – Nurture Your Physical Body (Healthy Eating and Supplements – page 49)

- **Emotional repression** – Solution: Secret Three – Face and Embrace Your Emotions (page 94); Holistic Health Tools – EmoTrance (page 158) and Mindfulness (page 147)

- **Poor diet** – Solution: Secret One – Nurture Your Physical Body (Healthy Eating and Supplements – page 49)

- **Relationship problems/isolation** – Solution: Secret Five – Develop and Deepen Your Relationships (page 127); Holistic Health Tools –

Mindfulness (page 147), EmoTrance (page 158) and The Work (page 163)

- **Nutritional deficiencies** – Solution: Secret One – Nurture Your Physical Body (Healthy Eating and Supplements – page 49)

- **Hypothyroidism** – Solution: Part Five (Hypothyroidism – page 356), (hypothyroidism can occur alongside adrenal fatigue and should not be missed); Holistic Health Tools – Emotional Freedom Technique (page 151) and The Work (page 163)

- **Depression** – Solution: Part Five (Depression – page 316), (depression is a common cause of low energy levels); Holistic Health Tools – Mindfulness (page 147), Values-based Goal Setting (page 166) and The Work (page 163)

- **Food intolerances** – Solution: Part Five (Food Intolerances – page 344); Holistic Health Tools – Emotional Freedom Technique (page 151)

- **Trauma** – Solution: Secret Three – Face and Embrace Your Emotions (page 94); Holistic Health Tools – Emotional Freedom Technique (page 151), EmoTrance (page 158) and Mindfulness (page 147)

- **Environmental toxicity** – Solution: Secret One – Nurture Your Physical Body (Healthy Environment and Sunlight – page 70)

- **Lack of physical activity** – Solution: Secret One – Nurture Your Physical Body (Physical Activity and Touch – page 67); Holistic Health Tools – Emotional Freedom Technique (page 151) and Values-based Goal Setting (page 166)

Step 4 • Start an adrenal support supplement programme

When used alongside step three, certain nutritional supplements can help to support the rejuvenation of the adrenal glands. My integrated medicine prescription for adrenal fatigue usually includes a combination of:

- **A multivitamin-mineral supplement**, plus **vitamin B$_5$** (500mg) to support adrenal health and replace nutrients depleted by stress and a stressful lifestyle.

- **Vitamin C with bioflavanoids** (3000mg a day) to support adrenal health.

- **Omega-3, 6 and 9** (taken in capsule or liquid form in a 2:1:1 ratio) to provide the body with health-promoting essential fatty acids.

- **Rhodiola[1] and Ashwagandha[2]** (dose as advised by manufacturers) is my preferred adrenal support formula, as it contains two adaptogenic herbs – rhodiola, also called Arctic root, and ashwagandha, or Indian ginseng. Adaptogenic means it helps the body to restore balance, fight fatigue and boost energy levels.

- **Ginseng** (dose as advised by manufacturers) is another adaptogen that has been used for thousands of years in traditional Chinese medicine as a tonic to help the body reach its full potential for health. There are a few different types of ginseng, but the ones most useful for helping recharge the adrenals are Siberian[3] and American ginseng.[4]

Step 5 • Consider other complementary approaches

While there is no definitive evidence that these can help you with your adrenal fatigue, some patients find the following useful in supporting their programme: acupuncture, homeopathy, massage, spiritual healing, yoga, traditional Chinese medicine and Ayurvedic medicine.

For recommended books see Resources.

Anxiety and panic disorders

Anxiety is a normal response to stress or danger. It increases our ability to focus, helps us prepare for action and can improve our performance. A certain amount of anxiety, on occasions and when appropriate, is very much part of being human. However, when anxiety is experienced intensely and/or when it interferes with your ability to carry out tasks and live life fully, then it becomes a problem.

Many of my female patients experience low-grade anxiety, a constant background worrying or a need to control, but few recognise it as anxiety, mainly because they have been living that way for many years. It's usually when the anxiety becomes unbearable, because of a significant stress or hormonal shift (such as entering the peri-menopause) that my patients then seek help. Interestingly, some of the most apparently 'together, dynamic and high achieving' women and men that I meet have chronic anxiety, usually dating back to childhood. Having an anxious parent or parents, experiencing abuse, trauma or neglect as a child, being brought up in an environment where you don't feel safe and having a temperament in which you are predisposed to worrying can all lead to the experience of anxiety. There are a number of different types of anxiety, all of which can overlap, including:

Generalised anxiety disorder – this is characterised by anxiety symptoms that are present much of the time and not related to any particular situations. It's experienced as an undercurrent of worry, and is often experienced by people with depression and phobias. This affects about 10 per cent of the population, two-thirds of whom are women.[1]

Panic disorder – this is marked by severe, often unpredictable, panic attacks. Symptoms are extreme and include the feeling of dying, excessive hyperventilation and the fear of losing control or going mad.

Phobic disorder – a phobia is a fear that is out of proportion to the situation that causes it and cannot be explained away. The person typically avoids the feared situation, since this helps to reduce the anxiety.

Post-traumatic stress disorder (PTSD) – this can start at any time after a traumatic incident in which you perceived yourself to be in danger, your life was being threatened or where you saw other people dying or being injured. Women are vulnerable to PTSD following childhood abuse, including sexual abuse, rape and traumatic childbirth. Symptoms include flashbacks and nightmares, intrusive thoughts and memories, insomnia, anger, numbness, depression, avoidant behaviour and being hypervigilant (see the section on trauma in Secret Three – Face and Embrace Your Emotions, page 94).

Obsessive compulsive disorder (OCD) – while 14 per cent of the population experience minor obsessive symptoms, about 0.1 per cent of the population actually has OCD. Symptoms of OCD include obsessive thoughts, which are often unpleasant, disturbing and, despite the person's best efforts, can't be stopped, which in itself adds to the stress. The obsessive thoughts can lead to compulsive, repetitive actions, for example repeated cleaning of the hands or checking that the door is locked. Although the action is not normally pleasurable, it reduces the experience of inner tension and decreases the obsessive thinking.

What are the risk factors?

The following are recognised as factors that increase the chances of you experiencing anxiety:

- Childhood trauma or abuse – physical, sexual, emotional, intellectual or spiritual

- Stress – either acute or chronic

- Temperament – some people are born with a tendency to worry more and experience more anxiety

- Genetics – there might be a genetically inherited vulnerability to anxiety

My integrated medical prescription for anxiety

In my experience, treating anxiety needs to go beyond just reducing the symptoms of anxiety. Of those patients who come to me with anxiety-related disorders, those that have experienced either complete or significant relief have made some significant changes, not only to the way they relate to themselves, their thoughts and their feelings, but they have also learnt meditation, simplified their lives and, in some cases, made major changes to the way in which they live their lives. Anxiety, like most health challenges, is an invitation to get connected to what truly matters.

Step 1 • Are you experiencing anxiety?

Your anxiety might well be obvious. However, some patients are so used to living with their symptoms that they don't recognise them as evidence of anxiety. Very much a condition affecting body and mind, anxiety has physical and emotional components, including:

Physical symptoms

- Butterflies in the stomach

- Sweating

- Tremor

- Diarrhoea

- Dry mouth

- Racing heart or palpitations

- Tightness or pain in chest

- Shortness of breath

- Abdominal discomfort

- Finding it hard to 'catch your breath'

- Dizziness

- Urge to pass urine

- Difficulty swallowing

Psychological symptoms

- Inner tension

- Insomnia

- Feeling worried or uneasy all the time

- Feeling tired

- Being irritable, agitated or quick to anger

- An inability to concentrate

- A fear that you are going 'mad'

- Feeling unreal and not in control of your actions (depersonalisation) or detached from your surroundings (derealisation)

Another symptom of anxiety is hyperventilation syndrome, which occurs when a person starts to breathe rapidly and shallowly. This in turn leads to various symptoms, such as tingling in the fingers and around the mouth, lightheadedness and possibly fainting. This pattern of breathing – without fully breathing out – also leads to a feeling of chest tightness. While extremely scary and stressful, hyperventilation syndrome is ultimately harmless, either settling down of its own accord or disappearing when you breathe into a paper bag.

If you can identify with any of these symptoms you should go to your GP to have your diagnosis confirmed. It is important to have various medical conditions also excluded, particularly if you suddenly develop anxiety out of the blue and are younger than 18 or older than 35. These other conditions include: hyperthyroidism, hypoparathy-roidism, hypoglycaemia, neurological illness, addictions and toxicity, as well as medication side-effects or withdrawal from medications, alcohol, stimulants such as cocaine and amphetamines, nicotine and caffeine.

Step 2 • Consider the medical options

Once the diagnosis of anxiety disorder has been made, your doctor will probably offer you medication.

For immediate treatment of your anxiety, you may be offered:

- **Benzodiazepines** – these are drugs to help you relax and feel less worried; brand names include Valium, Xanax and Ativan. However, you should only use this drug for two to four weeks. Some of the side-effects include feeling dizzy, making your memory worse, feeling drowsy or getting addicted to these drugs. About one-third of people taking benzodiazepines will experience the rapid return of their anxiety after stopping them.[2] In some cases this anxiety will be even worse than before. Because of their side-effects I really encourage you to stay well clear of benzodi-azepines. I have come across far too many women who have been taking them for years and cannot get off them. Follow my other recommendations instead.

- **Antihistamines** – these drugs help you relax and sleep.

- **Support and advice about helping yourself** – for example, your GP may put you in touch with a local support group where you can meet and talk to other people with anxiety disorder.

For longer-term treatment of your anxiety, you may be offered:

- **Psychological therapy** – for example, cognitive behaviour therapy. You'll usually have between 16 and 20 hours of therapy spread over 10 to 20 weeks.

- **Antidepressants** – for example, you may be prescribed a selective serotonin reuptake inhibitor (SSRI) such as paroxetine (Seroxat) or sertraline (Lustral), which help to increase levels of the good-mood brain chemical serotonin or, if that doesn't work, a serotonin and noradrenaline reuptake inhibitor (SNRI) such as venlafaxine (Efexor). SNRIs increase levels of two chemicals in the brain called serotonin and noradrenaline. The latter helps increase motivation. Antidepressants have been found to help about 50 per cent of the people who take them but you should give them at least 3 weeks to work.[3] If your symptoms haven't improved after 12 weeks of taking an antidepressant your doctor may prescribe a different one. If a drug is helping, you'll usually need to carry on taking it for at least six months. I rarely recommend antidepressants because I've found that an integrated medicine approach that addresses the underlying causes of anxiety works much better.

Step 3 • Address the underlying causes

While I am going to make recommendations to treat your anxiety symptoms using a variety of supplements, for lasting recovery from anxiety I encourage you to fill in the questionnaires in part one, section two, in order to identify possible root causes or contributors. In my experience, the ones to consider are:

- **Stress** – Solution: Secret Two – De-stress and Relax (page 77); Holistic Health Tools – Emotional Freedom Technique (page 151) and Mindfulness (page 147)

- **Sleep deprivation** – Solution: Secret One – Nurture Your Physical Body (Rest and Sleep – page 45)

- **Adrenal fatigue** – Solution: Part Five (Adrenal Fatigue – page 267); Secret Two – De-stress and Relax (page 77); Holistic Health Tools – Values-based Goal Setting (page 166) and Mindfulness (page 147)

- **Blood-sugar imbalance** – Solution: Secret One – Nurture Your Physical Body (Healthy Eating and Supplements – page 49)

- **Poor diet** – Solution: Secret One – Nurture Your Physical Body (Healthy Eating and Supplements – page 49)

- **Depression** – Solution: Part Five (Depression – page 316); Holistic Health Tools – Mindfulness (page 147), Values-based Goal Setting (page 166) and The Work (page 163)

- **Food intolerances** – Solution: Part Five (Food Intolerances – page 344); Holistic Health Tools – Emotional Freedom Technique (page 151)

- **Nutritional deficiencies** – Solution: Secret One – Nurture Your Physical Body (Healthy Eating and Supplements – page 49)

- **Environmental toxicity** – Solution: Secret One – Nurture Your Physical Body (Healthy Environment and Sunlight – page 70).

- **Addictions (nicotine, sugar, drugs and alcohol)** – Solution: Part Five (Addictions – page 260); Secret Four – Accept Yourself (page 113); Secret Three – Face and Embrace Your Emotions (page 94); Secret Five – Develop and Deepen Your Relationships (page 127); Holistic Health Tools – Mindfulness (page 147), Emotional Freedom Technique (page 151) and Values-based Goal Setting (page 166)

- **Trauma** – Solution: Secret Three – Face and Embrace Your Emotions (page 94); Holistic Health Tools – Emotional Freedom Technique (page 151), EmoTrance (page 158) and Mindfulness (page 147)

- **Low self-acceptance** – Solution: Secret Four – Accept Yourself (page 113); Secret Three – Face and Embrace Your Emotions (page 94); Secret Five – Develop and Deepen Your Relationships (page 127); Holistic Health Tools – Mindfulness (page 147), Emotional Freedom Technique (page 151) and Values-based Goal Setting (page 166)

Step 4 • Start an anxiety recovery supplement programme

When used alongside step three, certain nutritional supplements can help to alleviate many of the symptoms of anxiety. My integrated medicine prescription for anxiety usually includes a combination of:

- **A multivitamin-mineral supplement** – one study found that people taking a multivitamin-mineral supplement for a 28-day period experienced a significant reduction in anxiety and stress.[4]

- **Vitamin C with bioflavanoids** (1000mg) to support optimum health.

- **Fish oil**[5] (3000mg a day) might help to reduce anxiety levels.

- **Magnesium citrate**[6] (200mg twice daily or 400mg at night-time) may help to enhance stress resilience and reduce anxiety levels.

- **Valerian**[7] (300mg two to three times daily) – although this herb is traditionally used for insomnia, there are some studies that indicate it might help keep you calm in stressful situations.

- **L-theanine**[8] (100mg to 300mg a day) is an amino acid that works by increasing levels of a chemical in the brain called GABA, which in turn triggers relaxation.

- **Passion flower**[9] (250mg two to three times daily) has traditionally been used to calm the mind by increasing the levels of the brain neurotransmitter GABA.

Step 5 • Consider other complementary approaches

Not all of my patients want to deal with the underlying issues of their anxiety so for these people I usually recommend a medical device called the AlphaStim SCS. In a number of clinical trials it's been shown to significantly relieve the symptoms of depression, anxiety and insomnia in the majority of users and most of my patients have benefited considerably from using it.

If you want to learn how to manage your thinking and emotions more effectively you might want to choose human givens therapy, cognitive behavioural therapy, solution-focused brief therapy or acceptance and commitment therapy. I am a big fan of the latter, because it teaches people how to transform their relationship to their thoughts and feelings, while also committing to doing whatever is within their power to create a rich and meaningful life. Other therapies to consider include hypnotherapy, aromatherapy, spiritual healing, breathwork, massage, acupuncture, flower essences, life coaching and spiritual counselling. See Resources for details of all these complementary approaches.

Cancer

Cancer is one of the most feared and potentially devastating illnesses and it will affect one in three women. Breast cancer is by far the most common form, accounting for about one-third of cancer cases in women. After that bowel and lung cancer are the most common. While cancer treatment is beyond the scope of this book, integrated medicine has a significant role to play in supporting women who are going through cancer treatment.

What causes cancer?

The process by which cancer occurs is related to the failure of your body to repair damage to the DNA in its cells. Your DNA contains a set of instructions for your cells, telling them how to grow and divide. Cancer develops when any one of the following three processes happens:

- **Something causes a genetic mutation** – this might be inherited or caused by other factors such as hormones, viruses, chronic inflammation, ultraviolet (UV) light from the sun or cancer-causing chemicals (carcinogens) in your environment.

- **Something promotes rapid cell growth** – again this could be inherited or due to external factors.

- **Something causes the cancer to progress and spread** – again, this could be inherited or due to external factors.

What are the risk factors?

There are numerous factors and influences which can give rise to cancer, including: viruses and other infections, an unhealthy diet (high in sugar, processed foods and animal products, low in fruits, vegetables and fibre), smoking, the excessive consumption of alcohol, being overweight or obese, chronic inflammation, a sedentary lifestyle, hormone replacement therapy, the oestrogen contraceptive pill, radiation, genetic vulnerability (about 10 per cent of cancers are thought to be inherited), excessive exposure to UV light, geopathic stress (disruption or distortion of the earth's natural electromagnetic field), sick building syndrome, exposure to cancer-causing chemicals, immune system suppression and emotional trauma. Age is also a factor as the majority of people with cancer are aged 55 and over (although it can, of course, occur at any age). By the time the cancer is detected it's possible that up to one billion cancer cells are present and that the original cancer has been growing for up to ten years.

My integrated medical prescription for cancer

Upon receiving a diagnosis such as cancer, my advice is always to get a second opinion, so that you are absolutely confident and clear about what the diagnosis is. It is accepted practice to ask for a second opinion, so don't worry about upsetting your doctor! You can either ask them for a recommendation or you can do your own research and request that your doctor sends your medical notes to a doctor that you indentify. Either way, I really recommend that you do this.

Once that is done, the next step is to create a team of trusted people and professionals who will guide, support and encourage you during your healing journey. Next you need to become aware of all the options available to you – this means conventional, alternative and complementary. Each option needs to be explained, by a health-care professional who knows what they are talking about, and the pros and cons of each approach need to be shared with you.

With that information, your own intuition and the guidance of your support team you can create a holistic healthcare programme – one that honours your own needs, desires, expectations, past experiences, finances and biology, and achieves the greatest likelihood of success (however you define that), with the minimum of short- and long-term consequences. You will know that you have found the right programme and the right support team for you because you will feel empowered and hopeful.

While I do not have space in this book to go into detail about cancer, I would still like to share the advice that I give those of my patients who have been diagnosed with cancer and are looking for an integrated medical approach.

Step 1 • Do you have cancer?

If you are reading this it probably already means that you have a diagnosis. However, the following are just some of the signs and symptoms of cancer that are often missed or ignored.

Warning signs that would warrant an investigation to exclude cancer include a persistent cough, a change in appearance of a wart or mole, blood in the urine without any pain, unusual or persistent fatigue, an ulcer or sore that fails to heal, a persistent lump in the body, a change in bowel or bladder functioning, persistent abdominal pain, excessive bruising, persistent nose bleeds or low-grade fever. In a significant proportion of these cases the presence of these symptoms will not indicate cancer, but if you have any of them and are at all concerned you should see your GP.

Step 2 • What are the medical options?

As I've said, I'm unable to go into detail here, but the main orthodox medical approaches to cancer treatment are outlined below.

- **Chemotherapy** uses drugs to kill cancer cells.

- **Surgery** is used to remove the cancer or as much of the cancer as possible. This might be combined with chemotherapy and radiation therapy.

- **Radiation therapy** uses high-powered energy beams to kill cancer cells. Radiation treatment can come from a machine outside your body (external beam radiation) or it can be placed inside your body (brachytherapy).

- **Biological therapy** uses your body's immune system to fight cancer.

- **Hormone therapy** is used when certain cancers such as breast cancer are fuelled by the presence of hormones.

- **Targeted drug therapy** is designed to focus on specific abnormalities within cancer cells that allow them to survive.

Step 3 • Address the underlying barriers to cancer recovery

If you have cancer I would urge you to work with an integrated medical doctor who is experienced in treating cancer, as your programme will need to be tailored to you. In addition to this I encourage you to fill in the questionnaires in part one, section two, to help identify possible root causes, contributors and barriers to recovery from cancer. In my experience, the ones to consider are:

- **Poor diet** – Solution: Secret One – Nurture Your Physical Body (Healthy Eating and Supplements – page 49)

- **Environmental toxicity** – Solution: Secret One – Nurture Your Physical Body (Healthy Environment and Sunlight – page 70)

- **Parasites/viruses/candida** – Solution: Part Five (Dysbiosis – page 334); Holistic Health Tools – Emotional Freedom Technique (page 151)

- **Nutritional deficiencies** – Solution: Secret One – Nurture Your Physical Body (Healthy Eating and Supplements – page 49)

- **Excessive weight** – Solution: Secret One – Nurture Your Physical Body (Healthy Eating and Supplements – page 49); Part Five (Weight Loss – page 401); Holistic Health Tools – Emotional Freedom Technique (page 151) and The Work (page 163)

- **Stress** – Solution: Secret Two – De-stress and Relax (page 77); Holistic Health Tools – Emotional Freedom Technique (page 151) and Mindfulness (page 147)

- **Trauma** – Solution: Secret Three – Face and Embrace Your Emotions (page 94); Holistic Health Tools – Emotional Freedom Technique (page 151), EmoTrance (page 158) and Mindfulness (page 147)

- **Lack of physical activity** – Solution: Secret One – Nurture Your Physical Body (Physical Activity and Touch – page 67); Holistic Health Tools – Emotional Freedom Technique (page 151) and Values-based Goal Setting (page 166)

- **Weakened immune system** – Solution: Secret One – Nurture Your Physical Body (page 41); Secret Two – De-Stress and Relax (page 77); Holistic Health Tools – Emotional Freedom Technique (page 151) and Mindfulness (page 147)

Step 4 • Start a cancer support supplement programme

When used alongside step three and Western medicine approaches, certain nutritional supplements can help some of the symptoms of cancer and cancer treatment, as well as support your recovery from cancer. My integrated medicine prescription for cancer usually includes a combination of:

- **A multivitamin-mineral supplement** to provide your body with optimum levels of nutrients.

- **Vitamin C with bioflavanoids** (1000mg) to support healing and recovery.

- **Omega-3, 6 and 9** (taken in capsule or liquid form in a 2:1:1 ratio) to provide the body with hormone-balancing anti-inflammatory essential fatty acids.

- **Indole-3-Carbinol** (300mg daily), which can help the liver to detoxify excess oestrogen.[1] This is useful for breast cancer.

- **Acidophilus probiotic** to ensure that there are sufficient numbers of 'friendly' bacteria in the gut to help prevent deactivated oestrogen that has been excreted in the gut to be activated again by certain 'unfriendly' bacteria.

- **Ginger tea and Nux vomica**, the homeopathic remedy, taken regularly, can help with nausea.

- **A mix of organic mushroom tinctures**[2] or **Biobran MGN-3**,[3] a natural compound made from breaking down rice bran with enzymes from the shiitake mushroom, can both help boost a weakend immune system by activating the body's natural killer cells. See Resources.

- **Siberian ginseng**[4] (dose as advised by manufacturers) is good for fatigue and tiredness.

- **Hydrazine sulphate**,[5] which needs to be prescribed by a doctor, is an effective option for severe weight loss (cachexia).

- **Coriolus versicolor**[6] (1000mg three times a day), a mushroom extract which stimulates the immune system, and **astralagus**[7] (500mg three times daily) can help reduce the side-effects of chemotherapy. The latter should not be taken if you have a fever or acute infection.

- **Beta 1,3 glucan**[8] (10mg to 30mg daily) can help reduce the side-effects of radiation. You can also use **coriolus versicolor** as well.

Before taking any of these supplements you should check with your primary health professional.

Step 5 • Consider other complementary approaches

The majority of women with cancer, especially breast cancer, will use one or more complementary therapy approaches to support their treatment. The following are just a handful of those that my patients find useful, not just in terms of recovering from cancer, but to improve general health, vitality and mood: acupuncture, homeopathy, massage, spiritual healing, guided imagery, hypnotherapy, Brandon Bay's The Journey, yoga, reflexology, aromatherapy, traditional Chinese medicine and Ayurvedic medicine.

For recommended websites and books see Resources.

Cardiovascular disease

Cardiovascular disease is the number one cause of death in women. It refers to disease affecting the heart and circulatory system, and includes coronary heart disease (angina, heart attacks) and strokes. While traditionally regarded as being something that affects men, in Europe coronary heart disease alone kills 55 per cent of women, compared with only 43 per cent of men.[1] Research shows that most women think breast cancer is a greater threat to their health than coronary heart disease, yet statistically women are four times more likely to die of a heart problem than breast cancer. Heart disease and diseases of the blood vessels together claim nearly twice as many women's lives as all forms of cancer.[2]

What causes cardiovascular disease?

Coronary heart disease occurs when the coronary arteries that supply blood and oxygen to the heart become narrowed due to a process called atherosclerosis. This starts off with the cells lining the arteries becoming inflamed, which then leads to damage and the formation of a plaque containing fatty material called atheroma. If left untreated the arteries will become so narrowed that inadequate amounts of oxygen are delivered to the heart, resulting in oxygen deprivation and a condition called angina. If the blood supply is completely cut off, then a heart attack takes place.

Strokes affect 150,000 people in the UK each year. They are the third most common cause of death and the leading cause of disability in the UK.[3] A stroke is a brain attack, in which the blood supply to part of the brain becomes cut off. This most commonly occurs because of a blood clot or bleed. If the blood supply is interrupted for a small amount of time and all the symptoms resolve within 24 hours, then it is called a transient ischemic attack (TIA).

What are the risk factors?

There are many different contributors to heart disease, including poor diet, genetics, smoking (around 25 per cent of British women smoke and around 6,000 women die each year from coronary heart disease that's been brought on by smoking), high blood pressure, chronic inflammation, excess alcohol (more than two units a day), stress, mental illness (depression and anxiety), obesity, excess fibrinogen, high homocysteine, physical inactivity, social isolation, metabolic syndrome and diabetes.

My integrated medical prescription for cardiovascular disease

Integrated medicine has a lot to offer you. Pioneering work by Dr Dean Ornish, a heart disease specialist in America, has shown conclusively that heart disease symptoms will not only improve considerably with dietary change, regular physical activity and a programme of stress management, but also that they can actually reverse heart disease.[4] Many of the patients who come to me for advice are looking to come off the heart medication that they have been put on. This isn't always advisable, because it can lead to a worsening of symptoms. I much prefer to make the life changes first, prescribe appropriate supplements and then, once established, work with my patient's GP to reduce medications while monitoring the relevant vital signs and symptoms. For me, this is a good example of integrated medicine in action!

Step 1 • *Do you have cardiovascular disease?*

If you are reading this then you have probably already been diagnosed. However, if you don't have a diagnosis you might want to look through the following symptoms to see if you can associate with any of them:

Symptoms/signs of atherosclerosis – fainting, dizziness, leg pain that commences with walking and disappears after rest.

Symptoms/signs of angina – tightness in the chest, mild to severe chest pain, shortness of breath, although in addition to the classic symptoms associated with angina, women also tend to have less common symptoms, such as back pain, burning in the chest, abdominal discomfort, nausea and fatigue.

Symptoms/signs of a heart attack – mild to severe crushing or tight chest pain in the chest, which might radiate to the arms, back, neck or jaw, although women may experience more vague symptoms, such as stomach or jaw pain, or pain between the breasts, and other symptoms include sweating, dizziness, fainting, ringing in the ears, nausea and possibly vomiting.

Symptoms/signs of a stroke – numbness, weakness or paralysis on one side of the body (signs of this may be a drooping arm, leg or lower eyelid, or a dribbling mouth), slurred speech, difficulty finding words or understanding speech, sudden blurred vision or loss of sight, confusion, unsteadiness and severe headache.

If you are known to have any heart problems or suspect that you might have or are at risk of cardiovascular disease, I encourage you to start by arranging some tests. While most GPs will test your cholesterol and triglyceride levels, and make an assessment of your diet and lifestyle, there is convincing evidence that other markers of heart disease should also be explored. While it is beyond the scope of this book to go into them in detail, I recommend a blood test called the Comprehensive Cardiovascular Risk Assessment 2.0 from Genova Diagnostics (see Resources), which, in addition to assessing cholesterol levels, looks at:

- **hs C-reactive protein** – this is a marker of inflammation in the body and is considered to be one of the best predictors of heart disease

- **Homocysteine** – this is a toxic chemical that triggers inflammation and increases plaque formation in the walls of the artery

- **Lp(a)** – has a protective effect against heart disease

- **Fibrinogen** – elevated levels of this are associated with cardiovascular disease

Step 2 • Consider the medical options

Western medicine has a lot to offer you in terms of both preventing and treating heart disease and stroke. If you have a specific risk factor for heart disease, such as high cholesterol, diabetes, metabolic syndrome, weight gain and/or high blood pressure you should read the relevant section of this book and follow those instructions. The following are the recommended medical treatments for angina, for a heart attack and for a stroke.

Medications

FOR ANGINA

Glyceryl trinitrate (GTN) can be taken as tablets or a spray you put under your tongue to get quick relief from an angina attack. Its side-effects include headaches, flushing and dizziness. It should only be taken as and when you need it. If you are experiencing angina and continue to have discomfort or pain despite taking three doses over 15 minutes, you should phone for an ambulance immediately as you could be having a heart attack.

Beta-blockers are drugs that can help you have fewer angina attacks and stay active. They are usually the first treatment doctors give for stable angina. Some common beta-blockers are atenolol (Tenormin), bisoprolol (Cardicor), carvedilol (Eucardic), metoprolol (Lopresor) and propranolol (Inderal). The studies show that taking a beta-blocker will not only reduce the average number of angina attacks from three a week to less than one,[5] but you should also be able to exercise more, feel physically better and sleep better.[6] The most common side-effects are tiredness, dizziness, bad dreams and cold hands and feet. You should never stop taking beta-blockers suddenly as doing so can precipitate an angina attack or even a heart attack. I recommend that these are taken long term because of their benefits.

Calcium channel blockers,[7] **nitrates**[8] and **nicorandil**[9] also work for angina.

FOR A HEART ATTACK

Obviously the most important thing you can do if you or another person is having a heart attack is call 999 immediately. The quicker you get to hospital the better.

Aspirin should be chewed while you're waiting for an ambulance as this can help to thin your blood. Doing so reduces the chances of you having another heart attack and stroke by about one-third and dying from a heart attack or stroke by one-sixth.[10]

Thrombolytic or clot-busting drugs will probably be given to you in hospital, as these increase your chances of surviving your heart attack and being alive 12 years after your treatment.[11] As an alternative, and if you have been taken to a hospital where they offer it, you might be offered an operation to widen blocked arteries called a coronary angioplasty. It can help you survive a heart attack and reduce your chances of dying, having another heart attack or having a stroke between 6 to 18 months after your heart attack.[12]

Beta-blockers (mentioned above) can reduce your risk of dying after a heart attack. They may also lower your chances of having another heart attack.[13] As I have said, I recommend that these should be taken long term.

ACE inhibitors are drugs given after a heart attack, which can help you live longer and may prevent another heart attack.[14] These should also be taken long term.

FOR A STROKE

Call 999 immediately, as for a heart attack. While most people don't consider a stroke to be an emergency, it is.

If possible, a specialist stroke unit is the best place to be, as you're more likely to make a good recovery.[15]

Aspirin within two days of having an ischaemic stroke (the type that happens when a blood vessel is blocked) can reduce your chance of dying and also reduce the degree of disability you have afterwards. It also improves your chance of making a complete recovery.[16]

Thrombolytic (clot-dissolving) drugs can reduce your chances of being disabled after a stroke caused by a blood clot.[17] The sooner you get this treatment, the better it works. This is usually administered as a one-off treatment.

If you've had a stroke or a mini-stroke, there is a two in ten chance that you will have another one within five years.[18] Depending on what is relevant, your doctor will offer you medications to lower your cholesterol, blood pressure and stabilise an irregular heartbeat. In addition to this you should take an aspirin (75mg) every day if your stroke was due to a blockage in the blood supply to the brain. Studies have found that this will reduce the likelihood of you having another stroke, a heart attack or dying from a stroke or heart attack.[19]

Dipyridamole (Persantin, Persantin Retard), an additional blood thinning drug[20] should also be offered to you for a period of two years. This enhances the effects of aspirin. The most common concern with aspirin is its ability to cause bleeding from the stomach or intestines. However, this is rare and most doctors feel that the benefits outweigh the risks.

Step 3 • Address the underlying causes

While I am going to make recommendations to reduce the symptoms associated with cardiovascular disease using a variety of supplements, for long-lasting health and to potentially reverse atherosclerosis, for example, I encourage you to fill in the questionnaires in part one, section two, so as to help identify possible root causes or contributors to cardiovascular disease. In my experience, the ones to consider are:

- **Poor diet** – Solution: Secret One – Nurture Your Physical Body (Healthy Eating and Supplements – page 49)

- **Excessive weight** – Solution: Secret One – Nurture Your Physical Body (Healthy Eating and Supplements – page 49); Part Five (Weight Loss – page 401); Holistic Health Tools – Emotional Freedom Technique (page 151) and The Work (page 163)

- **Blood-sugar imbalance** – Solution: Secret One – Nurture Your Physical Body (Healthy Eating and Supplements – page 49)

- **Diabetes and metabolic syndrome** – Solution: Secret One – Nurture Your Physical Body (Healthy Eating and Supplements – page 49); Part Five (Diabetes – page 325; Metabolic Syndrome – page 368)

- **Stress** – Solution: Secret Two – De-stress and Relax (page 77); Holistic Health Tools – Emotional Freedom Technique (page 151) and Mindfulness (page 147)

- **Environmental toxicity** – Solution: Secret One – Nurture Your Physical Body (Healthy Environment and Sunlight – page 70)

- **Depression** – Solution: Part Five (Depression – page 316); Holistic Health Tools – Mindfulness (page 147), Values-based Goal Setting (page 166) and The Work (page 163), (if you have depression, you should seek help – one study in the *Journal of the American Medical Association* in 1993 found that just six months after a heart attack those who were depressed were six times more likely to have died than those who weren't)

- **Nutritional deficiencies** – Solution: Secret One – Nurture Your Physical Body (Healthy Eating and Supplements – page 49)

- **Addictions (smoking)** – Solution: Part Five (Addictions – page 260); Secret Four – Accept Yourself (page 113); Secret Three – Face and Embrace Your Emotions (page 94); Secret Five – Develop and Deepen Your Relationships (page 127); Holistic Health Tools – Mindfulness (page 147), Emotional Freedom Technique (page 151) and Values-based Goal Setting (page 166)

- **Lack of physical activity** – Solution: Secret One – Nurture Your Physical Body (Physical Activity and Touch – page 67); Holistic Health Tools – Emotional Freedom Technique (page 151) and Values-based Goal Setting (page 166)

- **Low self-acceptance** – Solution: Secret Four – Accept Yourself (page 113); Secret Three – Face and Embrace Your Emotions (page 94); Secret Five – Develop and Deepen Your Relationships (page 127); Holistic Health Tools – Mindfulness (page 147), Emotional Freedom Technique (page 151) and Values-based Goal Setting (page 166)

- **High blood pressure** – Solution: Part Five (Metabolic Syndrome – page 368)

- **High cholesterol** – Solution: Part Five (Metabolic Syndrome – page 368)

- **Emotional repression** – Solution: Secret Three – Face and Embrace Your Emotions (page 94); Secret Five – Develop and Deepen Your Relationships (page 127); Part Five (Tension Myoneural Syndrome – page 386)

Step 4 • Start a cardiovascular disease supplement programme

When used alongside step three, certain nutritional supplements can help to reverse and reduce the symptoms associated with cardiovascular disease. Because of the potential for negative interactions with your medications, before taking the supplements I suggest you check with your GP or check yourself online (see Resources). My integrated medicine prescription for cardiovascular disease usually includes a combination of:

- **A multivitamin-mineral supplement**.

- **Vitamin C with bioflavanoids**[21] (3000mg) to reduce inflammation and damage caused by free radicals in the body.

- **Fish oil**[22] (1000mg to 3000mg a day) to reduce inflammation, thin the blood and help lower cholesterol and triglycerides.

- **Glycine propionyl-L-carnitine hyduchloride**[23] (1000mg to 2000mg a day) to improve heart function and support energy production in the cells of the heart.

- **Coenzyme Q10** (100mg to 300mg a day) to help lower blood pressure and improve symptoms associated with angina and heart failure.[24]

- **Garlic** (900mg a day) to improve and help maintain heart and blood vessel health.[25]

- **Hawthorn** (300mg to 900mg a day), which may reduce mild blood pressure, increase the strength of heart contractions and increase circulation to the heart muscle.[26]

Based on the results from the Comprehensive Cardiovascular Risk Assessment 2.0 test that I mentioned in step one, you might also need to add:

For raised CRP

- **Fish oil** (3000mg to 10,000mg a day), **vitamin C with bioflavanoids** (1000mg to 3000mg a day), **vitamin E** (400IU a day) and **bromelain** (200mg three times a day).

For raised lipoprotein A

- **Flush-free niacin** (1500mg twice a day).

For raised homocysteine

- **Vitamin B$_{12}$** (800mcg to 2000mcg a day), **folic acid** (1mg to 10mg a day), **vitamin B$_6$** (20mg to 100mg a day) and **trimethylglycine** (TMG) (500mg to 1000mg daily).

For raised cholesterol

- See Metabolic Syndrome – page 368.

For raised blood glucose

- See Metabolic Syndrome (page 368) and Diabetes (page 325).

For raised fibrinogen

- As for raised CRP.

Step 5 • Consider other complementary approaches

In addition to changing your diet and increasing your levels of physical activity, you might also want to consider some of the following approaches to support you in your programme. While there is no definitive evidence that these can help you with your heart disease, some patients find the following useful in supporting their programme: acupuncture, homeopathy, massage, spiritual healing, yoga, traditional Chinese medicine and Ayurvedic medicine.

For recommended books and websites see Resources.

Cellulite

If I had a pound for every time I have been asked whether I know how to get rid of cellulite I would be a rich man! While cellulite isn't a medical term, the appearance of loose dimpled skin can often be a significant source of stress for many women and for that reason I have included it in this book. Most women suffer from cellulite around their hips and buttocks, but it can also affect the abdomen and upper arms.

What causes cellulite?

Cellulite seems to occur when fat cells within and under the skin become too large for the natural fibre compartments which hold them. These compartments start bulging, which in turn leads to uneven layers of fat underneath.

What are the risk factors?

While most women develop cellulite (about 90 per cent), there are some factors that make it even more likely.

- Genetics

- Hormone contraceptives

- Smoking

- Obesity

- Hormonal imbalance

- A sedentary lifestyle

- Poor diets and crash diets

My integrated medical prescription for cellulite

While I've never had a patient specifically come to me for advice on treating their cellulite, I have nonetheless been asked for advice many times. The first thing I say is that there isn't a cure, but there are certain things you can do to reduce the unsightly appearance and stop it getting worse.

Step 1 • Do you have cellulite?

You probably already know if you have cellulite or not. That said, it can be very mild and the only way you will know that it is present is if you pinch a big area of your skin, say on your thighs, and you see it in the pinched skin area. In more severe cases cellulite can make the skin appear rumpled and bumpy.

Step 2 • Consider the medical options

The most promising medical treatments for cellulite are lasers and radio frequency systems. While there are many different types, most systems work by breaking down fat deposits, increasing local circulation and promoting lymphatic drainage. While laser treatments do often improve the appearance of the skin, the results are usually only temporary, lasting up to six months. They also tend to be very expensive. I recommend to most of my patients that they try my integrated medical approach first, prior to using other treatments.

Step 3 • Address the underlying causes

While I am going to make recommendations to reduce the appearance of cellulite using a variety of supplements, for the best improvement I encourage you to fill in the questionnaires in part one, section
two, so as to help identify possible root causes or contributors to cellulite. In my experience, the ones to consider are:

- **Excessive weight** – Solution: Secret One – Nurture Your Physical
  Body (Healthy Eating and Supplements – page 49); Part Five
  (Weight Loss – page 401); Holistic Health Tools – Emotional
  Freedom Technique (page 151) and The Work (page 163)

- **Stress** – Solution: Secret Two – De-stress and Relax (page 77); Holistic Health Tools – Emotional Freedom Technique (page 151) and
  Mindfulness (page 147)

- **Poor diet** – Solution: Secret One – Nurture Your Physical Body
  (Healthy Eating and Supplements – page 49)

- **Addictions (smoking)** – Solution: Part Five (Addictions – page 260);
  Secret Four – Accept Yourself (page 113); Secret Three – Face and
  Embrace Your Emotions (page 94); Secret Five – Develop and
  Deepen Your Relationships (page 127); Holistic Health Tools –
  Mindfulness (page 147), Emotional Freedom Technique (page 151)
  and Values-based Goal Setting (page 166)

- **Self-acceptance** (if all else fails!) – Solution: Secret Four – Accept
  Yourself (page 113); Secret Three – Face and Embrace Your Emotions
  (page 94); Secret Five – Develop and Deepen Your Relationships
  (page 127); Holistic Health Tools – Mindfulness (page 147), Emotional Freedom Technique (page 151) and Values-based Goal Setting
  (page 166)

Step 4 • Start a cellulite supplement programme

When used alongside step three, certain nutritional supplements can
help to reduce the appearance of cellulite. My integrated medicine
prescription for cellulite would usually include:

- **A multivitamin-mineral supplement.**

- **Vitamin C with bioflavanoids** (1000mg) to reduce inflammation.

- **Omega-3, 6 and 9** (taken in capsule or liquid form in a 2:1:1 ratio) to provide the body with hormone-balancing anti-inflammatory essential fatty acids.

- **Alkaline mineral salts** – to counteract acidity from stress and a processed diet.

- **Conjugated linoleic acid** (dose as advised by manufacturers), which might help to slim the buttocks and thighs.

For the skin itself my patients seem to benefit from using one of the following two cellulite treatment systems:

- **Phytotec Cellulite System**, which consists of three plant-based gels that when applied daily to the affected area help to break up fat, reduce water retention and improve circulation – see Resources.

- **The Anti-Cellulite Body Blitz**, which uses seaweed mud to feed and nourish the tissues, break down fatty deposits and increase circulation. You receive this treatment while wrapped in a heated blanket and have a massage afterwards – see Resources.

Step 5 • Consider other complementary approaches

While there is no definitive evidence that these can help with your cellulite, some patients find the following useful in supporting their programme: deep massage, rebounding and acupuncture.

For recommended books see Resources.

Chronic fatigue syndrome and fibromyalgia

~

I have seen over a hundred women with chronic fatigue syndrome (CFS) or fibromyalgia and have come to really appreciate what a distressing illness this is. CFS is an umbrella term to describe a collection of symptoms, ranging from profound fatigue, muscle aches, digestive disturbance and sore throats, to recurrent viral infections, personality changes and difficulty concentrating, that interfere significantly with your ability to carry out everyday tasks. It is believed to affect 0.4 per cent of the population and twice as many women as men.

Fibromyalgia is related in many ways to chronic fatigue syndrome, but whereas fatigue is the dominant feature in CFS, pain and muscle soreness are the dominant features in fibromyalgia. In addition, fibromyalgia is frequently linked to a specific physical or emotional trauma, and the pain is relieved by massage and heat, whereas this doesn't happen with CFS.

What causes CFS and fibromyalgia?

The truth is no-one really knows. My own perspective is that, like most illnesses, CFS and fibromyalgia are a symptom of underlying imbalances and those imbalances vary amongst individuals. Put another way, the causes of CFS and fibromyalgia depend on the individual, but here are the factors and influences that, in my experience, can contribute to the symptoms of CFS and fibromyalgia:

- Toxicity – including heavy metal sensitivity

- Nutritional deficiencies

- Hormonal imbalances

- Low energy output from the mitochondria (the body's energy producer)

- Viral, mycoplasma and yeast infections

- Allergies – for example, to mould

- Psychological stress

- Repressed emotions

- Trauma – physical and emotional

- Metabolic disturbances

- Autonomic nervous system dysfunction

- Hypothalamic dysfunction

- Immune dysfunction

As you can see, there are a lot of them! I have worked mainly with patients with CFS and my own take on it is that it often follows a long period of stress and a triggering event, such as a viral infection. The bodymind eventually says 'no more' and shifts into a hyperaroused survival mode that won't switch off. This leads to many of the problems above, such as immune dysfunction and hormone imbalance.

What are the risk factors?

Because the medical profession has only just recently acknowledged CFS and fibromyalgia as diseases, the risk factors haven't been established yet.

My integrated medical prescription for CFS and fibromyalgia

My first piece of advice is to find yourself a health professional who is experienced in its treatment as it can be challenging to do it yourself, particularly as treatment, in my opinion, needs to be highly tailored to you as an individual. While most practitioners tend to focus either on a psychological or biological approach, my experience is that you need to address both in parallel, which is what my integrated medical programme is designed to do.

Step 1 • Do you have CFS or fibromyalgia?

Symptoms/signs of CFS – to be characterised as CFS your fatigue should be medically unexplained (in other words not caused by conditions such as anaemia), of recent onset (not lifelong), of at least six months' duration, not the result of ongoing exertion (overwork or athletic over-training), not substantially relieved by rest and causing a substantial reduction in previous levels of occupational, educational, social or personal activities.

Plus there must be *four or more* of the following symptoms: self-reported problems with short-term memory or concentration (cognitive defects), sore throat, tender neck (cervical) or armpit (axillary) glands, muscle pain (myalgia), headaches of a new type, pattern or severity, unrefreshing sleep, post-exertional malaise lasting more than 24 hours and multi-joint pain (arthralgia) without swelling or redness.

Other symptoms include palpitations, sweating, feeling faint or problems with balance, feeling sick and mood swings.

Symptoms/signs of fibromyalgia – these include widespread pain, chest pain, morning stiffness, fatigue, sleep disorders, anxiety, cognitive or memory impairment ('fibrofog'), depression and abdominal complaints.

If you have any of these symptoms or signs I encourage you to see your GP, who will need to consider, and where appropriate exclude, the following in order to make the diagnosis of CFS or fibromyalgia:

depression and anxiety, drug and alcohol abuse, eating disorders, underactive thyroid gland, hyperventilation, over-training, sleep apnoea syndrome (heavy snorers who periodically stop breathing in their sleep), infections, autoimmune disorders (such as Addison's disease), neuromuscular disease, malignancy, chemical sensitivities, carbon monoxide poisoning and heart, kidney and liver disease.

Step 2 • Consider the medical options

This won't take long, because Western medicine has at this moment in time very little to offer you. A doctor will probably recommend that you gradually increase the amount of physical activity that you take and provide you with a referral for cognitive behavioural therapy (CBT). This is a form of talking treatment that tries to change thinking and behaviour in a positive way. The studies show that it can help you feel better and enjoy life more when compared to normal standard care from a family doctor, relaxation therapy or support from a social worker.[1]

If you have symptoms of depression you will probably be offered an antidepressant medication such as fluoxetine (Prozac) or sertraline (Lustral). The trials to date do not warrant you taking antidepressants, plus they are associated with side-effects such as sweating, dry mouth, constipation, dizziness, stomach upsets, anxiety, sleeping trouble and headaches.

If you have fibromyalgia, in addition to painkillers such as paracteamol and non-steroidal anti-inflammatories (NSAIDS), you might be offered amitriptyline, which is is an antidepressant with some pain-relieving effects. It seems to help improve symptoms in about 30 per cent of those with fibromyalgia who take it.[2]

Step 3 • Address the underlying causes

While I am going to make recommendations to treat your fatigue and pain symptoms using a variety of supplements, for lasting resolution of these symptoms I encourage you to fill in the questionnaires in part one, section two, so as to help identify possible root causes or contributors to CFS and fibromyalgia. In my experience, the ones to consider are:

- **Adrenal fatigue** – Solution: Part Five (Adrenal Fatigue – page 267); Secret Two – De-stress and Relax (page 77); Holistic Health Tools – Values-based Goal Setting (page 166) and Mindfulness (page 147)

- **Viruses/candida/parasites** – Solution: Part Five (Dysbiosis – page 334); Holistic Health Tools – Emotional Freedom Technique (page 151)

- **Blood-sugar imbalance** – Solution: Secret One – Nurture Your Physical Body (Healthy Eating and Supplements – page 49)

- **Stress** – Solution: Secret Two – De-stress and Relax (page 77); Holistic Health Tools – Emotional Freedom Technique (page 151) and Mindfulness (page 147)

- **Emotional repression** – Solution: Secret Three – Face and Embrace Your Emotions (page 94); Secret Five – Develop and Deepen Your Relationships (page 127); Part Five (Tension Myoneural Syndrome – page 386)

- **Poor diet** – Solution: Secret One – Nurture Your Physical Body (Healthy Eating and Supplements – page 49)

- **Environmental toxicity** – Solution: Secret One – Nurture Your Physical Body (Healthy Environment and Sunlight – page 70)

- **Depression** – Solution: Part Five (Depression – page 316); Holistic Health Tools – Mindfulness (page 147), Values-based Goal Setting (page 166) and The Work (page 163)

- **Food intolerances** – Solution: Part Five (Food Intolerances – page 344); Holistic Health Tools – Emotional Freedom Technique (page 151)

- **Nutritional deficiencies** – Solution: Secret One – Nurture Your Physical Body (Healthy Eating and Supplements – page 49)

- **Hypothyroidism** – Solution: Part Five (Hypothyroidism – page 356); Holistic Health Tools – Emotional Freedom Technique (page 151) and The Work (page 163)

- **Trauma** – Solution: Secret Three – Face and Embrace Your Emotions (page 94); Holistic Health Tools – Emotional Freedom Technique (page 151), EmoTrance (page 158) and Mindfulness (page 147)

- **Low self-acceptance** – Solution: Secret Four – Accept Yourself (page 113); Secret Three – Face and Embrace Your Emotions (page 94); Secret Five – Develop and Deepen Your Relationships (page 127); Holistic Health Tools – Mindfulness (page 147), Emotional Freedom Technique (page 151) and Values-based Goal Setting (page 166)

Step 4 • Start a CFS or fibromyalgia supplement programme

When used alongside step three, certain nutritional supplements can help to alleviate many of the symptoms associated with CFS and fibromyalgia. My integrated medicine prescription for CFS/fibromyalgia usually includes a combination of:

- **A multivitamin-mineral supplement.**

- **Vitamin C with bioflavanoids** (1000mg).

- **Fish oil** (3000mg a day) to provide the body with health-promoting anti-inflammatory essential fatty acids.[3]

- **D-ribose**[4] (2g to 10g daily), **L-carnitine**[5] (3g daily), **magnesium**[6] (400mg daily) and **coenzyme Q10**[7] (100mg to 200mg daily) to support energy production in the body.

- **5-HTP** (50mg to 100mg three times a day) – in one study of 50 people with fibromyalgia, 5-HTP at these doses was found to significantly relieve pain, anxiety and tiredness and improve sleep.[8]

Step 5 • Consider other complementary approaches

In addition to my own Freedom Process (see Resources), the three main psychologically based approaches to CFS and fibromyalgia that I am aware of are the Lightening Process and Reverse Therapy. Another approach that claims a high success rate is called the Perrin Technique. The treatment is osteopathic and is based on the assumption that lymphatic drainage disturbance contributes significantly to CFS symptoms. For fibromyalgia I have had a number of patients report an excellent response after receiving treatment using the Neurostructural Integration Technique, a gentle approach to bodywork that releases tension and pain from the body.

For details of these approaches, plus recommended books and websites, see Resources.

Codependency

At least 80 per cent of the women who come to see me in my clinic are codependent. Although previously used to describe someone who would perpetuate another person's addictions, the term is now used to describe an adult whose emotional management style, patterns of behaviour and ways of relating to themselves and others have failed to mature and develop since childhood. Although not strictly a disease, I have included it in this book because it represents a significant barrier to emotional health and happiness for a lot of women (and men). It's also a significant driving factor for addictions.

What causes codependency?

According to Barry and Janae Weinhold in their pioneering book *Breaking Free of the Codependency Trap*, codependency is not a disease, but a pattern of dependency, neediness and low self-esteem caused primarily by traumatic bonding breaks within the first six months of life, which prevents the development of a secure healthy attachment. To put it bluntly, this happens when our need for nurturing, protection, safety and emotional mirroring as children was, for whatever reason, not met. This is particularly the case when children are used, usually unconsciously, to meet the emotional needs of their parents.

What's liberating about this perspective is that it does not view codependency as a disease that you are stuck with, but as a series of limiting emotional and behavioural patterns that are preventing you from having a healthy relationship with yourself and with others. Therefore, the key to recovery is to learn new patterns of relating to emotions, to yourself and to others. Codependency is, in my view, an opportunity to replace a false self and a less-than-satisfying life with a deeply fulfilling life rooted in an authentic sense of self and loving, intimate relationships.

What are the risk factors?

Essentially if you were brought up in a less-than-nurturing family environment then the likelihood of you having a degree of codependency is high. If one or more of your parents were addicts, then the chances are even higher.

My integrated medical prescription for codependency

There is a theory that says it takes one month for every year that you have been alive to recover from codependency. So if you are 36 it will take about three years! It does, of course, depend a lot on your level of commitment and various other factors, but I have seen in my own experience that this appears to be true. The key to recovering from codependency is to start facing and embracing reality – and, in particular, to start allowing yourself to feel your feelings, get in touch with your needs and live a values-based life. It's not easy, but many people have walked this path and transformed their quality of life by following variants of the suggestions that I am about to share with you.

Step 1 • Are you codependent?

Acknowledging the fact that codependency might be a dynamic that is affecting you and your relationships is the first step in doing something about it. If you haven't done this already I encourage you to fill in the codependency questionnaire in part one, section two. In addition to that, you could take a look at the website of Codependents Anonymous (CODA), which has a list of the characteristics and patterns of codependency. See Resources.

Step 2 • Consider the medical options

The subject of codependency is not one to take to your doctor, because it's highly unlikely he or she will have heard of it or will understand it. That said there are numerous health professionals and treatment centres who do understand what it is and, importantly, how to support you in recovering from it.

The first port of call for help would be a counsellor or psychotherapist trained to work with people who have codependency. Ideally this should not only involve individual therapy, but couples therapy as well. See Resources.

If your symptoms of codependency are severe, and impairing your ability to live a healthy and functional life, then you might want to consider going into a codependency treatment programme. The two that I am most familiar with and recommend are the Bridge to Recovery in Bowling Green, Kentucky, USA, and the Survivors Workshop at the Meadows in Wickenburg, Arizona, USA. Another alternative is one-to-one, or couple intensives, or workshops with the authors of *Breaking Free of the Codependency Trap*, Barry and Janae Weinhold. For more information on these see Resources.

Step 3 • Address the underlying causes

Developing new emotional, relating and behavioural patterns doesn't happen overnight, unfortunately. As to how you recover from codependency, that will depend very much on you, as everyone has their unique path. However, most codependency authorities would include some or all of the following elements in their recovery programme:

- **Self-acceptance** – Solution: Secret Four – Accept Yourself (page 113); Secret Three – Face and Embrace Your Emotions (page 94); Secret Five – Develop and Deepen Your Relationships (page 127); Holistic Health Tools – Mindfulness (page 147), Emotional Freedom Technique (page 151) and Values-based Goal Setting (page 166)

- **Emotional healing** – Solution: Secret Three – Face and Embrace Your Emotions (page 94); Holistic Health Tools – Mindfulness (page 147), Emotional Freedom Technique (page 151) and EmoTrance (page 158)

- **Trauma** – Solution: Secret Three – Face and Embrace Your Emotions (page 94); Holistic Health Tools – Emotional Freedom Technique (page 151), EmoTrance (page 158) and Mindfulness (page 147)

- **Stress** – Solution: Secret Two – De-stress and Relax (page 77); Holistic Health Tools – Emotional Freedom Technique (page 151) and Mindfulness (page 147)

- **Addictions** – Solution: Part Five (Addictions – page 260); Secret Four – Accept Yourself (page 113); Secret Three – Face and Embrace Your Emotions (page 94); Secret Five – Develop and Deepen Your Relationships (page 127); Holistic Health Tools – Mindfulness (page 147), Emotional Freedom Technique (page 151) and Values-based Goal Setting (page 166)

Creating healthy boundaries

Boundaries are important when addressing codependency. A boundary is an invisible line or space that you create in order to protect yourself and maintain an authentic sense of self without offending others. It is made up of your sense of worth, your identity, your rights, and your right to express and defend your rights. Having a healthy boundary allows me to have a real sense of who I am, to know where you end and I begin, and it alerts me to when others are intruding on my boundaries. This is crucial to healthy self-care. For example, if someone touched you inappropriately or got too close to you without permission that's a physical boundary violation. However, if you don't have a healthy boundary in place you probably wouldn't notice it. If someone told you that your idea about something was rubbish, that's an intellectual boundary violation.

Essentially, to lead a healthy life and experience healthy relationships we need to understand where our boundaries are; take responsibility for the things within our own boundaries; and allow other people to take responsibility for the things within their boundaries. The concept of boundaries can be a bit tricky to grasp, but it's of absolute importance when progressing to mature adulthood.

Healing shame

Shame is the inner experience and deeply felt sense of being flawed and unloveable as a human being. In contrast with guilt, in which you feel bad about something that you did, with shame you feel you are bad. In my experience working with people with codependency, shame resides at the core of their codependency and is a major driver of addictions, low self-esteem and inability to form healthy relationships. One of the most liberating pieces of healing work they can do is to either release or learn how to contain that shame. For recommended books see Resources.

Step 4 • Consider joining a support group

I'm a big fan of Codependents Anonymous (CODA), a support group and fellowship of men and women who are committed to creating healthy and intimate relationships through sharing their experience, strength and hope. The members of CODA will be facing similar struggles to the ones you are encountering, so by listening to their own challenges and solutions you can pick up a lot of advice and support. CODA is a spiritually based programme of recovery from codependency and addictions, and the informal meetings are based on the 12-step model of Alcoholics Anonymous. For more information see Resources.

Constipation

~

Constipation is a major challenge, and source of physical and emotional distress, to many women, with twice as many women reporting being constipated compared to men. About five in ten women strain at the toilet at least a quarter of the time, compared with about four in ten men.[1] Another study found that about one in ten women have constipation for more than 12 weeks a year.[2]

Constipation can be defined as a difficulty and/or infrequency in the passage of stool. Being constipated is not only uncomfortable, but it can lead to the build up of toxins, which in turn can trigger inflammatory and autoimmune diseases. One study found that women who had fewer than three bowel movements a week – which is the medical definition of constipation – had four times the risk of breast disease than those who had one or more bowel movements a day.

What causes constipation?

There are numerous different causes, including dehydration, insufficient fibre, inactivity, stress, parasites, medications (such as painkillers), candida, dysbiosis, magnesium deficiency, underactive thyroid, diverticulitis and, rarely, cancer. Interestingly, women tend to experience constipation in the week prior to their period. This is thought to be due to the retention of fluids that normally allow the stool to soften and pass through.

What are the risk factors?

The likelihood of you experiencing constipation is increased if you are older, sedentary or pregnant. In addition to this, a diet low in fibre and being dehydrated can contribute to constipation.

My integrated medical prescription for constipation

Most women with constipation will have tried laxatives and, while they work, they are just a quick fix. The real key to lasting recovery from constipation is to address its underlying causes. Here is what I recommend if you are constipated.

Step 1 • Are you constipated?

As I've said, the medics define someone who has less than three bowel movements a week as constipated, but my personal perspective is that it really depends on you. As a general rule of thumb, if you feel that your bowel movements or constipation is in any way limiting your ability to enjoy optimum health, then I would go ahead and treat your constipation using the following recommendations.

Step 2 • Consider the medical options

The most effective conventional medical approach to constipation is the use of laxatives. There are several types of laxatives, including those that make your stool softer, those that stimulate your bowels and those that make your stools bigger and easier to push along and out of the body. Of those available, the research has found that laxatives containing polyethylene glycol, such as Idrolax and Movicol, are probably the most effective.[3] They work by encouraging your bowels to add water to your stools, which in turn makes them softer. As I mentioned before, it's really important that you address the underlying cause of your constipation as well and I would also avoid using these laxatives long term, because in my experience the bowel can become dependent on them.

Step 3 • Address the underlying causes

While I am going to make recommendations to treat your constipation using a variety of supplements, for lasting resolution of constipation I encourage you to fill in the questionnaires in part one, section two, in order to identify possible root causes or contributors. In my experience, the ones to consider are:

- **Poor diet** – Solution: Secret One – Nurture Your Physical Body (Healthy Eating and Supplements – page 49)

- **Stress** – Solution: Secret Two – De-stress and Relax (page 77); Holistic Health Tools – Emotional Freedom Technique (page 151) and Mindfulness (page 147)

- **Food intolerances** – Solution: Part Five (Food Intolerances – page 344); Holistic Health Tools – Emotional Freedom Technique (page 151)

- **Nutritional deficiencies** – Solution: Secret One – Nurture Your Physical Body (Healthy Eating and Supplements – page 49)

- **Hypothyroidism** – Solution: Part Five (Hypothyroidism – page 356); Holistic Health Tools – Emotional Freedom Technique (page 151) and The Work (page 163)

- **Parasites/candida** – Solution: Part Five (Dysbiosis – page 334); Holistic Health Tools – Emotional Freedom Technique (page 151)

- **Lack of physical activity** – Solution: Secret One – Nurture Your Physical Body (Physical Activity and Touch – page 67); Holistic Health Tools – Emotional Freedom Technique (page 151) and Values-based Goal Setting (page 166)

- **Depression** – Solution: Part Five (Depression – see page 316); Holistic Health Tools – Mindfulness (page 147), Values-based Goal Setting (page 166) and The Work (page 163)

- **Medications** – if you are taking any medications you should read the information that came with them to see if they cause constipation.

Step 4 • Start a constipation supplement programme

When used alongside step three, certain nutritional supplements can help to alleviate constipation. My integrated medicine prescription for constipation usually includes a combination of:

- **Flaxseed oil**[4] (1 to 2 tablespoons a day) helps to lubricate the colon so that the stool can move along it more easily.

- **Acidophilus probiotic**[5] (dose as advised by manufacturers) to repopulate the bowel with 'friendly' bacteria, which in turn support a healthy digestion.

- **Psyllium**[6] (5g twice daily) is a bulk-forming laxative and is what I usually recommend as an alternative to conventional laxatives. It helps to soften your stools.

- **Oxygenated magnesium** (dose as advised by manufacturers) is the product I recommend most for constipation as it also helps to treat candida, which can cause constipation.

Step 5 • Consider other complementary approaches

While there is no definitive evidence that these can help you with your constipation, some patients find the following useful in supporting their programme: colonic hydrotherapy, Western herbal medicine, acupuncture, homeopathy, massage, yoga, traditional Chinese medicine and Ayurvedic medicine.

For recommended books and websites see Resources.

Depression

Depression affects 121 million people worldwide and it is expected that half of all women will suffer depression at some point in their lives, with an estimated 9.5 per cent of women experiencing a depressive episode in any given year. The prevalence of depression is rising every year and depression is predicted to be the world's second most common disabling disease (after heart disease) by 2020. Rather than thinking of depression as a psychological illness, I prefer to describe it as a whole-person illness; a disorder of mind, body and soul that influences every aspect of your life, including thoughts, feelings, behaviour and relationships. This, in my experience, more accurately describes the truth about depression.

What causes depression?

The answer you get will depend on who you talk to. A doctor will probably say it's related to a genetically inherited vulnerability and an imbalance in your brain biochemistry; a nutritionist might say it's because of nutrient deficiencies, hormonal imbalances and/or food intolerances; a counsellor may say it's due to addictions, low self-acceptance or trauma; and a cognitive behavioural therapist might say it's down to the negative, 'black and white' way you interpret your life circumstances. So who's right? From my own experience of having worked with hundreds of people with depression, all of these various factors can play a part to differing degrees in people's mood problems. The key, and the road to emotional health, is to work out which are relevant to you.

What are the risk factors?

The following are recognised risk factors for depression:

- Having biological relatives with depression
- Having family members who have taken their own life
- Stressful life events, such as the death of a loved one or experiencing abuse (physical, emotional, intellectual, sexual and spiritual)
- Having depression as a youngster
- Illness, such as cancer, heart disease, Alzheimer's or HIV/AIDS
- Long-term use of certain medications, such as some drugs used to control high blood pressure, sleeping pills or, occasionally, birth control pills
- Certain personality traits, such as having low self-esteem and being overly dependent, self-critical or pessimistic
- Alcohol, nicotine and drug abuse
- Having recently given birth
- Being in a lower socioeconomic group

My integrated medical prescription for depression

Many of my female patients come to me with depression and at least 50 per cent of those are taking antidepressants. However, most are interested in addressing the underlying cause of their depression without drugs. I do not immediately take my patients off medications until the foundations of a new integrated medical treatment programme for depression are in place. It is vital, in my experience, that some time is spent identifying what factors (there are usually a couple) are contributing to the depression. For example, about six in ten people who stop taking their antidepressants after a few months get depressed again within a year, because they haven't dealt with the underlying causes. Once my patient is stable with her programme then I will look to help them gradually withdraw from their antidepressants. Some can do this without any problem, others may experience side-effects. Again, in my experience if you are addressing the underlying causes of depression, eating a healthy diet and taking the appropriate supplements, the latter is much less likely to happen.

Step 1 • Are you experiencing depression?

The brief screening questionnaire in part one, section two, is designed to alert you to the possibility that you might be experiencing depression. If you answer yes to the question it poses or you can associate with any of the descriptions that I have provided above then you should consult with your doctor to confirm the diagnosis and exclude medical causes of depression. These include post-viral illness, cancer (for example, cancer of the pancreas can present as depression), sleep apnoea, thyroid disease, Addison's disease, Cushing's disease, hyperparathyroidism, systemic lupus erythematosus, multiple sclerosis, stroke, addiction, alcohol abuse and alcohol withdrawal, stimulant withdrawal and the side-effects of certain medications such as steroids, cimetidine, blood pressure-lowering medication, anxiolytics and digoxin.

Your GP will probably then assess the severity of your depression. To find out how bad your depression is, your doctor first looks for one of the three key symptoms:

- Feeling sad or low most of the time

- Losing interest in things you used to enjoy

- Having no energy or feeling really tired

A depressed person will have at least one of these symptoms on most days, most of the time, for two weeks.

If you have a key symptom, your doctor will consider how many, if any, of the following symptoms you also have:

- Problems sleeping or sleeping too much

- Poor concentration or difficulty making decisions

- Low self-confidence

- Poor or increased appetite

- Thoughts of suicide

- Agitation or sluggishness

- Feelings of guilt for no reason

A doctor usually decides that someone with four of these symptoms has mild depression, someone with five or six symptoms has moderate depression, and someone with seven has severe depression.

In depression, women, when compared to men, also tend to report more frequent bodily symptoms, such as fatigue, and appetite and sleep disturbances.

Step 2 • Consider the medical options

Research has substantiated what many patients and health professionals working in the field of depression have suspected for a long time – that antidepressants are not the answer to depression. They certainly have their role to play for some people and you might want to consider them, for example, if you have severe depression, but for longstanding recovery from depression the integrated medical approach, which usually involves a psychological talking therapy, is now the preferred way forward.

If you have mild depression, it's unlikely that your GP will recommend antidepressants. However, he or she will recommend exercise and also a self-help programme based on a talking treatment called cognitive behaviour therapy. You'll probably be given some leaflets or books about this and your doctor or a nurse will see you regularly to find out how you're getting on.

If you have moderate depression your doctor may advise you to take an antidepressant called a selective serotonin reuptake inhibitor (SSRI). People with depression are more likely to stick with taking an SSRI than with taking the older types of antidepressant. SSRIs include fluoxetine (Prozac), fluvoxamine (Faverin), paroxetine (Seroxat), sertraline (Lustral) and citalopram (Cipramil). Possible side-effects of SSRIs include tiredness, dizziness, problems with sweating, nausea, headaches and dry mouth. SSRIs can cause withdrawal symptoms if you stop taking them suddenly or if your dose is reduced. The most common withdrawal symptoms are dizziness, sickness, headaches, a feeling that the room is spinning, and numbness or tingling feelings. Others are sweating, anxiety and problems sleeping.

I firmly believe that the majority of people with mild to moderate depression do not need antidepressants. One very important review of the studies relating to antidepressants and their effectiveness found that antidepressants do help severely depressed people, but for people with mild to moderate depression the effect is entirely due to the placebo effect – in other words belief and expectation.[1] For this reason, although there are some exceptions, I encourage most of my patients to try the remaining steps before using antidepressants.

Step 3 • Address the underlying causes

While I am going to make recommendations to treat your symptoms relating to depression using a variety of supplements, for lasting recovery from depression I encourage you to fill in the questionnaires in part one, section two, in order to identify possible root causes or contributors. In my experience, the ones to consider are:

- **Addictions** – Solution: Part Five (Addictions – page 260); Secret Four – Accept Yourself (page 113); Secret Three – Face and Embrace Your Emotions (page 94); Secret Five – Develop and Deepen Your Relationships (page 127); Holistic Health Tools – Mindfulness (page 147), Emotional Freedom Technique (page 151) and Values-based Goal Setting (page 166)

- **Stress** – Solution: Secret Two – De-stress and Relax (page 77); Holistic Health Tools – Emotional Freedom Technique (page 151) and Mindfulness (page 147)

- **Trauma** – Solution: Secret Three – Face and Embrace Your Emotions (page 94); Holistic Health Tools – Emotional Freedom Technique (page 151), EmoTrance (page 158) and Mindfulness (page 147)

- **Adrenal fatigue** – Solution: Part Five (Adrenal Fatigue – page 267); Secret Two – De-stress and Relax (page 77); Holistic Health Tools – Values-based Goal Setting (page 166) and Mindfulness (page 147)

- **Blood-sugar imbalance** – Solution: Secret One – Nurture Your Physical Body (Healthy Eating and Supplements – page 49)

- **Poor diet** – Solution: Secret One – Nurture Your Physical Body (Healthy Eating and Supplements – page 49)

- **Environmental toxicity** – Solution: Secret One – Nurture Your Physical Body (Healthy Environment and Sunlight – page 70), (mercury toxicity is a rare cause of depression that shouldn't be missed)

- **Food intolerances** – Solution: Part Five (Food Intolerances – page 344), (food intolerances to wheat and sugar are especially common); Holistic Health Tools – Emotional Freedom Technique (page 151)

- **Nutritional deficiencies** – Solution: Secret One – Nurture Your Physical Body (Healthy Eating and Supplements – page 49)

- **Parasites/candida** – Solution: Part Five (Dysbiosis – page 334); Holistic Health Tools – Emotional Freedom Technique (page 151)

- **Hypothyroidism** – Solution: Part Five (Hypothyroidism – page 356); Holistic Health Tools – Emotional Freedom Technique (page 151) and The Work (page 163)

- **Lack of physical activity** – Solution: Secret One – Nurture Your Physical Body (Physical Activity and Touch – page 67); Holistic Health Tools – Emotional Freedom Technique (page 151) and Values-based Goal Setting (page 166)

- **Low self-acceptance** – Solution: Secret Four – Accept Yourself (page 113); Secret Three – Face and Embrace Your Emotions (page 94); Secret Five – Develop and Deepen Your Relationships (page 127); Holistic Health Tools – Mindfulness (page 147), Emotional Freedom Technique (page 151) and Values-based Goal Setting (page 166)

Step 4 • Start a depression recovery supplement programme

When used alongside step three, certain nutritional supplements can help to alleviate many of the symptoms of depression. My integrated medicine prescription for depression usually includes a combination of:

- **A multivitamin-mineral supplement** as deficiencies of vitamin C, various B vitamins, folic acid, magnesium and zinc are associated with an increased incidence and severity of depression.

- **Folic acid** (400mcg to 800mcg) as studies suggest that between 15 per cent and 38 per cent of people with depression have low folic levels in their bodies and those with very low levels tend to be the most depressed.[2] One study involving 127 people with severe depression found that folate supplements at a dose of 500mcg significantly improved the effectiveness of fluoxetine (Prozac) in women, but not men.[3]

- **Vitamin C with bioflavanoids** (1000mg) as an antioxidant and to support health.

- **Chromium** (600mcg a day), particularly if your depression is associated with weight gain, heavy arms/legs, cravings for sweets/carbohydrates and a feeling of grogginess. A trial conducted with Cornell University found that eight weeks of treatment with chromium resulted in a significant improvement in depression of 65 per cent of those on chromium versus 33 per cent of those on a placebo.[4]

- **Fish oil** (3000mg to 10,000mg), because there is some preliminary evidence that omega-3 essential fatty acids might help reduce depression symptoms and enhance the effectiveness of antidepressants.[5]

As an alternative to antidepressants, some patients prefer to take a natural supplement to help lift their mood. The ones that I tend to use with my patients are either 5-HTP or St John's wort.

- **5-HTP** (50mg to 100mg twice a day) is the precursor amino acid to the feel-good mood neurotransmitter serotonin. 5-HTP is produced commercially by extraction from the seeds of the African plant *Griffonia simplicifolia*, and its mood-stabilising effects are believed to result from its ability to increase the production of serotonin levels in the brain. One trial found that 5-HTP was equally effective as the antidepressant fluvoxamine.[6]

- **St John's wort** (300mg three times daily, standardised to 0.9mg hypericin) is the most well studied of all the alternative, natural antidepressants. In Germany, more than 50 per cent of patients with mild or moderate depression, anxiety and sleep disorders are treated with St John's wort. In a double-blind trial using standard 20mg per day amounts of fluoxetine (Prozac), St John's wort extract in the amount of 400mg twice daily was equally effective at relieving depression in people aged 60 to 80 years.[7] This herb also has immune-stimulating and female hormone-balancing properties, and is effective in relieving the symptoms associated with seasonal affective disorder (depression related to lack of sunshine during the winter months). You shouldn't take St John's wort if you are taking the oestrogen contraceptive pill, antidepressants, warfarin, digoxin, MAO inhibitors or if you have a diagnosis of manic depression.

Step 5 • Consider other complementary approaches

- **An online depression recovery course** is a free resource that provides you with a complete psychological programme for recovering from depression. See Resources.

- **Alphastim SCS** is a medical device I usually recommend to patients who don't want to deal with the underlying issues of their depression. It's been shown in a number of clinical trials to significantly relieve the symptoms of depression, anxiety and insomnia in the majority of users, and most of my patients have benefited considerably from using it. For more information visit www.mindbodyproducts.com.

- **A lightbox** can help patients with seasonal affective disorder. Regular exposure to full-spectrum lighting can result in a significant improvement within just a couple of weeks. See Resources.

- **Complementary therapies** such as cognitive behavioural therapy, acceptance and commitment therapy, solution-focused brief therapy, acupuncture, music therapy, art therapy, hypnotherapy, homeopathy, Bach Flower Remedies, spiritual healing, yoga, t'ai chi and meditation have helped some patients with depression.

For recommended books, therapies and websites see Resources.

Diabetes

⁓

Diabetes is one of the major health challenges of our time, affecting over 2.3 million people in the UK,[1] and it's getting more common – in 1994, two in a hundred women had diabetes, compared with between three and four out of a hundred in 2003.[2] One report estimated that 500,000 women in the UK have diabetes, but don't know it.[3]

In most healthy people blood-sugar levels are stable, but the blood sugars of someone with diabetes increase beyond normal levels, because of disruption in the use or production of insulin, a hormone that helps to transport glucose into the cells of the body. The high blood-sugar levels cause damage in two primary ways. The first is glycation, in which the glucose (sugar) reacts with proteins in the body rendering them non-functional, leading to possible inflammation, nerve damage, heart problems and blindness. The second is oxidative damage, in which an excessive amount of chemicals called free radicals are generated in the body, also leading to widespread damage to many of the major organs in your body, including your heart, blood vessels, nerves, eyes and kidneys.

Having diabetes significantly increases the chances of you developing chest pain (angina), heart attack, stroke, narrowing of the arteries (atherosclerosis) and high blood pressure, skin and gum infections, kidney damage (nephropathy), damage to nerves causing tingling, pain, burning or numbness (neuropathy), damage to your eyes (diabetic retinopathy), as well as increased risk of developing cataracts and glaucoma, foot damage (reduced blood flow and increased risk of infection) and osteoporosis. Keeping your blood-sugar level close to normal most of the time can dramatically reduce the risk of these complications.

What causes diabetes?

There are two types of diabetes, each of which has different causes.

Type I diabetes occurs when the body is unable to produce enough insulin to maintain a stable blood-sugar level. This is an autoimmune disease in which the body attacks and destroys the beta cells in the pancreas that make insulin. This might be due to a combination of genetic vulnerability and a triggering event such as an infection. It has also been suggested that some people with a cow's milk allergy have antibodies that are capable of cross-reacting with the pancreas's beta cells. Type I diabetes accounts for about 5 to 10 per cent of cases. Because type I diabetics can no longer make insulin, insulin replacement therapy is essential.

Type II diabetes occurs when the body progressively becomes resistant to the effects of insulin. Unlike type I diabetes, which tends to appear before the age of 40, this tends to appear after 40. Type II diabetes is associated with being overweight, excessive consumption of sugar, stimulants and refined foods, genetic predisposition, sedentary lifestyle and malnutrition.

What are the risk factors?

Your risk of developing type I diabetes increases if you have a parent or sibling who has type I diabetes.

In type II diabetes the following are recognised risk factors:

- Metabolic syndrome (see page 368)

- Being overweight

- Inactivity

- Family history – if a parent or sibling has type II diabetes you are more likely to develop it

- Race – African Americans, Latinos, Native Americans, Asian Americans, Afro-Caribbeans and Asians are more likely to develop type II diabetes

- Age – as you get older, especially after age 45, you are more likely to develop type II diabetes

- Prediabetes – your blood-sugar level is higher than normal, but not high enough to be classified as diabetic

- Gestational diabetes – if you developed gestational diabetes when pregnant or gave birth to a baby weighing more than nine pounds, you are more likely to develop type II diabetes

My integrated medical prescription for diabetes

The good news is that if you are prediabetic or in the early stages of type II diabetes, by making significant changes to your diet and lifestyle you can halt the progression of the disease, prevent the complications I discussed earlier and even (in the case of prediabetes) prevent it from becoming diabetes. It is, however, very important that you work with an integrated medical doctor or health professional who is experienced in helping people with diabetes as the exact nature of the treatment depends on a lot of different factors, including what type of diabetes you have, whether it's type I or type II, the stage of your disease (for example the treatment for people with early type II is different to late stage type II) and whether complications are present or not.

If you have type I diabetes the treatment is always insulin. However, some of the supplements below might help to offset potential complications and damage to the body. If you have type II diabetes, it is important to both increase insulin sensitivity and protect the body from damage related to glycation and oxidative stress.

If you are already receiving treatment for diabetes and do decide to implement some of my suggestions, it's important you tell your GP and monitor your blood-sugar levels, especially if you are already taking insulin.

Step 1 • Do you have diabetes or prediabetes?

Quite often diabetes might be picked up as a coincidental finding if you are being investigated for another health problem. Many people with prediabetes or early stage type II diabetes won't have any symptoms and that is why it can be so hard to detect. For those that do have symptoms the most common ones are:

- Polyuria – the need to urinate frequently
- Polydipsia – increased thirst and fluid intake
- Polyphagia – increased appetite

More specifically, symptoms for type I diabetes include:

- Extreme thirst
- Dry mouth
- Frequent urination
- Loss of weight
- Weakness or fatigue
- Blurred vision

Symptoms for type II diabetes include:

- Blurred vision
- Cuts or sores that take a long time to heal
- Itching skin or yeast infections
- Excessive thirst
- Dry mouth
- Frequent urination
- Leg pain

Type I diabetics can also present as an emergency due to extremely high levels of blood glucose. This might cause a variety of symptoms, including nausea, vomiting, fever, stomach pain and a sweet, fruity smell on your breath. If you have any of these symptoms you should see your GP, who will arrange to take a blood sample. There are a number of tests that can be performed. They include:

- **Random glucose test** – glucose levels are taken at a random time on two occasions and any figure above 11.1mmol/L is a diagnosis of diabetes (mmol/L = millimoles per litre).

- **Fasting glucose test** – glucose levels are measured after an overnight fast and on two different days, with a figure above 7.0mmol/L being a diagnosis of diabetes.

- **Oral glucose tolerance test** – this can be carried out if the diagnosis is still unclear after these tests or if you have symptoms or risk factors associated with diabetes. It is the most reliable test for diagnosing diabetes. You will be asked to fast overnight and then blood samples are taken from you before, and two hours after, consuming a glucose-containing drink. A two-hour blood glucose level above 11.1mmol/L is a diagnosis of diabetes. A level below 7.8mmol/L is normal. If the level falls between these values you have what is called impaired glucose tolerance. This is a prediabetes state, in which you are at a higher risk of developing heart disease and diabetes.

If you are diagnosed as having diabetes, your doctor will want to arrange other tests to check on your thyroid, liver, kidneys and cholesterol.

Step 2 • Consider the medical options

In type I diabetes the treatment is replacement insulin. Your doctor will prescribe insulin as an injection to help you keep the fluctuations in your blood sugar as close to normal as possible. Doing so should enable you to live a healthy life with minimum complications. Most insulin is genetically engineered and very similar to the insulin that your body produces (or used to produce). The exact dosing schedule will be personalised by your doctor or nurse to meet your unique requirements.

The biggest challenge in using insulin therapy is trying to keep your blood-sugar levels in a normal range. If you take too much insulin you could get hypoglycaemia, in which your blood-sugar levels drop to low. If you don't take enough insulin you might get hyperglycaemia in which your blood-sugar levels go to high.

In type II diabetes you will be given advice on losing weight, dietary and lifestyle changes and also be offered one or more medications to help control your blood-sugar levels.

Metformin is one of the most commonly prescribed.[4] It works by causing your liver to make less glucose and by making your muscles increase their use of glucose. Unlike some other diabetes drugs it doesn't usually cause weight gain. Side-effects include nausea, diarrhoea and a rare condition called lactic acidosis. The latter most commonly occurs in people over the age of 65 or those who have an existing heart or kidney problem.

Sulphonylurea is a group of medications that may be recommended instead of or in addition to metformin. These drugs can help because they stimulate your pancreas to put more insulin into your bloodstream. Side-effects include weight gain and an increased risk of developing a low blood-sugar level.[5]

While both of the medications are invaluable to women with type II diabetes, I find that most of my patients who follow steps three and four can either reduce their dose or stop them completely. This should, however, only be done while being supervised by a health professional.

In addition to taking medications:

- Monitoring your blood-sugar levels is very important. Your doctor or diabetes nurse will tell you how often you need to check your blood-sugar level using a pin-prick glucose test. It's usually between one and four times a day.

- Another test your GP will arrange from time to time (every three to six months) is called haemoglobin A1c (HbA1c for short). Its level gives your doctor an idea of your average blood glucose level over the previous few weeks. Haemoglobin A1c is a chemical found in your blood. Keeping your haemoglobin A1c below 7.5 per cent indicates that you are much less likely to get complications.[6]

- You will also be invited to have a yearly check-up with your GP in order to make sure that you stay as healthy as possible and that if complications are occurring they are picked up and addressed quickly.

Step 3 • Address the underlying causes

While type I diabetes definitely needs to be treated using insulin, for type II diabetes and also prediabetes it is possible to halt the progression and reduce the risk of complications by addressing the underlying causes and contributors. To help you with this I encourage you to fill in the questionnaires in part one, section two, in order to identify possible root causes or contributors. In my experience, the ones to consider are:

- **Excessive weight** – Solution: Secret One – Nurture Your Physical Body (Healthy Eating and Supplements – page 49); Part Five (Weight Loss – page 401); Holistic Health Tools – Emotional Freedom Technique (page 151) and The Work (page 163)

- **Blood-sugar imbalance** – Solution: Secret One – Nurture Your Physical Body (Healthy Eating and Supplements – page 49)

- **Stress** – Solution: Secret Two – De-stress and Relax (page 77); Holistic Health Tools – Emotional Freedom Technique (page 151) and Mindfulness (page 147)

- **Poor diet** – Solution: Secret One – Nurture Your Physical Body (Healthy Eating and Supplements – page 49)

- **Food intolerances** – Solution: Part Five (Food Intolerances – page 344); Holistic Health Tools – Emotional Freedom Technique (page 151)

- **Nutritional deficiencies** – Solution: Secret One – Nurture Your Physical Body (Healthy Eating and Supplements – page 49)

- **Lack of physical activity** – Solution: Secret One – Nurture Your Physical Body (Physical Activity and Touch – page 67); Holistic

Health Tools – Emotional Freedom Technique (page 151) and Values-based Goal Setting (page 166)

- **PCOS** – Solution: Part Five (Addictions – page 260), (smoking increases the likelihood of you developing heart and circulation problems considerably); Secret Four – Accept Yourself (page 113); Secret Three – Face and Embrace Your Emotions (page 94); Secret Five – Develop and Deepen Your Relationships (page 127); Holistic Health Tools – Mindfulness (page 147), Emotional Freedom Technique (page 151) and Values-based Goal Setting (page 166)

Step 4 • Start a diabetes support supplement programme

When used alongside step three, certain nutritional supplements can help you to achieve a normal blood glucose, and also prevent and possibly reverse the complications associated with diabetes. Because these suggestions may influence your blood-sugar levels, you must inform your GP and monitor your blood sugar carefully. My integrated medicine prescription for prediabetes and diabetes would usually include:

- **A multivitamin-mineral supplement**, plus a total daily dose of magnesium (500mg), which is involved in insulin production and utilisation. In one study supplementation with a multiple vitamin and mineral preparation for one year reduced the risk of infection in people with diabetes by more than 80 per cent, compared with a placebo.[7]

- **Vitamin C with bioflavanoids** (1000mg to 3000mg) to reduce inflammation, act as an antioxidant and help reduce diabetes-associated complications.[8]

- **Evening primrose oil** (4g per day) has been found in double-blind research to improve nerve function and to relieve pain symptoms of diabetic neuropathy.[9]

- **Chromium** supplements (200mcg three times daily) have been found in some, but not all, studies to be effective in restoring normal insulin function in people with type II diabetes.[10]

- **Gymnema sylvestre** (400mg daily) is a plant extract that appears to stimulate insulin production. This has been found to reduce insulin requirements in people with type I diabetes and also help normalise blood-sugar levels in people with type II diabetes.[11]

- **Alpha lipoic acid** (800mg per day) is a powerful antioxidant, which improves insulin sensitivity, and prevents and treats diabetic neuropathy, as well as reducing damage to blood vessels.[12]

Step 5 • Consider other complementary approaches

While there is no definitive evidence that these can help you with your diabetes, some patients find the following useful in supporting their programme: acupuncture, homeopathy, massage, spiritual healing, yoga, traditional Chinese medicine and Ayurvedic medicine.

For recommended books and websites see Resources

Dysbiosis

Dysbiosis refers to a condition in which the normal healthy population of beneficial bacteria in the intestines has been disrupted, leaving it open to the overgrowth of yeast, fungi, parasites and potentially harmful strains of bacteria. This intestinal imbalance then adversely affects other important organ systems via toxic stress and by interfering with nutrient absorption and utilisation.

What causes dysbiosis?

One intriguing theory is that some people with irritable bowel syndrome (IBS) actually have a type of dysbiosis called small intestinal bacterial overgrowth (SIBO). The entire gastrointestinal tract contains over 500 different species of bacteria, the highest frequency of which reside in the colon (at least 1,000,000,000 bacteria per ml of fluid), with much lower numbers in the small intestine (less than 10,000 bacteria per ml of fluid). SIBO occurs when abnormally large numbers of bacteria (at least 100,000 bacteria per ml of fluid) are present in the small intestine and the types of bacteria resemble those normally found in the colon rather than the small intestine. Typical symptoms of SIBO are not too dissimilar to those of IBS and they include abdominal pain, flatulence, abdominal bloating and distension and diarrhoea. Occasionally patients with SIBO have chronic constipation rather than diarrhoea. When the overgrowth is severe and prolonged, the bacteria may interfere with the digestion and/or absorption of food, and vitamin and mineral deficiencies may develop.

What are the risk factors?

The following increase the likelihood of experiencing dysbiosis:

- History of antibiotic use
- Birth control pill use
- Steroid use
- Low fibre intake
- High sugar/processed food intake
- Excessive alcohol consumption
- Stress

My integrated medical prescription for dysbiosis

Because dysbiosis is underdiagnosed, the first challenge is to consider it as a diagnosis and then find a practitioner with the expertise to help you. If you are considering dysbiosis as a possible contributor to your symptoms, my recommendation is to work with a nutritional therapist or integrated medical doctor. The real key to successful treatment is to identify which bacteria, parasites and yeasts are growing, and then, having done so, to treat them while also addressing other issues, such as low stomach acid levels, low digestive enzyme levels and deficiencies in certain probiotics.

Step 1 • Do you have dysbiosis?

If you scored more than ten on the dysbiosis questionnaire in part one, section two, then the next step is to book an appointment with a nutritional therapist or integrated medical doctor who can arrange a test called the Comprehensive Digestive Stool Analysis with Parasitology (CDSAP) 2.0 test (see Resources). This will tell you what type of dysbiosis you are experiencing (if any), how well you are digesting and absorbing your food, whether you have blood in your stool, how your intestinal immune function is doing, and what antibiotic and anti-fungal preparations, both herbal and drug, you should use to treat the dysbiosis. It's an invaluable test.

Once the results come back your practitioner will be able to use the information to decide whether you have a fungal dysbiosis, a bacterial dysbiosis and/or a parasite dysbiosis. Usually it's a combination. As a general rule of thumb, if you do have any of these you will need to treat them for a *minimum* of six months and maybe up to 12 months. While your practitioner will tailor a programme to you, here is an overview of how I go about treating the patients who come to see me.

Step 2 • Consider the medical options

Fungal dysbiosis treatment
To treat a fungal dysbiosis, such as infection with candida albicans, requires a commitment to changing your diet, taking supplements and/or medications, and tackling the underlying causes. In a nutshell, if fungal dysbiosis is diagnosed, I recommend:

- For a minimum of six weeks avoid all sugar, including fruit juices, fruits, honey, molasses, fructose, maple syrup, corn syrup, chocolate and sucrose, and all foods containing yeast, such as dried fruit, peanut butter, chocolate, cakes, wheat, dairy produce, mushrooms, mouldy cheese and tomato ketchup.

- After six weeks, I ask my patients to cautiously reintroduce one or two portions of fresh fruit a day – apples and pears tend to be best tolerated.

- Consider taking a herbal anti-fungal. The CDSAP 2.0 test will tell you which ones will work. Ones to consider include: mycopril (a fatty acid derived from coconut oil), grapefruit seed extract, berberine, oregano and garlic.

- To support your immune system, try taking a mix of organic mushroom tinctures or Biobran MGN-3 (a natural compound made from breaking down rice bran with enzymes from the shiitake mushroom). Both of these can help to build a healthy immune system by activating the body's natural killer cells. See Resources.

- Consider taking an anti-fungal medication. This will need to be prescribed by a doctor, and because they have the potential for side-effects you will need to be monitored. The most effective anti-fungals in my experience are sporanox (itraconazole), nizoral (ketoconazole) and diflucan (fluconazole), Lamisil (Terbinafine HCL) and nystatin.

- Take an oxygenated magnesium product. This is what I use with at least 80 per cent of my patients who have a confirmed diagnosis of fungal dysbiosis and, as long as the underlying imbalances are being treated, I find it to be very successful in treating fungal dysbiosis. See Resources.

- I also like to alkalise the body with alkaline mineral salts, and support the bowels and liver with a variety of nutrients and supplements, such as milk thistle, artichoke and psyllium husks.

Parasite dysbiosis treatment

This should only be done under supervision of an integrated medical doctor or nutritional therapist. In practice, most people with parasite infections need to be treated with anti-parasite medications. The results of the CDSAP 2.0 test will guide your doctor in choosing which medication to use. However, the most common and effective ones include: metronidazole, paromomycin and doxycycline.

You can sometimes strike it lucky with herbal anti-parasite formulas, such as oregano, black walnut hull, fenugreek, goldenseal, grapefruit seed extract and wormwood. However, you really need the CDSAP 2.0 results to guide you.

Once the parasites have been successfully treated – you should know because you feel significantly better – you should consider precautions to prevent a further parasite infection. Here are a couple of tips:

- When travelling take a lactobacillus probiotic supplement and an anti-parasite formula, to prevent infection

- Drink clean, pure water

- Avoid raw or undercooked beef, chicken, pork and fish

- Avoid fruit and vegetables that are not properly washed, and don't eat the skin of fruits

- Wash your hands after handling pets or working outdoors

- Never let your pets lick your face or your plates

- Worm your pets regularly

Bacterial dysbiosis treatment

The successful treatment of bacterial dysbiosis, the most common of which is small intestinal bacterial overgrowth (SIBO), relies on eating a specialised diet similar to the one mentioned in fungal dybisosis, plus taking anti-bacterial treatments (medicinal and herbal) and pro-biotics or prebiotics. An improvement in irritable bowel syndrome (IBS) symptoms while taking antibiotics is a strong indicator that bac-terial overgrowth might be a contributor to IBS.

One of the most immediate ways to improve the symptoms asso-ciated with SIBO is to reduce your carbohydrate intake. Ingested car-bohydrates are fermented by the bacteria in the small intestine and in turn produce toxic waste products such as organic acids (acetic acid, lactic acid) and hydrogen sulphide (H_2S), all of which are potentially toxic in increased amounts and can lead to an acidification of the body. Your diet should therefore be low in sugars, cereals and grains, and low in fruit and starchy vegetables, such as potatoes. Because this diet is fairly restrictive, you should really see a nutritional therapist who can help to create a healthy eating programme for you.

- The most common drug of choice for treating SIBO is neomycin and metronidazole.

- Herbal treatment options include grapefruit seed extract, garlic, ginger, olive leaf extract, berberine and Echinacea. The exact ones you need to use will be determined by the CDSAP 2.0 results.

- To prevent fungal overgrowth I recommend taking either an anti-fungal medication and probiotic or an oxygenated magnesium product and acidophilus probiotic as well. See Resources.

Eczema

While mild eczema doesn't tend to cause that much physical or emotional distress for some women, for others severe eczema or eczema that is located on exposed parts of the body, such as the face, breasts, legs or hands, can be a source of misery and even trigger depression and anxiety. Eczema is essentially inflamed itchy skin.

What causes eczema?

The two main types of eczema are atopic and contact dermatitis. The first tends to present early in childhood, is related to allergies and is made worse following exposure to various foods, dust and pollen. The second is an allergic response to an irritant such as soaps, metals, wool, cosmetics, jewellery, feathers, plants and environmental pollutants.

What are the risk factors?

There are many possible causes of eczema, including genetic inheritance, stress, vitamin and mineral deficiencies, candida, food intolerances, constipation or gut health imbalance, low levels of stomach acid, and deficiency or inability to process essential fatty acids. The following are known to worsen the symptoms and signs associated with eczema: long, hot baths or showers, dry skin, stress, sweating, low humidity, soaps, sand, dust and cigarette smoke.

My integrated medical prescription for eczema

One of the limitations of the conventional medical approach to dealing with eczema is the one-pointed focus on treating the eczema, without paying attention to the underlying causes. In integrated medicine it's even more important to address the underlying causes, for example constipation or food intolerances, since this can lead to a complete resolution of the problem.

Step 1 • Do you have eczema?

Skin with eczema may be itchy, pink or red, dry and flaky, broken and bleeding and/or thick and tough. If the skin becomes infected you might experience crusty yellow blisters, bumps filled with pus, and wet, oozing areas of skin where the blisters have burst. Eczema is especially common in the natural creases of the body, such as behind the knees and inside the elbow.

If you have any of these symptoms and signs you should go to your GP who can usually make a diagnosis for you. If he or she thinks it might be due to allergies, they will probably give you a referral to a dermatologist (skin specialist) in order to find out exactly what it is you are intolerant to.

Step 2 • Consider the medical options

To treat the symptoms of eczema most doctors will offer you a moisturiser to reduce the itchiness and appearance of dryness, and also a steroid ointment or cream, which will help reduce the irritation, itching and inflammation. Ointments are best when the eczema is very dry, and creams or lotions are good when the eczema is weeping. While they work, if used repeatedly at high dosages they can lead to a thinning of the skin. The key is to use the lowest strength steroid that is most effective for the shortest period of time. While I don't tend to recommend using steroid creams or ointments as the mainstay of treating eczema, they can be very useful for treating flare-ups, while you wait for the effects of more natural approaches to kick in.

Step 3 • Address the underlying causes

While I am going to make recommendations to treat your eczema symptoms using a variety of supplements, for lasting resolution I encourage you to fill in the questionnaires in part one, section two, in order to identify possible root causes or contributors. In my experience, the ones to consider are:

- **Food intolerances** – Solution: Part Five (Food Intolerances – page 344), (the most common culprits are wheat, cows' milk, eggs, citrus fruits and chocolate); Holistic Health Tools – Emotional Freedom Technique (page 151)

- **Poor diet** – Solution: Secret One – Nurture Your Physical Body (Healthy Eating and Supplements – page 49)

- **Nutritional deficiencies** – Solution: Secret One – Nurture Your Physical Body (Healthy Eating and Supplements – page 49)

- **Lack of digestive enzymes/stomach acid** – Solution: Secret One – Nurture Your Physical Body (Healthy Eating and Supplements – page 49)

- **Constipation** – Solution: Secret One – Nurture Your Physical Body (Healthy Eating and Supplements – page 49); Part Five (Constipation – page 312)

- **Candida** – Solution: Part Five (Dysbiosis – page 334); Holistic Health Tools – Emotional Freedom Technique (page 151)

- **Stress** – Solution: Secret Two – De-stress and Relax (page 77); Holistic Health Tools – Emotional Freedom Technique (page 151) and Mindfulness (page 147)

- **Allergy causing substances** – Solution: as far as you can, avoid substances such as soaps, metals, wool, cosmetics, jewellery, feathers, plants and environmental pollutants

Step 4 • Start an eczema supplement programme

When used alongside step three, certain nutritional supplements may help to alleviate the symptoms of eczema, although the research evidence for their effectiveness is not that strong. The key in my experience is to address the underlying causes discussed above. My integrated medicine prescription for eczema would usually include:

- **A multivitamin-mineral supplement,** plus an additional daily dose of **zinc** (30mg three times daily), **beta-carotene** (10,000IU twice daily) and to support skin healing, **vitamin E** (400IU daily for one month).

- **Vitamin C with bioflavanoids** (1000mg to 3000mg) to reduce inflammation.

- **Fish oil** (3000mg to 10,000mg a day) to provide anti-inflammatory essential fatty acids.

- **Acidophilus probiotic** to ensure that there are sufficient numbers of 'friendly' bacteria in the gut, as this helps to reduce gut-related inflammation that may contribute to eczema.

Step 5 • Consider other complementary approaches

As an alternative to steroids and moisturisers such as E45, I usually recommend a range of products produced by a company called Elena's Nature Collection. They offer a range of all-natural shampoos, soaps, oils and creams, which when used together can help to support the skin's healing and regeneration. I find them to be particularly effective for relieving eczema. See Resources.

While there is no definitive evidence that these can help you with your eczema, some patients find the following useful in supporting their programme: acupuncture, homeopathy, colonic hydrotherapy, spiritual healing, yoga, traditional Chinese medicine and Ayurvedic medicine.

For recommended books see Resources.

Food intolerances

~

Food intolerance is a word that is used to describe a range of detrimental responses to a specific food or food ingredient. It can include allergic reactions which involve the immune system (such as peanut allergy or coeliac disease); reactions resulting from enzyme deficiencies (such as lactose intolerance, which affects 70 per cent of the world's population, but much fewer people of North European descent – about 2 per cent); sensitivities to certain types of food (such as yeast in people with candida); or pharmacological reactions (such as caffeine or sugar sensitivity). The most common food intolerances are due to cows' milk and cheese, wheat, gluten (found in wheat, rye, barley and oats), corn, beef, yeast, eggs, garlic, nuts, seeds, kiwi and soya.

What causes food intolerances?

Some food intolerances, for example lactose intolerance, are genetically inherited, whereas many others arise because of an overconsumption of certain food products (for example bread) combined with a condition called leaky gut syndrome. This is a condition in which the spaces in between the cells that line the intestines become irritated, inflamed and, as the name suggests, leaky. This allows undigested food to pass through into the blood, the body reacts to these 'foreign invaders' and the immune system is activated, leading to widespread inflammation and food allergies or sensitivities.

What are the risk factors?

While there are no definitive risk factors, the following appear likely to increase the probability of suffering from food intolerances:

- Impaired gut immunity (IgA is a specific type of antibody made in the gut in response to the presence of potential invaders)

- Intestinal infections – yeast, candida and parasites

- Excess alcohol

- NSAIDS/steroids

- Bowel disease

- Stress

- Lack of stomach acid and digestive enzymes

My integrated medical prescription for food intolerances

I suspect that food intolerances are probably overdiagnosed in a lot of people, particularly those with anxiety and food addictions, but underdiagnosed in people with chronic health complaints that can't be fully explained. As a general rule of thumb, however, if my patients experience symptoms that involve the digestive system, I will consider food intolerances as a possible cause and offer them testing. If the test comes back positive, it's not just simply a case of avoiding those foods, it's just as important to address the underlying factors that triggered the food intolerances in the first place.

Step 1 • Do you have food intolerances?

A score of ten or more on the food intolerance questionnaire in part one, section two, may indicate that food intolerances are contributing to your symptoms. One of the classic ways to identify what foods might potentially be contributing to your symptoms is to go on an elimination diet. This restricted diet removes all of the most allergenic foods (such as wheat and dairy) from your diet for a ten-day period and then reintroduces them at defined intervals, usually every couple of days, while monitoring whether any symptoms return. This can be very useful, but in practice most people struggle to do it and for that reason I tend to stick with blood tests.

IgG Elisa blood test

As its name suggests this blood test measures levels of IgG antibodies in relation to various different foods. This is helpful to know because about 80 per cent of food allergies are mediated by IgG. Some companies now offer a testing kit that allows you to discover what you are intolerant to in the comfort of your own home. All they need from you is a small sample of blood, which you can collect yourself. They will then analyse it and tell you which foods you are reacting to. The limitation of this test is that if you have leaky gut, the likelihood of you developing IgG antibodies to foods that you consume regularly is highly probable anyway. For that reason I prefer to use the food allergen cellular test (FACT), described below. See Resources.

Food allergen cellular test

This test measures levels of the inflammatory chemicals released from white blood cells when they are exposed to various food allergens. The nice thing about this test is that it will pick up IgG and IgA immune responses, as well as other non-immune responses. This makes it the allergy test of choice. The only downside, apart from cost, is that you will need to have blood taken from you in order to have the test done. See Resources.

Step 2 • Consider the medical options

Western medicine doesn't really recognise food intolerances as a contributor to ill-health, so it is unlikely that your GP will be able to help or advise you. If you have an allergy to food then he or she will be able to refer you to an allergy specialist. A food allergy refers to an immune system response to one or more proteins within a specific food. The classical true allergy is type I or immediate-onset allergy. In this case a food substance, such as peanut or prawn, triggers an immediate release of histamine and other inflammatory chemicals from a group of antibodies called IgE. These give rise to symptoms including an itchy red rash, shortness of breath, wheezing and swelling of the lips, mouth and throat, stomach cramps, vomiting and diarrhoea. The reactions can be severe and life-threatening. Your doctor will probably arrange for a radioallergosorbent (RAST) test, which looks for the presence of food-specific IgE in the blood, and then make recommendations based on that.

Step 3 • Address the underlying causes

While I am going to make recommendations to reduce the negative impact of food intolerances on your health, for lasting resolution of non-genetic food intolerances I encourage you to fill in the questionnaires in part one, section two, in order to identify possible root causes or contributors. In my experience, the ones to consider are:

- **Leaky gut syndrome** – Solution: avoid alcohol and treat with nutritional supplementation (see step four below for suggested supplements)

- **Stress** – Solution: Secret Two – De-stress and Relax (page 77), (stress suppresses the body's immune system); Holistic Health Tools – Emotional Freedom Technique (page 151) and Mindfulness (page 147)

- **Dysbiosis (fungal/parasites/bacteria)** – Solution: Part Five (Dysbiosis – page 334)

- **Poor diet** – Solution: Secret One – Nurture Your Physical Body (Healthy Eating and Supplements – page 49)

- **Lack of digestive enzymes/stomach acid** – Solution: Secret One – Nurture Your Physical Body (Healthy Eating and Supplements – page 49)

- **Trauma** – Solution: Secret Three – Face and Embrace Your Emotions (page 94); Holistic Health Tools – Emotional Freedom Technique (page 151), EmoTrance (page 158) and Mindfulness (page 147),

(occasionally, although rarely, food intolerances and allergies are caused by a certain food being present at the same time as you went through a trauma – negative association is formed with that food leading to a reaction when eaten)

Step 4 • Start a food intolerance supplement programme

When used alongside step three, certain nutritional supplements can help to alleviate many of the symptoms associated with food intolerances. My integrated medicine prescription for food intolerances would usually include:

- **A multivitamin-mineral supplement**.

- **Vitamin C with bioflavonoids** (1000mg to 3000mg) to reduce inflammation and the allergy response.

- **Omega-3, 6 and 9** (taken in capsule or liquid form in a 2:1:1 ratio) to provide the body with anti-inflammatory essential fatty acids.

- **L-glutamine** (5g just before bedtime), an amino acid powder that can help to repair the lining of the small intestine (leaky gut).

- **Butyric acid** (1200mg a day) feeds the cells of the intestinal lining and is essential in maintaining the integrity of the gastro-intestinal wall.

- **A comprehensive digestive enzyme formula** should be taken with each main meal if you get bloating or wind after eating and/or have undigested food in your stool.

- **Acidophilus probiotic** to ensure that there are sufficient numbers of 'friendly' bacteria in the gut as this helps to support healthy gut and immune function.

- **Betaine hydrochloride** can help to improve stomach acid levels. See Resources.

Step 5 • Consider other complementary approaches

Once you have your test results back, you should ideally avoid or limit your consumption of the intolerance-evoking foods for at least three months. Then, having taken the supplements above, you might either choose to remain off the foods which you can't tolerate or re-introduce them back into your diet on a rotating basis, for example every third day.

Here are some alternatives to the main foods that my patients have intolerances to:

- Cows' dairy produce – goat milk, sheep milk, almond milk, rice milk

- Wheat – rye, barley, oat cakes, quinoa, buckwheat, millet

- Gluten – rice, quinoa, buckwheat, millet, corn, potato flour, sago, tapioca

For recommended books see Resources.

Headaches and migraines

~

Headaches and migraines are a real problem for women. While 80 per cent of women will get episodic, tension-type headaches from time to time, about one in 50 women will get chronic tension headaches.[1] The condition counts as chronic if you get tension headaches more than 15 days a month for at least three months. Separate to headaches are migraines, which affect 15 per cent of the population and women three times more frequently than men.[2]

What causes headaches and migraines?

There are many different types of headaches each of which have different causes:

- Tension headaches are, as the name suggests, caused by a build-up of stress and tension in and round the head, neck and back

- Migraines are caused by altered blood flow to the brain – when you have an attack the blood vessels in your brain open up (dilate), allowing more blood to flow through them

- Headaches can be sometimes related to exercise, sex or bouts of coughing, but it's not clear what causes this

What are the risk factors?

The risk factors for tension headaches include:

- Anxiety

- Depression

- Stress

- Sleep disturbances

- Obesity

- Overuse of caffeine

- Overuse of pain medication

- Neck and/or back problems

- Allergies and snoring

The risk factors for migraines include:

- Hormonal disturbances

- Genetic factors

- Stress

- Food intolerances

- Sleep deprivation

- Fatigue

- Eye strain

- Excessive intake or withdrawal from caffeine, alcohol, sugar and drugs

- Low blood sugar

- Excessive exercise

- Nutritional imbalances

Some women report that their migraines start shortly before or after the onset of their period.

My integrated medical prescription for headaches/migraines

Because it's so important to receive an accurate diagnosis before treating headaches and especially migraines symptomatically, I encourage you to see your GP in order to get a diagnosis first. However, because of its focus on dealing with the underlying problems, integrated medicine has a lot to offer you.

Step 1 • What type of headache do you have?

There are many different types of headaches, so to help you work out what type you have, I invite you to read through the following:

- If your headaches are dull and achy, the most likely headache type is a tension headache. They usually feel like a tight band around your head. They can last from 20 minutes to a few days.

- If your headaches are throbbing and severe and/or accompanied by nausea, vomiting, or sensitivity to light or sound, you probably are experiencing a migraine. In six out of ten cases, migraines affect only one side of your head. The pain may worsen with routine activity. A migraine typically lasts from 4 to 72 hours.

- If you have headaches that have lasted more than 15 days a month for at least three months then you probably have a chronic tension headache. You may feel steady pain on one or both sides of your head. Sometimes the pain is described as a dull ache or a tight band of pressure around the head. The signs, symptoms and time frame vary depending on the specific type of chronic daily headache.

- If you have taken pain medication more than two or three days a week, your headache might be a rebound headache, caused by medication overuse. The pain often starts in the early morning, when it is most severe, and then eases as the day continues.

You might want to consider keeping a headache diary for a few weeks. This will help your GP decided whether you have chronic tension headache or another kind of headache, such as migraine, as well as making it easier to identify trigger factors or patterns.

Step 2 • Consider the medical options

Most tension headaches are easily treated with over-the-counter medications, including aspirin, ibuprofen and paracetamol. You should be aware, though, that if you have to take painkillers more than two or three times a week for a headache, they might actually be making it worse, because of the rebound effect I mentioned in step one. Your doctor might also offer you an antidepressant such as amitriptyline or Mirtazapine, both of which have been found to result in fewer, shorter and less painful headaches. I personally would encourage you to follow my recommendations before resorting to these.

If you are diagnosed with a migraine, you will be offered painkillers such as aspirin and ibuprofen, as well as general advice such as resting in a quiet room, avoiding migraine triggers such as alcohol, bright light, foods containing monosodium glutamate (MSG), dehydration, very cold foods and so on, massaging the affected area, taking small amounts of caffeine and holding a hot or cold compress to your head. The most effective groups of medications for migraine appear to be triptans. They work by helping to make the blood vessels in the brain narrower. They appear to help six out of ten women who take them.[3] All triptans have side-effects, including pins and needles and feelings of warmth in different parts of the body, dizziness, flushing or neck pain, but they are usually short-lived.

Step 3 • Address the underlying causes

While I am going to make recommendations to treat and prevent the pain of your headache or migraine using a variety of supplements, for lasting resolution I encourage you to fill in the questionnaires in part one, section two, in order to identify possible root causes or contributors. In my experience, the ones to consider are:

- **Stress** – Solution: Secret Two – De-stress and Relax (page 77); Holistic Health Tools – Emotional Freedom Technique (page 151) and Mindfulness (page 147)

- **Tiredness** – Solution: Secret One – Nurture Your Physical Body (Rest and Sleep – page 45); Secret Two – De-stress and Relax (page 77); Holistic Health Tools – Emotional Freedom Technique (page 151) and Mindfulness (page 147); Part Five (Adrenal Fatigue – page 267)

- **Nutritional deficiencies** – Solution: Secret One – Nurture Your Physical Body (Healthy Eating and Supplements – page 49), (especially magnesium, B_6 and essential fatty acids)

- **Blood-sugar imbalance** – Solution: Secret One – Nurture Your Physical Body (Healthy Eating and Supplements – page 49)

- **Poor diet** – Solution: Secret One – Nurture Your Physical Body (Healthy Eating and Supplements – page 49)

- **Food intolerances** – Solution: Part Five (Food Intolerances – page 344); Holistic Health Tools – Emotional Freedom Technique (page 151)

- **Depression** – Solution: Part Five (Depression – page 316); Holistic Health Tools – Mindfulness (page 147), Values-based Goal Setting (page 166) and The Work (page 163)

- **Excessive intake or withdrawal from caffeine, nicotine, sugar, alcohol or drugs** – Solution: Secret One – Nurture Your Physical Body (Healthy Eating and Supplements – page 49); Part Five (Addictions – page 260)

- **Poor posture, eye strain and neck or back problems** – Solution: seek advice from an osteopath, chiropractor or Alexander Technique therapist

Step 4 • Start a headache and migraine supplement programme

When used alongside step three, certain nutritional supplements can help to alleviate and prevent many of the symptoms of headaches and migraines. My integrated medicine prescription for headaches and migraines would usually include:

- **A multivitamin-mineral supplement**, plus a total daily dose of **vitamin B**$_6$ (50mg) and **magnesium**[4] (600mg). There is some evidence to suggest that the latter can help alleviate migraine headaches and prevent tension headaches.

- **Fish oils** (3000mg a day) may help to reduce the symptoms associated with migraines.[5]

- **Butterbur**[6] (75mg twice a day) or **feverfew**[7] (dose as advised by manufacturers) are both herbs which have been found to reduce the severity, duration and frequency of migraines.

- **5-HTP** (50mg to 100mg three times daily) is an amino acid that helps to produce the good-mood brain neurotransmitter serotonin. Several studies have found that it can help prevent migraine and tension-type headaches.[8]

Step 5 • Consider other complementary approaches

While there is no definitive evidence that these can help you with your headaches or migraines, some patients find the following useful in supporting their programme: acupuncture, meditation, homeopathy, massage, spiritual healing, yoga, traditional Chinese medicine and Ayurvedic medicine.

For recommended books see Resources.

Hypothyroidism

~

An estimated one in ten women suffer from hypothyroidism, an underfunctioning of the thyroid gland, and the majority don't know that they have it.[1] Women are at the greatest risk, developing thyroid problems seven times more often than men, with the risk increasing with age and for those with a family history of thyroid problems. If left untreated, thyroid imbalances can leave people at risk of heart disease, infertility and osteoporosis.

Your thyroid is a butterfly-shaped gland that curves around your windpipe. The cells that make up the thyroid gland combine the mineral iodine with the amino acid L-tyrosine to create two hormones: thyroxine (T4) and the biologically more active triiodothyronine (T3). Once released by the thyroid gland these hormones travel throughout the body and regulate the enzymes involved in controlling the rate at which bodily functions occur. If thyroid hormone levels are high everything speeds up – your heart quickens, you lose weight and you find it hard to switch off. If the thyroid hormone levels are too low everything slows down – you become constipated, tired and mentally slow.

An underactive thyroid or hypothyroidism occurs when the thyroid gland fails to make sufficient thyroid hormone to meet the body's demand. This gives the classic hypothyroid symptoms of low energy, low temperature, extreme tiredness, intolerance to cold weather, mental drowsiness, weight gain, depression, low libido, thinning hair and constipation.

What causes hypothyroidism?

There are many different factors that can affect thyroid function. The most common is an autoimmune disease called Hashimoto's disease, in which antibodies are produced and directed towards your thyroid gland by your body's immune system. This might be triggered by a virus infection or possibly happen due to a genetic vulnerability. Other known causes include mineral deficiencies, such as iodine, selenium and zinc, a tumour of the pituitary gland, certain medications, such as lithium (used to treat some kinds of depression), amiodarone (used to treat abnormal heart rhythms) and interferon (used to treat hepatitis), and thyroid surgery.

What are the risk factors?

The following are known to increase the likelihood of your developing hypothyroidism:

- Over 50 years of age

- A parent or grandparent with an autoimmune disease

- Radioactive iodine treatment or anti-thyroid medications

- Radiation treatment to your neck or upper chest

- Thyroid surgery (partial thyroidectomy)

- Pregnancy – about five in a hundred pregnant women get an underactive thyroid after they have their baby, but it usually clears up after a few months

My integrated medical prescription for hypothyroidism

Hypothyroidism is one of the first things I consider in my female patients who complain of fatigue, low mood and weight gain, because a positive result for it comes back so often.

Step 1 • Do you have hypothyroidism?

If you haven't already, I encourage you to fill in the thyroid questionnaire in part one, section two, a score of ten or more indicates that hypothyroidism may be contributing to your symptoms.

To assess your thyroid function you will need to get a blood test done – see Resources. Most doctors will measure for various blood markers, including TSH (thyroid stimulating hormone), T4 (thyroid hormone) and T3 (active thyroid hormone), as well as antimicrosomal and anti-thyroglobulin antibodies (to check for an autoimmune cause). Ideally you should also have your free T3 and free T4 tested too, as these indicate the actual amounts of thyroid hormones that are available to exert their influence on the cells of the body. In the presence of hypothyroidism symptoms, the following are strongly suggestive of a diagnosis of hypothyroidism:

- Free T3 levels of less than 260 pg/ml

- Free T4 levels of less than 0.7

- And/or TSH levels above 2.0 to 3.0 (this low level is controversial and not universally accepted)

If you would like your levels to be checked you can do this via a nutritional therapist or integrated medical doctor who can arrange a Total Thyroid Screen Test via Genova Diagnostics – see Resources.

Step 2 • Consider the medical options

If your blood tests indicate that you have hypothyroidism, your doctor will start you on thyroid hormone drug replacement therapy, the goal of which is to relieve symptoms and to provide sufficient thyroid hormone to decrease elevated TSH levels to within the normal range. Conventional treatment almost always begins with synthetic T4 drugs such as levothyroxine. Sometimes a synthetic form of T3 might also be used in combination with T4. An alternative preferred by some people is armour thyroid, a prescription medication that contains desiccated thyroid derived from the thyroid gland of the pig. Some people reportedly do better on this, possibly because it contains a mix of T4 (80 per cent) and T3 (20 per cent). The best preparation and at which dose often depends on the individual.

Side-effects of levothyroxine include anxiety and it can trigger a fast and irregular heart beat in older people. If you have already been through the menopause, taking too much levothyroxine can cause thinning of the bones (osteoporosis). This can happen to women who've been taking high doses of levothyroxine for ten years.[2]

In addition to the approaches above, there are a number of nutritional ways to support healthy thyroid function.

Step 3 • Address the underlying causes

While I am going to make recommendations to resolve your hypothyroid symptoms using a variety of supplements, for lasting resolution I encourage you to fill in the questionnaires in part one, section two, so as to help identify possible root causes or contributors to hypothyroidism. In my experience, the ones to consider are:

- **Adrenal fatigue** – Solution: Part Five (Adrenal Fatigue – page 267), (adrenal fatigue and hypothyroidism tend to go hand in hand, so addressing any adrenal problems is a good idea, as is checking your cholesterol level, as thyroid deficiency can cause raised cholesterol); Secret Two – De-stress and Relax (page 77); Holistic Health Tools – Values-based Goal Setting (page 166) and Mindfulness (page 147)

- **Stress** – Solution: Secret Two – De-stress and Relax (page 77); Holistic Health Tools – Emotional Freedom Technique (page 151) and Mindfulness (page 147)

- **Poor diet** – Solution: Secret One – Nurture Your Physical Body (Healthy Eating and Supplements – page 49)

- **Environmental toxicity** – Solution: Secret One – Nurture Your Physical Body (Healthy Environment and Sunlight – page 70)

- **Food intolerances** – Solution: Part Five (Food Intolerances – page 344), (if you are diagnosed with autoimmune disease, you should also assess the possibility of food intolerances being a trigger – wheat, dairy and soya are the usual culprits); Holistic Health Tools – Emotional Freedom Technique (page 151)

- **Nutritional deficiencies** – Solution: Secret One – Nurture Your Physical Body (Healthy Eating and Supplements – page 49)

- **Lack of physical activity** – Solution: Secret One – Nurture Your Physical Body (Physical Activity and Touch – page 67); Holistic Health Tools – Emotional Freedom Technique (page 151) and Values-based Goal Setting (page 166)

Step 4 • Start a thyroid support supplement programme

When used alongside step three, certain nutritional supplements can help to alleviate many of the symptoms associated with hypothyroidism. My integrated medicine prescription for hypothyroidism would usually include:

- **A multivitamin-mineral supplement**, including selenium, iron, zinc, copper and the B vitamins, to help ensure that your thyroid hormones are achieving their maximal effect within the body.

- **Vitamin C with bioflavonoids** (1000mg a day) to reduce inflammation

- **Fish oil** (3000mg a day) to increase the body's sensitivity to thyroid hormones and decrease inflammation, which in turn might contribute to the autoimmune attack on the thyroid gland.

- **L-tyrosine** (500mg twice a day) is an energising amino acid that gets used in the synthesis of thyroid hormones.

- **Kelp** (dose as advised by manufacturers) is a potent source of iodine and is useful if a deficiency of iodine is suspected,[3] but do not take if you have Hashimoto's thyroiditis as it will aggravate it.

If you have autoimmune thyroiditis, the treatment must be conventional. Synthetic T4 (synthroid), either with or without synthetic T3 (usually called Cytomel), is the best treatment and this must be done under the supervision of a doctor. Some doctors, however, will not treat this if the TSH, T4 and T3 are normal.

Step 5 • Consider other complementary approaches

While my dietary recommendations in Secret One – Nurture Your Physical Body will apply to you if you have hypothyroidism, you should be aware that there are certain foods that support and interfere with thyroid function.

Foods that interfere with the release of thyroid hormone and with the conversion of T4 to T3 include soya, walnuts, peanuts, almonds, millet, pine nuts, cabbage, mustard and apples, and foods from the brassica family, such as cabbage and turnips. Intake of these should be limited. However, when these are cooked the compounds that cause thyroid imbalance are deactivated.

Foods that help stimulate thyroid hormone production and the conversion of T4 to T3 include egg yolk, seaweeds (kelp and dulse), mushrooms, garlic, seafood and wheatgerm. Coconut oil is also thyroid-stimulating and should be used to cook with.

You might also want to consider the following complementary therapies to support your programme: acupuncture, homeopathy, massage, spiritual healing, yoga, traditional Chinese medicine and Ayurvedic medicine.

For recommended books see Resources.

Irritable bowel syndrome

Irritable bowel syndrome (IBS) is a common and very frustrating health condition affecting one in five women in the UK.[1] The average age of onset is between 20 and 29, and women are thought to be affected twice as often as men. The majority of people with IBS, about 95 per cent, will not seek medical help for their symptoms.

What causes IBS?

Having worked with a lot of women with IBS, the three main causes in my experience are:

- Repressed emotions (see Tension Myoneural Syndrome, page 386)
- Candida and/or parasites
- Food intolerances

What are the risk factors?

There might be a genetic link, but being female is also a factor.

My integrated medical prescription for IBS

My number one challenge as an integrated medical doctor is to establish what the underlying cause of my patients' IBS symptoms are, because this is the key to lasting resolution of the symptoms.

Step 1 • Do you have irritable bowel syndrome?

IBS is associated with a number of symptoms which vary both in their frequency and severity. The following criteria are used by most doctors to assess the possibility of IBS as a diagnosis.

If you have experienced abdominal discomfort or pain for at least 12 (not necessarily consecutive) weeks in the last year and if your discomfort or pain is accompanied by two or more of the following features, then you may have IBS:

- Your pain or discomfort is relieved after you have a bowel movement

- When your pain or discomfort starts, you have a change in your usual number of bowel movements (either more or fewer)

- When your pain or discomfort starts, you have either softer or harder stools than usual

In addition to the above, other symptoms of IBS include:

- Abnormal bowel frequency (more than three per day or less than three per week)

- Abnormal stool passage, including straining, urgency or the feeling that you have not completely emptied your rectum after a bowel movement

- Abnormal stool form (lumpy/hard or loose/watery stool)

- Passage of mucus in or on the stool

- Abdominal bloating, distension or swelling

Another important step in making the diagnosis of IBS is to exclude the possibility of you having another health problem masquerading as IBS. To help you and your doctor decide whether this is a possibility, read through the following list of 'red flags'. If you have any of the following you will need to undergo further investigation:

- Did your symptoms start after the age of 45?

- Did your symptoms start shortly after taking antibiotics?

- Are you anaemic and/or do you have blood in your stools?

- Do you experience nausea, vomiting and/or fever?

- Are you anorexic?

- Do you have a family history of colonic carcinoma, inflammatory bowel disease or coeliac disease?

- Do you have a fever?

- Do you have symptoms that are progressively getting worse?

- Do you have a change in the pattern of symptoms or are you getting new symptoms?

- Do you wake at night because of your symptoms?

- Are you experiencing unexplained weight loss?

- Do you have diarrhoea that won't stop and/or are you dehydrated?

If any of these apply to you please tell your GP as he or she will need to exclude the following: malabsorption (coeliac disease), gastrointestinal cancer, inflammatory bowel disease (ulcerative colitis and Crohn's disease), infection (parasites and bacteria), lactose intolerance, thyroid problems and diverticulosis.

Once these have been excluded and the diagnosis of IBS made, the next step is to identify the underlying cause of your IBS symptoms.

Step 2 • Consider the medical options

Because IBS is so readily treated using an integrated medical approach that deals with the underlying causes, I rarely recommend medication. However, there are circumstances when it has its uses.

To help with the pain your doctor will probably offer you an antispasmodic medication, such as mebeverine (Colofac IBS), alverine (Spasmonal), hyoscine (Buscopan) and dicycloverine (Merbentyl). These drugs help to stop or reduce the spasms by relaxing the walls of the bowel.[2] The latter two are particularly associated with side-effects, including constipation, dry mouth, flushing and dry skin. I sometimes recommend taking these to my patients in order to manage pain *while* they are addressing the underlying causes.

If you have diarrhoea your doctor will probably recommend loperamide. This drug works by stopping your bowels going into spasm. It may also help reduce the urge to go to the toilet.[3] Side-effects include stomach cramps, bloating, itchy skin and dizziness. If it causes abdominal pain at night you might want to consider halving the dose and taking it twice daily. If you have diarrhoea, I do recommend taking loperamide, but it is essential that you see your GP to make sure that nothing else is causing the diarrhoea. Taking an acidophilus probiotic might help to stop the diarrhoea.

If you have constipation your doctor will probably offer you a fibre-containing laxative such as ispaghula husk, which absorbs water and swells up in the gut. Brand names include Fybogel, Isogel and Ispagel. These fibre supplements help reduce IBS symptoms in about two-thirds of people who take them. However, they can make the abdominal pain and bloating worse in other people.[4] They should always be taken with extra water. Fibre supplements are useful in the short term, but in the long term it is much more important to get your fibre from eating a healthy diet (see Secret One, page 49).

If all of the above fail to help then your GP might prescribe a tricyclic antidepressant medication, such as mitriptyline, clomipramine, doxepin (Sinequan) or trimipramine (Surmontil). In addition to treating any underlying depression and anxiety, these will help to reduce pain and diarrhoea.[5] Side-effects include dry mouth, constipation and dizziness, but I would stay well clear of antidepressants, as you will not need them if you deal with the underlying causes of IBS.

Step 3 • Address the underlying causes

While I am going to make recommendations to treat your IBS symptoms using a variety of supplements, for lasting resolution of IBS I encourage you to fill in the questionnaires in part one, section two, in order to identify possible root causes or contributors. In my experience, the ones to consider are:

- **Repressed emotions** – Solution: Secret Three – Face and Embrace Your Emotions (page 94); Holistic Health Tools – Mindfulness (page 147) and EmoTrance (page 158); Part Five (Tension Myoneural Syndrome – page 386)

- **Parasites/candida** – Solution: Part Five (Dysbiosis – page 334); Holistic Health Tools – Emotional Freedom Technique (page 151)

- **Food intolerances** – Solution: Part Five (Food Intolerances – page 344); Holistic Health Tools – Emotional Freedom Technique (page 151)

- **Stress** – Solution: Secret Two – De-stress and Relax (page 77); Holistic Health Tools – Emotional Freedom Technique (page 151) and Mindfulness (page 147)

- **Poor diet** – Solution: Secret One – Nurture Your Physical Body (Healthy Eating and Supplements – page 49)

- **Lactose intolerance** – avoiding lactose (present in milk and some other dairy products) may help reduce IBS symptoms[6] in people with IBS who are lactose intolerant

Step 4 • Start an IBS supplement programme

When used alongside step three, certain nutritional supplements can help to alleviate many of the symptoms of IBS. My integrated medicine prescription for IBS would usually include:

- **Aloe vera juice** (dose as advised by manufacturers) is my first choice of supplement for the majority of non-emotionally induced IBS patients. While there is a lack of convincing evidence to substantiate its use, there is a lot of anecdotal evidence to suggest that it can help reduce some of the symptoms associated with IBS, including diarrhoea and constipation, gut pain, bloating and wind.

- **Acidophilus probiotic** (dose as advised by manufacturers) has been found in some studies to significantly improve symptoms and quality of life in patients with IBS.[7] Probiotic therapy, primarily in the form of *Lactobacillus acidophilus*, is most useful for people with dysbiosis. It's important to purchase a well-known brand and to take it for at least six months.

- **Psyllium** is a high-fibre, bulk-forming laxative that might help to improve your bowels and reduce the symptoms of IBS.[8]

- **Peppermint oil** (dose as advised by manufacturers), with or without caraway oil, can act as a natural anti-spasmodic.[9] If taken as capsules, they should be enteric-coated so that they dissolve in the intestines rather than the stomach. As an alternative, try drinking peppermint tea after your meal.

Step 5 • Consider other complementary approaches

While there is no definitive evidence that these can help you with your IBS, some patients find the following useful in supporting their programme: hypnotherapy, acupuncture, homeopathy, massage, spiritual healing, yoga, traditional Chinese medicine and Ayurvedic medicine.

For recommended books see Resources.

Metabolic syndrome

Metabolic syndrome affects 25 per cent of the British population and is a big risk factor for heart disease, stroke, high blood pressure, polycystic ovary syndrome, Alzheimer's disease and type II diabetes.[1] Metabolic syndrome (or syndrome X as it is also known), is not a disease, but a collection of metabolic imbalances and a by-product of obesity, chronic inflammation and stress. The most common features of metabolic syndrome, and the tell-take signs that you might be affected by it, are:

- Excess body fat around the middle

- High levels of fats in the blood that are known to be associated with disease

- Reduced levels of the 'good' fat high-density lipoprotein (HDL) cholesterol

- Raised blood pressure

- Blood that has an increased tendency to clot

What is the cause of metabolic syndrome?

At the heart of metabolic syndrome is insulin resistance. Insulin is a hormone produced by specialised cells in the pancreas in response to raised blood sugar. One of insulin's main jobs is to drive glucose, plus other nutrients, into the cells of the body, especially muscle cells. Insulin resistance is said to be occurring when those same cells lose their sensitivity to insulin. Why this happens is still unclear, but the research shows that a combination of genetic factors, obesity, inactivity, high cortisol levels due to stress, and a diet high in sugar and refined foods are all significant players. Of these, obesity is considered to be the most significant issue.

While most people tend to think of the rolls of fat that they carry around their waist as inert, the truth is quite the opposite. Researchers find that fat is a living tissue that is constantly influencing the rest of the body through hormones called adipokines. In addition to regulating appetite and metabolic rate, these hormones also influence inflammation. This is important to know because the fatter you are, the greater the number of hormones produced and the higher the level of inflammation within the body. This is a problem, because it is this chronic low-grade inflammation in the body which makes the body more resistant to the effects of insulin.

As your cells become resistant to insulin, blood-sugar level increases and the pancreas is forced to produce more insulin to compensate. The higher insulin levels result in more glucose being stored as fat, plus they prevent cells from breaking down fat. This double whammy makes it very hard to lose weight. In fact, if you really struggle to lose weight, this might be the reason why!

The result is your waistline gets bigger, your levels of good (HDL) cholesterol go down, inflammation levels rise, blood pressure goes up (due to retained sodium and constricting blood vessels) and the blood becomes thicker. Before you know it metabolic syndrome has crept up on you and you are a walking time bomb for more serious disease.

What are the risk factors?

The following increase your chance of developing metabolic syndrome:

- Age (although some research shows that about one in eight schoolchildren have three or more components of metabolic syndrome)

- Obesity, particularly abdominal obesity or having an apple rather than a pear shape

- Diabetes, particularly a family history of it or you have it during pregnancy

- Other health problems such as high blood pressure, cardiovascular disease or polycystic ovary syndrome

My integrated medical prescription for metabolic syndrome

Because metabolic syndrome isn't a specific disease I consider it whenever I meet with a patient who is overweight or is known to have a raised cholesterol level or raised blood pressure. The real key to addressing it is to focus on dealing with the underlying insulin resistance using lifestyle and dietary changes, and supplements.

Step 1 • Do you have metabolic syndrome?

Because metabolic syndrome can progress to heart disease and cancer, diagnosing it early and treating it fully gives you a great opportunity to prevent an inevitable deterioration in health. If you haven't done so already, I encourage you to complete the metabolic syndrome questionnaire in part one, section two. If you score greater than ten you should ask your integrated medical doctor or nutritional therapist to order a Metabolic Syndrome Profile from Genova Diagnostics (see Resources). It measures insulin, glucose, cholesterol and triglyceride levels.

While guidelines differ slightly as to what results constitute metabolic syndrome, one set of criteria indicates that a diagnosis can be made if you have three or more of the following[2]:

- Your waist measures more than 35in/89cm (40in/102cm for men)

- The level of fats called triglycerides in your blood is 1.7 mmol/L before breakfast

- Your level of good (HDL) cholesterol is less than 1.3 mmol/L (1 mmol/L for men)

- The level of glucose in your blood is more than 6 mmol/L before breakfast

- Your blood pressure is 130/85 or higher

Step 2 • Consider the medical options

It is possible that your doctor might not have heard of metabolic syndrome, because it is a relatively new diagnostic criteria. However, your doctor will be able to provide advice on addressing raised cholesterol and blood pressure (see below) and prediabetes (insulin resistance), which is covered in the diabetes section on page 325.

Medications
For raised blood pressure
If your blood pressure is raised (greater than 140/90) you will be provided with advice on lifestyle changes and diets. You might also be offered some medications to lower your blood pressure.

- If you are aged 55 years or over, or of African or Caribbean descent, you will probably be offered a drug called a calcium channel blocker or a diuretic.

- If you are younger than 55 and not of African or Caribbean descent you will probably be offered a drug called an ACE inhibitor. If you can't take an ACE inhibitor, for example because it makes you cough, then you will probably be offered an angiotensin II receptor blocker (ARB).

If your blood pressure does not come under control using one of these medications (and it often doesn't) then you will be offered a second one.

- If you are already taking a calcium channel blocker or a diuretic you will probably be offered an ACE inhibitor or an ARB.

- If you're taking an ACE inhibitor or an ARB and you need another drug, you will be offered a calcium channel blocker or a diuretic.

While blood pressure medications are essential for many women with high blood pressure, unless it is very high I always encourage my patients to try my integrated medical prescription for three months prior to starting them because of their side-effects, which can include dizziness, headaches, swollen ankles, muscle cramps and kidney problems.

For raised cholesterol

About two in three women have a total cholesterol level that exceeds the optimum level, which is generally regarded as being less than 5 millimoles per litre (mmol/L). Your total cholesterol count is the combination of the levels of good high-density lipoprotein cholesterol and bad low-density lipoprotein cholesterol in your blood. If it is above this, in addition to being given advice on dietary and lifestyle change, you will probably be offered a medication called a statin. The main statins are: atorvastatin (Lipitor), fluvastatin (Lescol), pravastatin (Lipostat), rosuvastatin (Crestor) and simvastatin (Zocor, Zocor Heart-Pro, Simzal). All of these are effective at lowering cholesterol and reducing the risk of developing heart disease and stroke.[3] They work by interfering with the liver's production of cholesterol. Side-effects include headaches, fatigue, muscle pain, liver damage and kidney damage.

With most of my patients I will help them to lower their cholesterol using dietary and lifestyle changes, and supplements, before taking a cholesterol-lowering medication. If we haven't succeeded in getting their cholesterol down below 5 mmol/L within six months then I will recommend a statin.

If you decide to take cholesterol-lowering drugs, you should consider supplementing with Coenzyme Q10 (100mg a day), as statins interfere with the body's synthesis of this important heart nutrient.

Step 3 • Address the underlying causes

While I am going to make recommendations to lower your blood pressure and cholesterol using a variety of supplements, I encourage you to fill in the questionnaires in part one, section two, in order to identify possible root causes or contributors. In my experience, the ones to consider are:

- **Excessive weight** – Solution: Secret One – Nurture Your Physical Body (Healthy Eating and Supplements – page 49); Part Five (Weight Loss – page 401); Holistic Health Tools – Emotional Freedom Technique (page 151) and The Work (page 163)

- **Blood-sugar imbalance** – Solution: Secret One – Nurture Your Physical Body (Healthy Eating and Supplements – page 49)

- **Stress** – Solution: Secret Two – De-stress and Relax (page 77); Holistic Health Tools – Emotional Freedom Technique (page 151) and Mindfulness (page 147)

- **Poor diet** – Solution: Secret One – Nurture Your Physical Body (Healthy Eating and Supplements – page 49)

- **Nutritional deficiencies** – Solution: Secret One – Nurture Your Physical Body (Healthy Eating and Supplements – page 49)

- **Lack of Physical Activity** – Solution: Secret One – Nurture Your Physical Body (Physical Activity and Touch – page 67); Holistic Health Tools – Emotional Freedom Technique (page 151) and Values-based Goal Setting (page 166)

Step 4 • Start a metabolic syndrome supplement programme

When used alongside step three, certain nutritional supplements can help to address the underlying causes of metabolic syndrome. My integrated medicine prescription for metabolic syndrome would usually include:

- **Chromium polynicotinate** (400mcg to 1000mcg a day), which is essential to insulin and helps to drive blood glucose into the body's cells. A number of studies have found that supplementation of chromium can improve insulin sensitivity, cholesterol levels and blood-sugar levels.[4]

- **Fish oil** (3000mg a day), because its active components, EPA and DHA, are known to help burn fat and improve the efficiency with which the body uses glucose. When used in high enough dosages fish oil can also help reduce the low-grade inflammation that is often seen in people with metabolic syndrome.[5]

- **Alpha-lipoic acid** (100mg a day) is an antioxidant that can improve insulin resistance and increase glucose uptake into muscle cells.[6]

- **Coenzyme Q10** (30mg a day) may help to improve the function of insulin-producing cells in the pancreas, as well as lower blood pressure and raise HDL cholesterol levels.[7]

If you have a high blood pressure, you might want to consider adding:

- **Garlic**, which is highly regarded for its ability to improve, and maintain, heart and blood vessel health. In addition to this, it is believed to have a mild blood pressure-lowering effect when taken in doses of at least 900mg a day.[8]

- **Coenzyme Q10** (100mg one to three times a day) is a powerful antioxidant that protects the body from free radicals, regularises heart rhythm and lowers blood pressure.[9] You need to take this for at least two months to see an effect.

If there has been little improvement after six weeks I might then add in one or more of the following:

- **Hawthorn** (100mg to 300mg three times a day of a dose standardised to contain about 2 to 3 per cent flavonoids or 18 to 20 per cent procyanidins). The flowers and berries of this plant have been used for hundreds of years to reduce mild blood pressure, increase the strength of heart contractions, increase circulation to the heart muscle and slow the heart rate.[10] Several weeks or months are required for the full effects of hawthorn supplementation to become evident.

- **Arginine** (2g three times a day for a month, then reducing to 1g three times a day) is an amino acid that is known to make nitric oxide, a substance that allows blood vessels to dilate, thus leading to reduced blood pressure.[11]

If you have a high cholesterol level, you might want to consider adding:

- **No-flush niacin** (1000mg twice daily) can help to lower LDL cholesterol and raise HDL cholesterol.[12]

- **Plant sterols** impair uptake of cholesterol from the gut and can lower total and LDL cholesterol.[13] They should be taken with food.

Step 5 • Consider other complementary approaches

While there is no definitive evidence that these can help you with metabolic syndrome, some patients find the following useful in supporting their programme: acupuncture, homeopathy, spiritual healing, yoga, traditional Chinese medicine and Ayurvedic medicine.

For recommended books see Resources.

Osteoporosis

~

Osteoporosis is a progressive disease in which the bones gradually become weaker, causing changes in posture and making the individual extremely susceptible to bone fracture. More than half of all women between the ages of 45 and 70 will have some degree of osteoporosis, and a third of women will get one or more broken bones due to osteoporosis. In the UK osteoporosis leads to more than 200,000 broken bones a year.[1]

What causes osteoporosis?

From about the age of 35, old bone is broken down faster than new bone is made and the process speeds up as you get older. In some women this happens more quickly, resulting in your bones becoming thinner and more likely to break. At menopause, when oestrogen levels drop, bone loss in women increases dramatically. Decreased oestrogen production during menopause is the leading cause in women of osteoporosis.

What are the risk factors?

There are many different factors that can increase your risk of developing osteoporosis, including:

- Being female – particularly if you are slender and small-framed

- Getting older

- Race – particularly if you are white or of Southeast Asian descent

- Family history – having a parent or sibling with osteoporosis or a family history of fractures

- Exposure – to nicotine, excess alcohol, excess caffeinated fizzy drinks, steroid medications or thyroid medications

- Low lifetime exposure to oestrogen – infrequent menstrual periods or menopause before age 45

- Health problems – eating disorders, diabetes, depression, alcoholism, inflammatory bowel disease or coeliac disease

- Low calcium intake

- Sedentary lifestyle

- Stress

My integrated medical prescription for osteoporosis

In my experience most women (and men) don't attach too much importance to looking after the health of their bones and yet by making some changes to your life, you will not only reduce the risk of developing or experiencing a deterioration in osteoporosis, but importantly you will significantly reduce the chances of developing a bone fracture later on in life.

Step 1 • Do you have osteoporosis?

Osteoporosis is called the silent disease, because it has few symptoms and signs. Late stage signs include loss of height, a hunched back or spinal deformity, back pain and fracture without trauma.

If you are unsure as to whether you have osteoporosis, you could contact your GP to arrange a DXA scan, which measures bone density at various parts of the body and tells you how strong your bones are.

The second test, which will need to be done privately, is Osteoporosis Risk Assessment, which measures bone turnover, i.e. how quickly your bone is rebuilding itself. It's also a good way to monitor your treatment. See Resources.

Step 2 • Consider the medical options

Once upon a time you would have been offered hormone replacement therapy (HRT) by your doctor, but thankfully that is no longer recommended for osteoporosis, because of its side-effects (see Menopause, page 238).

Medications

If you have been diagnosed as having osteoporosis you will probably be offered a class of drugs called bisphosphanates, the two main ones being alendronate (Fosamax) and risedronate. Taking either of these increases the chances of your bones staying stronger for longer, and they also reduce the likelihood of you breaking a bone in your body.[2] They are associated with some mild side-effects such as stomach pain, bloating, indigestion, feeling sick, diarrhoea or constipation, but more serious side-effects include irritation, swelling and possible ulceration of the oesophagus, and severe pain in the joints, muscles and bones.

Unless the osteoporosis is severe, I usually advise my patients to try the rest of my recommendations first before starting these drugs, because of their side-effect profile. Most of my patients are unwilling to take them anyway.

Step 3 • Address the underlying causes

While I am going to make recommendations to treat osteoporosis using a variety of supplements, I encourage you to fill in the questionnaires in part one, section two, so as to help identify possible root causes or contributors to osteoporosis. In my experience, the ones to consider are:

- **Lack of physical activity** – Solution: Secret One – Nurture Your Physical Body (Physical Activity and Touch – page 67); Holistic Health Tools – Emotional Freedom Technique (page 151) and Values-based Goal Setting (page 166)

- **Inadequate exposure to the sun** – Solution: Secret One – Nurture Your Physical Body (Healthy Environment and Sunlight – page 70)

- **Excessive weight** – Solution: Secret One – Nurture Your Physical Body (Healthy Eating and Supplements – page 49); Part Five (Weight Loss – page 401); Holistic Health Tools – Emotional Freedom Technique (page 151) and The Work (page 163)

- **Eating disorder** – Solution: Secret One – Nurture Your Physical Body (Healthy Eating and Supplements – page 49); Holistic Health Tools – Emotional Freedom Technique (page 151) and The Work (page 163)

- **Stress** – Solution: Secret Two – De-stress and Relax (page 77); Holistic Health Tools – Emotional Freedom Technique (page 151) and Mindfulness (page 147)

- **Poor diet** – Solution: Secret One – Nurture Your Physical Body (Healthy Eating and Supplements – page 49)

- **Environmental toxicity** – Solution: Secret One – Nurture Your Physical Body (Healthy Environment and Sunlight – page 70)

- **Hormonal imbalance** – Solution: Part Five (Hypothyroidism – page 356, and Adrenal Fatigue – page 267); Part Four (Menopause – page 238)

- **Acidity** – Solution: Secret One – Nurture Your Physical Body (Healthy Eating and Supplements – page 49, and Rest and Sleep – page 45); Secret Two – De-stress and Relax (page 77)

Step 4 • Start an osteoporosis supplement programme

When used alongside step three, certain nutritional supplements can help to slow the progress, prevent and maybe even reverse osteoporosis. My integrated medicine prescription for osteoporosis would usually include:

- **A multivitamin-mineral supplement**, although in addition to this you should also ensure that you take a daily total of 1200mg **calcium**[3] (ideally as calcium citrate, calcium aspartate or calcium chelate), 1mg or 2mg of **boron citrate**; 2 to 10mg of **vitamin K**,

600mg of **magnesium** (oxide, citrate or chelate) and 800IU of **vitamin D3**. The latter helps to absorb calcium from the intestine.[4]

- **Vitamin C with bioflavonoids** (1000mg a day), as this will help the manufacture of collagen, a constituent of bone.

- **Omega-3, 6 and 9** (taken in capsule or liquid form in a 2:1:1 ratio) to provide the body with hormone-balancing, anti-inflammatory essential fatty acids.

- **Alkaline mineral salts** (dose as advised by manufacturers) to help reverse acidity of the body due to processed diet and stress. See Resources.

- **Natural progesterone cream** is used by some integrated medicine doctors to treat osteoporosis associated with a relative deficiency in progesterone.[5] This should only be used under medical supervision. See Resources.

Step 5 • Consider other complementary approaches

While there is no definitive evidence that these can help treat osteoporosis, some patients find the following useful in supporting their programme: swimming, t'ai chi, qi gong, acupuncture, homeopathy, spiritual healing, yoga, traditional Chinese medicine and Ayurvedic medicine.

For recommended books see Resources.

Rheumatoid arthritis

Rheumatoid arthritis affects approximately 400,000 people in the UK, the majority of whom are women.[1] The condition usually starts between the ages of 20 and 50. It involves an autoimmune response in which the body's immune system turns against itself – namely the joints and connective tissue structures, which support and surround the joints. This, if left untreated or inadequately treated, leads to significant pain, disability and deformity.

What causes rheumatoid arthritis?

Rheumatoid arthritis occurs when the body's immune systems and white cells attack the lining of the joints (synovium). The resulting inflammation causes a release of proteins which, over time, results in damage to the cartilage, bones, tendons and ligaments. This can lead to swelling and deformity, and eventually a loss of function.

What are the risk factors?

Factors that might increase the chances of you developing rheumatoid arthritis include:

- Being a woman – women develop it more often than men

- Age – it most commonly occurs between the ages of 20 and 50

- Genetics – if a family member has it

- Smoking

My integrated medical prescription for rheumatoid arthritis

Rheumatoid arthritis responds very well to an integrated medical approach, especially one that includes stress management, which is often a trigger for flare-ups in symptoms.

Step 1 • Do you have rheumatoid arthritis?

Rheumatoid arthritis usually begins with irritation and inflammation of the synovial membrane, causing pain, stiffness and swelling. The inflamed membrane responds by sending out enzymes that cause the cartilage of the joint to break down. The cartilage is then replaced with fibrous tissue that can calcify and form bony knobs that may fuse the joint and restrict movement. Symptoms include warmth, redness, pain, stiffness (often improving during the day) and the development of roundish rheumatoid nodules. Multiple joints may be involved.

If you have any of these you should see your GP, who will examine you and arrange testing. After doing this, if you have four or more of the following then it is very likely that you have rheumatoid arthritis:

- Morning stiffness in your joints that lasts for more than an hour

- Swelling and inflammation in three or more joints that lasts for more than six weeks

- Swelling and inflammation in your hand joints or wrists that lasts for more than six weeks

- Symptoms in the same joints on both sides of your body that last for more than six weeks

- Rheumatoid nodules (firm lumps under your skin)

- Rheumatoid factor in the blood (many people with rheumatoid arthritis have this protein in their blood)

- X-rays showing changes in your joints

Step 2 • Consider the medical options

Depending on the severity of your symptoms, and other factors such as your age and health, your doctor will offer you a variety of drugs to reduce inflammation and limit damage to your body.

Medications

For pain you will probably be offered non-steroidal anti-inflammatory drugs, such as ibuprofen and voltarol. However, because of their long-term side-effects, such as stomach irritation, gastro-intestinal bleeding and possible joint degeneration, they are not ideally taken for more than a week at a time.

The main class of drugs that you will be offered is called disease-modifying anti-rheumatic drugs (DMARD). They can prevent your joints from wearing down, and help to ease your pain and swelling.[2] Examples include methotrexate, sulfasalazine and infliximab. While all of these can help to reduce pain and swelling, and slow down the disease, they have significant side-effects, including: acne, blisters on the skin and mouth, tiredness and, rarely, damage to your liver and lungs.

Unless my patients' symptoms are severe, I usually recommend these after trying the rest of my suggestions or use them in conjunction with other approaches. There are some doctors who believe that rheumatoid arthritis is caused by a bacteria, which, when treated with antibiotics, causes a complete resolution of symptoms. I believe that there is some truth in this, but rather than resorting to antibiotics I much prefer to use dietary changes and supplements first – as most women respond positively to this – and then consider the use of antibiotics.

Step 3 • Address the underlying causes

While I am going to make recommendations to treat your arthritis symptoms using a variety of supplements, for lasting resolution I encourage you to fill in the questionnaires in part one, section two, so as to help identify possible root causes or contributors to arthritis. In my experience, the ones to consider are:

- **Viruses/bacteria/parasites/candida** – Solution: Part Five (Dysbiosis – page 334); Holistic Health Tools – Emotional Freedom Technique (page 151)

- **Blood-sugar imbalance** – Solution: Secret One – Nurture Your Physical Body (Healthy Eating and Supplements – page 49)

- **Stress** – Solution: Secret Two – De-stress and Relax (page 77); Holistic Health Tools – Emotional Freedom Technique (page 151) and Mindfulness (page 147)

- **Poor diet** – Solution: Secret One – Nurture Your Physical Body (Healthy Eating and Supplements – page 49)

- **Environmental toxicity** – Solution: Secret One – Nurture Your Physical Body (Healthy Environment and Sunlight – page 70)

- **Depression** – Solution: Part Five (Depression – page 316), (women with rheumatoid arthritis have an increased risk of developing depression); Holistic Health Tools – Mindfulness (page 147), Values-based Goal Setting (page 166) and The Work (page 163)

- **Food intolerances** – Solution: Part Five (Food Intolerances – page 344); Holistic Health Tools – Emotional Freedom Technique (page 151)

- **Nutritional deficiencies** – Solution: Secret One – Nurture Your Physical Body (Healthy Eating and Supplements – page 49)

- **Low self-acceptance** – Solution: Secret Four – Accept Yourself (page 113); Secret Three – Face and Embrace Your Emotions (page 94); Secret Five – Develop and Deepen Your Relationships (page 127); Holistic Health Tools – Mindfulness (page 147), Emotional Freedom Technique (page 151) and Values-based Goal Setting (page 166)

Step 4 • Start a rheumatoid arthritis supplement programme

When used alongside step three, certain nutritional supplements can help to alleviate some of the symptoms and damage associated with rheumatoid arthritis. My integrated medicine prescription for rheumatoid arthritis would usually include:

- **A multivitamin-mineral supplement.**

- **Vitamin C with bioflavonoids** (1000mg to 3000mg a day) to reduce inflammation and pain.

- **Fish oil**[3] (3000mg to 10,000mg a day) to provide the body with hormone-balancing, anti-inflammatory, essential fatty acids.

- **GLA** (up to 2.8g of borage oil a day) may help to relive rheumatoid arthritis symptoms.[4]

- **Bromelain** (200mg three times a day) is a powerful natural anti-inflammatory. It is most effective when taken with DLPA (an amino acid painkiller) and astaxanthin (an antioxidant).[5] See Resources.

- **Plant sterols** (dose as advised by manufacturers) can help to calm the immune system response and reduce inflammation.

- **Alkaline mineral salts** help to reverse the tissue acidity that is often found with rheumatoid arthritis.

Step 5 • Consider other complementary approaches

To help you manage your pain more effectively I recommend using either the portable electromagnetic device Magnessage or the Pain Ease microcurrent patch, both of which stimulate healing and reduce the amount of pain and inflammation (see Resources). Other complementary medicine approaches to consider include: Western herbal medicine, acupuncture, homeopathy, spiritual healing, yoga, traditional Chinese medicine and Ayurvedic medicine.

For recommended books see Resources.

Tension myoneural syndrome

~~~

While you probably haven't heard of tension myoneural syndrome (TMS), I find this condition to be relatively common among patients who have chronic or recurring pain, and are also highly perfectionist and self-critical. TMS (previously known as tension myositis syndrome) refers to a group of emotionally induced conditions which include chronic or recurring back, neck, limb and leg pain, carpel tunnel syndrome and fibromyalgia. The pioneer of this work is Dr John Sarno, Professor of Clinical Rehabilitation Medicine at New York University Hospital Medical School and author of the books *Healing Chronic Back Pain*, *The Mindbody Prescription* and *The Divided Mind*.

What causes TMS?

Dr Sarno proposes that throughout life we accumulate psychological tension, in the form of grief, anger, anxiety, emotional pain and rage, within our unconscious mind in response to the pressures placed upon us. These pressures are from three places:

- Stresses and strains of everyday issues, such as home and work responsibilities

- Childhood experiences

- Self-imposed pressures resulting from certain personality traits, such as being highly sensitive, overly nice, self-sacrificing and/or self-critical, or being a people-pleaser or perfectionist

Because we are afraid to feel these emotions, they are repressed and placed where we're not aware of them, in the unconscious mind. At the time this seems like a good idea as it allows us to survive the situation, maintain an outward calmness and get on with life. However, the accumulated emotional upset, conflicts and anger build up and become rage, which seeks to come through into our awareness. Fearing being overwhelmed by this reservoir of rage, our subconscious mind, via the brain, restricts blood flow to various muscles and nerves. This lack of oxygen and build up of waste materials results in muscle pain, tension and spasms. According to TMS theory, this very real physical pain is designed to distract us, and keep unpleasant thoughts and feelings from rising into the conscious mind. Although the pain can be very debilitating, it does not cause any permanent damage and can disappear quickly without any lasting effects.

My integrated medical prescription for TMS

Because TMS is a relatively new diagnosis and certainly not one that's accepted yet by Western medicine, many women are quite rightly sceptical about it. My advice to you is to follow my suggestions and to discover for yourself whether TMS is real or not.

Step 1 • Do you have TMS?

I use the following questionnaire to help identify my patients who might have TMS as the root cause of their pain. As long as other causes of pain, such as fractures, tumours, infections, rheumatoid arthritis, cancer, severe disc herniations and other major structural problems are excluded, a score of ten or more is highly suggestive of TMS. The following questionnaire assumes that you are already suffering from chronic (greater than six months duration) or recurring back and neck pain.

If the answer is yes to any of the following give yourself a score of two for that question:

- Have you noticed a relationship between your pain and your emotional state/stress level just prior to the onset or flare up of pain? ☐

- Are you conscientious, driven, self-critical, a people-pleaser, an overly nice/helpful/non-confrontational person and/or perfectionist? ☐

- Do you have pain that has been thoroughly investigated, but for which you have not been given a definitive diagnosis? ☐

- Do you have a history of irritable bowel syndrome, migraines, tension headaches, heartburn, carpel tunnel syndrome, repetitive strain injury, peptic ulcers, hives, Raynaud's phenomenon, teeth grinding, frequent urination (not related to any medical condition), tinnitus or dizziness not related to neurological disease? ☐

- Does the pain persist and/or recur despite treatment with conventional and complementary therapy approaches? ☐

If the answer is yes to any of the following give yourself a score of one for that question:

- Does your pain shift around your body and/or tend to hurt more at night, first thing in the morning or at weekends ? ☐

- Did the pain come on during or just after a psychologically traumatic event(s)? ☐

- Have you found that massage helps your pain significantly or that you are quite sensitive to massage in certain areas of your neck and back? ☐

- When you get upset or stressed does the pain significantly increase in intensity? ☐

- Have you noticed the pain improving when you have another stress-related problem? ☐

- Does the pain improve with distraction or when on holiday? ☐

- Do you have a history of physical, emotional and/or sexual abuse? ☐

- Do you tend to suppress your anger? ☐

Total ☐

If you score over ten, I would then encourage you to contact a TMS-trained health professional who can support you through the rest of the programme that I am about to suggest. See Resources.

Step 2 • Consider the medical options

Your doctor probably won't have heard of TMS. However, it is very important that prior to making the diagnosis you have been fully assessed and investigated to exclude the causes of back pain that I mentioned earlier.

Step 3 • Address the underlying causes

Earlier I mentioned Dr Sarno's theory that TMS is caused by repressed emotions and I have certainly found that to be true. My own six-week TMS Recovery Programme focuses on addressing the following four barriers to healing and recovery:

- **Emotional repression** – Solution: Secret Three – Face and Embrace Your Emotions (page 94); Secret Four – Accept Yourself (page 113); Holistic Health Tools – Emotional Freedom Technique (page 151), EmoTrance (page 158) and Mindfulness (page 147)

- **Low self-acceptance** – Solution: Secret Four – Accept Yourself (page 113); Secret Three – Face and Embrace Your Emotions (page 94); Secret Five – Develop and Deepen Your Relationships (page 127); Holistic Health Tools – Mindfulness (page 147), Emotional Freedom Technique (page 151) and Values-based Goal Setting (page 166)

- **Stress** – Solution: Secret Two – De-stress and Relax (page 77); Holistic Health Tools – Emotional Freedom Technique (page 151) and Mindfulness (page 147)

- **Trauma** – Solution: Secret Three – Face and Embrace Your Emotions (page 94); Holistic Health Tools – Emotional Freedom Technique (page 151), EmoTrance (page 158) and Mindfulness (page 147)

Step 4 • Start My TMS Solutions Programme

Unlike most of my integrated medicine programmes, my TMS Solutions Programme involves a purely psychological and emotional approach. This is because the key to permanent recovery from TMS is to understand and accept, with your whole body and mind, that your pain has an emotional cause and that your recovery therefore needs to be emotionally focused. Your pain is real, it is caused by mild oxygen deprivation, but the root cause is emotional.

How this is achieved depends on the individual. For example I have come across individuals who have experienced a complete recovery from their pain just by reading one of Dr Sarno's books. Others have experienced a significant improvement in their pain by attending TMS-focused lectures. However, there are many people with TMS for whom this alone doesn't work, for those I offer my own approach called the TMS Solutions Programme, which consists of four steps:

Step One: Increasing Your Understanding of TMS
This involves learning about TMS, your relationship to emotions and how your emotions are influencing your health. Much of the material covered in Secret Three – Face and Embrace Your Emotions is relevant to this step.

Step Two: Discovering and Resolving any Underlying Trauma/Conflict
This appears to be the real key for some people to recover from TMS. In my experience many people with TMS experienced a trauma or conflict prior to the onset of their pain. If the pain was out of the blue, a trauma usually happened within a 72-hour time period prior to onset. If the pain was of a gradual onset or is recurring, then the trauma usually occurred 6 to 18 months prior to the first onset of the pain. The key to resolving the trauma or conflict is to isolate it and

then process it using one of a number of different approaches. This is best done in a consultation with me or one of my colleagues. See Resources

Step Three: Learning New Ways to Process Emotion and Manage Stress

Many people with TMS repress and suppress a variety of emotions, usually anger and sadness. Learning how to get in touch with those emotions and process them differently, as well as learning a variety of stress reduction approaches is important to maintain emotional health and prevent the TMS pain from returning.

Step Four: Increasing your Level of Self-Acceptance

Whilst this is not unique to people with TMS, many people have a low level of self-acceptance. Learning new ways to relating yourself with greater kindness, acceptance and respect helps to bring about a much more peaceful way of being.

In addition to having a TMS consultation with myself or a colleague, you can work through each of the steps by purchasing my TMS workbook. See Resources.

Vaginal thrush

Thrush is a very common problem for women and seven in ten say they have had thrush at some time in their lives.[1] Thrush is the second most common cause of an inflamed vagina (vaginitis), the most common being bacterial vaginosis, an infection caused by bacteria.

What causes thrush?

Thrush is an infection caused by a yeast called *Candida albicans*, which normally lives on the skin and around the vaginal area. The immune system and the 'friendly' bacteria that live on the skin and in the vagina as well usually keep them in check. Candida thrives in warm, moist airless conditions, which is why the vagina, groin and mouth are most commonly affected. While most bouts of thrush are caused by *Candida albicans*, about one in ten are caused by other strains of candida, such as *Candida glabrata*, which doesn't respond so well to anti-thrush treatment

What are the risk factors?

The following are associated with an increased risk of developing thrush:

- Antibiotics (they probably kill 'friendly' bacteria in the vagina)

- The contraceptive pill and intrauterine device

- Diabetes (the high blood-sugar levels provide food for candida)

- A high-sugar diet (as above)

- Perfumed soaps, vaginal deodorants, douches, disinfectants and scented bubble baths (these can irritate or damage the delicate tissues of the vagina and vulva, and alter the naturally acidic pH of the vagina)

- Periods (changes in vaginal secretions and the presence of menstrual blood increase the likelihood of developing thrush for some women)

- Pregnancy (changes in hormones create high-sugar levels in vaginal secretions)

- Sex (if your partner has thrush or if you have sex without adequate lubrication)

- Tight trousers, synthetic knickers or tights (these prevent air from circulating, creating a warm, moist place for thrush to develop)

- Weak immune system (stress, illness, poor nutrition, HIV, fatigue or serious injury can make you more vulnerable to thrush)

My integrated medical prescription for vaginal thrush

If you experience repeated bouts of thrush, I would really recommend that you follow through on the following suggestions, as my patients find they considerably reduce the frequency of vaginal thrush episodes.

Step 1 • Do you have vaginal thrush?

The most common symptom of thrush is a discharge from your vagina. This is usually thick and white (a bit like cottage cheese, although some women get a discharge that is watery). The area outside your vagina may also feel sore and itchy. The skin might be red and cause you discomfort. You may find it hurts or burns when you pass urine or have sex.

If you are experiencing these symptoms for the first time or are unsure as to what is causing them you should go to your GP who can take a swab and examine you properly. A lot of women feel they can diagnose and treat thrush themselves, especially if they've had it before, but research has shown that one in two women who diagnose themselves as having thrush do not actually have it.

Step 2 ● Consider the medical options

If your doctor has been able to make the diagnosis of thrush or if you know it is thrush, you might want to consider the following treatments. Most of my patients prefer to take the tablets because they are more convenient.

Medications
Anti-fungal tablets offer two main choices: fluconazole, which is taken as a single dose, or itraconazole, which is taken as two doses over the course of one day. You can get these treatments on prescription and you can also buy fluconazole from pharmacies without a prescription. Side-effects are uncommon, but always read the product label and leaflet for full information.

Topical anti-fungals include pessaries and creams impregnated with anti-yeast medicines such as clotrimazole, econazole, fenticonazole, or miconazole. Commonly, a single large dose inserted into the vagina is sufficient to clear a bout of thrush. However, you may also want to rub some anti-yeast cream onto the skin around the vagina (the vulva) for a few days, especially if it is itchy. You can get topical treatments on prescription or you can buy them at pharmacies without a prescription.

Step 3 ● Address the underlying causes

While I am going to make recommendations to treat your thrush symptoms using a variety of supplements, for lasting resolution of thrush, I encourage you to fill in the questionnaires in part one, section two, in order to identify possible root causes or contributors. In my experience, the ones to consider are:

- **Candida** – Solution: Part Five (Dysbiosis – page 334); Holistic Health Tools – Emotional Freedom Technique (page 151)

- **Blood-sugar imbalance** – Solution: Secret One – Nurture Your Physical Body (Healthy Eating and Supplements – page 49)

- **Stress** – Solution: Secret Two – De-stress and Relax (page 77); Holistic Health Tools – Emotional Freedom Technique (page 151) and Mindfulness (page 147)

- **Poor diet** – Solution: Secret One – Nurture Your Physical Body (Healthy Eating and Supplements – page 49)

- **Food intolerances** – Solution: Part Five (Food Intolerances – page 344); Holistic Health Tools – Emotional Freedom Technique (page 151)

- **Nutritional deficiencies** – Solution: Secret One – Nurture Your Physical Body (Healthy Eating and Supplements – page 49)

Step 4 • Start an anti-thrush supplement programme

When used alongside step three, certain nutritional supplements can help to alleviate many of the symptoms of thrush. My integrated medicine prescription for thrush would usually include:

- **Probiotic pessary** (dose as advised by manufacturers) – these are an effective and natural alternative to anti-fungal pessaries. They work by introducing 'friendly' bacteria into the vagina through an applicator. See Resources.

- **Oral acidophilus probiotic** (dose as advised by manufacturers) to ensure that there are sufficient numbers of 'friendly' bacteria in the gut, which is important as it helps to prevent intestinal thrush from growing.[2]

Step 5 • Consider other complementary approaches

While there is no definitive evidence that these can help with your thrush, some patients find the following useful in supporting their programme: homeopathy, Western herbal medicine, traditional Chinese medicine and Ayurvedic medicine.

For recommended books see Resources.

Varicose veins

The word 'varicose' comes from the Latin root 'varix', which means 'twisted', and varicose veins are very common, affecting about one-third of women.[1] They are essentially dilated, tortuous veins, usually of the legs, that can cause considerable discomfort when inflamed. Because they do tend to get worse, they should be treated sooner rather than later.

What causes varicose veins?

The purpose of veins is to return blood to the heart, but unlike arteries, which have blood moved through them because of the pumping action of the heart, veins require a pumping action from the muscles surrounding them. To ensure that the blood flows in one direction, towards the heart, veins contain one-way valves. If those valves don't work or if the vein wall is in any way weakened, then blood will accumulate within the veins, leading to varicose veins.

What are the risk factors?

In addition to a genetically inherited weakness, other risk factors include:

- Being overweight

- Physical inactivity

- High-sugar, high-fat, low-fibre diet

- Prolonged periods of sitting or standing

- Constipation

- Hormonal imbalances

- Nutritional deficiencies

My integrated medical prescription for varicose veins

It's important to be realistic about what can be achieved if you do already have varicose veins! In my experience natural approaches, including supplements and lifestyle changes, can help prevent them from getting worse, but if they are causing severe problems or are cosmetically unsightly you will probably have to choose injections or surgery.

Step 1 • Do you have varicose veins?

Varicose veins are pretty easy to recognise. They are dark purple or blue in colour and may appear twisted and bulging. They most commonly appear on the back of the calves or inside the leg. When they become symptomatic they can cause:

- Itching around your veins

- An achy or heavy feeling in your legs

- Burning, throbbing, muscle cramping and swelling in your lower legs

- Skin ulcers near your ankle

Step 2 • Consider the medical options

The two main forms of medial treatment are injections and surgery.

Injections

Injections involve having a liquid injected into the varicose vein. The chemicals in the liquid damage the lining of the vein, causing it to collapse inwards and form a scar. This blocks off the vein and the vein fades within a few weeks. Injections help to improve appearance and relieve aching.[2] However, one study found that 50 per cent of people who have injections get new veins appearing within five years, compared to 30 per cent with surgery.[3] Side-effects include pain, itchy rash, blood clots, bruising, inflammation and reddish/brown stains on the surface of the skin.

Surgery

Surgery to remove varicose veins has been found to improve the way the legs look and reduce symptoms such as aching and heaviness.[4] The research has found that if varicose veins are removed by stripping, then you have less chance of them coming back than if the veins are tied off, but not removed. Surgery is usually more effective than injections, but it is associated with more side-effects, including post-operative pain, infections, numb patches on the legs, inflammation, brown stains on the legs and interference with normal daily function.[5] One study found that the average time taken off from work following surgery for varicose veins was 20 days.[6]

Step 3 • Address the underlying causes

While I am going to make recommendations to reduce the symptoms associated with varicose veins, for the best results, I encourage you to fill in the questionnaires in part one, section two, in order to identify possible root causes or contributors. In my experience, the ones to consider are:

- **Excessive weight** – Solution: Secret One – Nurture Your Physical Body (Healthy Eating and Supplements – page 49); Part Five (Weight Loss – page 401); Holistic Health Tools – Emotional Freedom Technique (page 151) and The Work (page 163)

- **Nutritional deficiencies** – Solution: Secret One – Nurture Your Physical Body (Healthy Eating and Supplements – page 49)

- **Lack of physical activity** – Solution: Secret One (Physical Activity and Touch – page 67); Holistic Health Tools – Emotional Freedom Technique (page 151) and Values-based Goal Setting (page 166)

Step 4 • Start a varicose vein supplement programme

When used alongside step three, certain nutritional supplements can help to alleviate the symptoms associated with varicose veins. My integrated medicine prescription for varicose veins would usually include:

- **Vitamin C with bioflavonoids** (1000mg to 3000mg a day) to reduce inflammation and pain.[7]

- **Omega-3, 6 and 9** (taken in capsule or liquid form in a 2:1:1 ratio) to provide the body with anti-inflammatory essential fatty acids.

- **Horse chestnut** (dose as advised by manufacturers), a herb commonly prescribed in Germany for venous problems, might help to reduce swelling and strengthen the valves of the veins.[8]

- **Bromelain** (200mg three times a day) is a natural anti-inflammatory and also helps to prevent blood clots.[9]

Step 5 • Consider other complementary approaches

While there is no definitive evidence that these can help you with your varicose veins, some patients find the following useful in supporting their programme: acupuncture, acupressure, reflexology, Western herbal medicine, homeopathy, yoga, traditional Chinese medicine and Ayurvedic medicine.

For recommended books see Resources.

Weight loss

Trying to lose weight, or more accurately lose fat, is a national pastime. One report found that British women spend an average of six months a year counting calories and more than a fifth are on a permanent diet throughout their lifetime. The average diet will last just five weeks, with most giving up either through 'lack of willpower' or because they felt worse being on a diet. For women looks are the most important reason for dieting, with over half reporting that they diet to wear fashionable clothes, and a third of those surveyed said they watched their weight in a bid to feel more attractive.[1]

Being overweight or obese (56 per cent of women are overweight or obese[2]) increases the risk of numerous health problems, including cancer (endometrial, breast and colon), heart disease, stroke, infertility, oestrogen-contraceptive pill failure, type II diabetes, high blood pressure, arthritis and gall bladder disease.[3]

What causes weight gain?

While there is no doubt that genetic factors, daily calorie consumption and levels of physical activity all play their part in obesity and weight gain, in my experience many of the women I see who want advice on losing weight are emotional eaters – that is they use food to make themselves feel better and to manage stress. Other causes or contributors include insulin resistance, food addiction, food intolerances, hypothyroidism, sleep deprivation, medications, nutritional deficiencies and hormonal fluctuations.

What are the risk factors?

The risk factors for obesity include:

- Being female (women have a lower muscle mass than men and a lower average metabolic rate, which means you burn less calories per day compared to men)

- Genes (your genetic make-up plays a role in how efficiently your body converts food into energy, the amount of body fat you store and where it is stored)

- Family history (especially if one or both of your parents are obese)

- Age (as you get older you tend to be less active, you lose muscle mass and you will experience a decrease in your rate of metabolism)

My integrated medical prescription for weight loss

At the heart of my own approach to weight loss is a personalised nutrient-dense diet, consisting mainly of foods that have a high proportion of nutrients (including vitamins, minerals, fibre and phytochemicals) to calories. It also deals with the underlying barriers to lasting weight loss, such as emotional eating and stress, weight promoting habits (lack of physical activity, sleep deprivation and poor eating choices), insulin resistance, food cravings, prescription drugs and health problems (including hyperthyroidism and food intolerances). The key to its success in helping my patients lose weight and then maintain that weight loss is the fact that it helps identify what is preventing you from losing weight, plus it supports you in making food choices that are designed to reduce low-grade inflammation and blood-sugar imbalances, which are responsible for many of the negative health effects related to obesity.

Step 1 • Are you overweight?

There are plenty of ways to work out whether you are overweight or obese. The quick test is to pinch your skin just below your belly button, if you can pinch more than one inch you might benefit from losing weight. If you go to your GP they will measure your body mass index (BMI). It helps to work out whether your weight is healthy or not by taking your height (in centimetres or feet) and then dividing it by your weight (in kilograms or pounds). See Resources for an online BMI calculator. The table below shows what your score indicates:

BMI	WHAT IT INDICATES
Less than 18.5	underweight
18.5 to 24.9	healthy weight
25 to 29.9	overweight
30 or more	obese

There are a couple of limitations with this, though. Firstly muscle weighs more than fat, so if you are muscular you might show up as overweight, when in fact you are really at a healthy weight. I also believe weight is not the best indicator of health. For example, it is better to be fit and slightly overweight than a normal weight and unfit.

An alternative to BMI, and the method I prefer, is weight to hip ratio, which is as important as BMI, because it's not just how much fat you carry that influences your health, but also where you carry your fat. Women who are 'apple-shaped', with a lot of fat around their waist and chest, are more likely to develop heart disease and diabetes, for example, when compared with women who are 'pear-shaped' and who carry weight on their hips and buttocks.

For example, if your waist is 35 inches and your hips are 38 inches, your waist to hip ratio is 0.92. Your risk of developing heart disease and diabetes increases significantly if:

- You are apple-shaped

- Your waist-hip ratio is more than 0.9

Step 2 • Consider the medical options

If you present to your GP and ask them to support you in losing weight, or if he or she suggests it, in theory you should be offered a combination of a low-calorie diet, an exercise programme, psychotherapy or support in making these changes and perhaps drugs and surgery. In reality most women avoid asking their GP about weight loss, because they know for most of them it's not their area of expertise! However, there might be circumstances in which your weight is a significant threat to your physical and emotional health, and your GP might refer you to a weight loss specialist.

Medications

Medical options for supporting weight loss include medications, which need to be combined with dietary changes and exercise.

Orlistat (Xenical) – this drug reduces the amount of fat you absorb from food. While it does support weight loss and it can help lower cholesterol and elevated blood-sugar levels,[4] it is associated with a variety of side-effects, such as diarrhoea, wind and oily leakage from bowels, and it reduces the absorption of vitamin D, vitamin E, vitamin K and beta-carotene (vitamin A).

Rimonabant (Accomplia) – this is an appetite suppressant that helps to reduce feelings of hunger. Again, it can help a weight-loss programme, but its side-effects are significant – it doubles the likelihood of you becoming depressed, and it can also cause nausea, dizziness and headaches.[5]

Sibutramine (Reductil) – this drug is also an appetite suppressant. Its side-effects are a dry mouth, constipation, raised blood pressure and insomnia.[6]

I recommend to all my patients that they stay well away from these medications, simply because safe, effective weight loss can be achieved without them.

Surgery

If you have severe obesity you might be offered one of the following operations: gastric bypass (making the stomach smaller), gastric banding and biliopancreatic diversion. All of these are associated with significant risks and do nothing to address the underlying issues. They should only be used as an absolute last resort.

Step 3 • Address the underlying causes

While I am going to make recommendations for supplements that will support your weight loss, at the heart of my weight loss programme is secret one – nurture your physical body. In this part of the book I provide advice on what and what not to eat, as well as physical activity, sleep, rest and a healthy environment, all of which are essential to healthy weight loss. As long as you are also addressing the underlying barriers to healthy weight loss (below) and following my instructions in secret one, you should experience a weight loss of between 2 and 4lb per week. My preference for you is that you see these dietary and lifestyle changes as a new way of being, rather than a diet that you want to do for a couple of months. If you take this attitude you are so much more likely to not only achieve your target weight, but keep the excess fat off. To support you in this, I encourage you to fill in the questionnaires in part one, section two, in order to identify possible barriers to successful weight loss. In my experience, the ones to consider are:

- **Stress** – Solution: Secret Two – De-stress and Relax (page 77); Holistic Health Tools – Emotional Freedom Technique (page 151) and Mindfulness (page 147)

- **Emotional eating** – Solution: Secret One – Nurture Your Physical Body (Healthy Eating and Supplements – page 49); Secret Three – Face and Embrace Your Emotions (page 94); Secret Two – De-stress and Relax (page 77); Holistic Health Tools – Emotional Freedom Technique (page 151) and Mindfulness (page 147)

- **Habits** – Solution: Secret One – Nurture Your Physical Body (Healthy Eating and Supplements – page 49); Holistic Health Tools – Emotional Freedom Technique (page 151) and Values-based Goal Setting (page 166)

- **Poor diet** – Solution: Secret One – Nurture Your Physical Body (Healthy Eating and Supplements – page 49)

- **Metabolic syndrome** – Solution: Part Five (Metabolic Syndrome – page 368)

- **Lack of physical activity** – Solution: Secret One – Nurture Your Physical Body (Physical Activity and Touch – page 67); Holistic Health Tools – Emotional Freedom Technique (page 151) and Values-based Goal Setting (page 166)

- **Eating disorders** – Solution: Secret One – Nurture Your Physical Body (Healthy Eating and Supplements – page 49); Secret Four – Accept Yourself (page 113); Secret Three – Face and Embrace Your Emotions (page 94); Secret Five – Develop and Deepen Your Relationships (page 127); Part Five (Addictions – page 260); Holistic Health Tools – Mindfulness (page 147), Emotional Freedom Technique (page 151) and Values-based Goal Setting (page 166)

- **Low self-acceptance** – Solution: Secret Four – Accept Yourself (page 113); Secret Three – Face and Embrace Your Emotions (page 94); Secret Five – Develop and Deepen Your Relationships (page 127); Holistic Health Tools – Mindfulness (page 147), Emotional Freedom Technique (page 151) and Values-based Goal Setting (page 166)

- **Food intolerances** – Solution: Part Five (Food Intolerances – page 344); Holistic Health Tools – Emotional Freedom Technique (page 151)

- **Nutritional deficiencies** – Solution: Secret One – Nurture Your Physical Body (Healthy Eating and Supplements – page 49)

- **Hypothyroidism** – Solution: Part Five (Hypothyroidism – page 356); Holistic Health Tools – Emotional Freedom Technique (page 151) and The Work (page 163)

- **Sleep deprivation** – Solution: Secret One – Nurture Your Physical Body (Rest and Sleep – page 45); Holistic Health Tools – Emotional Freedom Technique (page 151)

Step 4 • Start a weight loss support supplement programme

When used alongside step three, certain nutritional supplements can help to support healthy weight loss. My integrated medicine prescription for weight loss would usually include:

- **Easy-3** (dose as advised by manufacturer) If you don't eat at least 5 portions of fruit and vegetables a day, then I highly recommend you take a whole food supplement such as Easy-3. While nothing compares to real fruits and vegetables, whole food supplements contain concentrated whole foods, such as tomatoes, broccoli sprouts, berries and apples. These whole foods are dried, ground up, put into powders and then drunk as a smoothie or sprinkled on food. Unlike isolated vitamins and minerals, whole foods supplements retain all the phyto-nutrients and fibre of fruits and vegetables. See Resources.

- **Potato protein extract (PI2)** stimulates the release of a chemical called cholecystokinin, which creates the feeling of fullness and satisfaction. It is best taken about an hour before eating to help manage hunger and appetite.[7] Because it triggers feelings of fullness it is particularly helpful if you have a tendency to overeat or feel peckish all of the time. I recommend my patients take one capsule of the product Full? Stop! before meals as this contains the potato protein extract PI2. See Resources.

- **Chromium GTF** (400mcg to 1000mcg a day) is good for helping to balance blood-sugar swings, treat insulin resistance and prevent carbohydrate-sugar cravings.[8] It is best taken between meals on an empty stomach.

- **Alpha-lipoic acid** (100mg three times a day) is a powerful antioxidant that helps to combat damaging free radicals, as well as helping to increase the uptake of glucose into muscle cells and improve insulin sensitivity.[9] This makes it a useful aid to blood-sugar balance and appetite management. L-carnitine is an amino acid that increases the metabolism of fat. It works by helping to shuttle fatty acids into the mitochondria of cells where they are burnt for energy, so it is great for encouraging fat loss. The dose for this is also 100mg three times a day.

- **Conjugated Linolenic Acid CLA** (1000mg 3 times a day) is particularly appropriate for people who struggle to manage their weight and yo-yo between weight loss and weight gain. A 2005 study published in the US Journal of Nutrition looked at the effect of CLA on body fat mass and fat regain after dieting. Of the 134 subjects tested those with the highest body fat mass lost the most weight. In addition, the subjects did not regain any of the fat over the full two-year testing period, avoiding the yo-yoing effects of weight loss and regain.[10]

- **5-HTP** (100mg to 300mg daily) is an amino acid that helps to produce the good-mood brain neurotransmitter serotonin. If you experience cravings or are an emotional eater, you might want to consider taking this. 5-HTP is best taken in combination with the nutrients B3, B6, folic acid, zinc and biotin as these are important cofactors for the pathway the body uses to make serotonin. The most effective way to take 5-HTP is on an empty stomach with a small carbohydrate snack such as an oatcake or rice cake. This ensures maximum absorption of the 5-HTP and helps it to get transported into the brain where it is most needed.

Step 5 • Consider other complementary approaches

In addition to considering the suggestions I have made, the following have also been found to help women maintain a lower weight:

- Having long-term contact with a health professional or a therapist
- Going to a self-help group
- Getting support from family or partner
- Being very focused on losing weight and keeping it off

The latter might mean weighing yourself every day, and following a plan about what you eat and how much exercise you take, although personally I'm not a fan of weighing yourself every day, as it can become obsessive and also take the focus away from healthy living to an excessive focus on weight loss.

Other supportive approaches that you might want to consider include cognitive behavioural therapy, motivational interviewing, life coaching, acupuncture, homeopathy, yoga, traditional Chinese medicine and Ayurvedic medicine.

For recommended books and for details of my weight loss seminars and consultation services see Resources.

Resources

Health practitioners – UK

If you need some help and advice in overcoming a health challenge, I recommend that you contact one of the following organisations:

Integrated Medical Practice
This is my own clinic
W: www.drmarkatkinson.com
T: 0845 0946450

British Society for Ecological Medicine
For doctors who practise allergy, environmental and nutritional medicine
W: www.ecomed.org.uk
T: 0207 100 7090

British Society of Integrated Medicine
For doctors who practise integrated medicine
W: www.bsim.org.uk
T: 01962 718000

British College of Integrated Medicine
Offers training programmes to doctors and nurses in integrated medicine.
W: www.integratedmedicine.org.uk
T: 0845 8909131

Complementary Medical Association

The world's largest membership organisation for complementary
therapists

W: www.the-cma.org.uk

T: 0845 1298434

British Naturopathic Association

The professional body for naturopaths

W: www.naturopaths.org.uk

T: 0870 7456984

British Association for Applied Nutrition and Nutritional Therapy

The professional body for nutritional therapists

W: www.bant.org.uk

T: 0870 6061284

Health practitioners – worldwide

Australasian Integrative Medical Association

Provides a list of general practitioners and/or specialists who are
members of the association and who practise some form of integrative
medicine

W: www.aima.net.au

T: (03) 86990582

New Zealand Natural Medicine Association

Provides a list of health professionals dedicated to the promotion of
integrative healthcare

W: www.nznma.com

T: 64 9 4432066

South African Society of Integrated Medicine

Provides a list of registered health practitioners, who practise, or have
an interest in, integrative medicine

W: www.integrativemedicine.co.za

T: 27-21-885 1010

American Association of Integrative Medicine
Provides a list of health professionals dedicated to the promotion of integrative healthcare
W: www.aaimedicine.com
T: 417-881-9995

American Holistic Medical Association
Provides a list of health professionals dedicated to the promotion of holistic healthcare
W: www.holisticmedicine.org
T: 425-967-0737

Supplement companies – UK

Higher Nature
One of the UK's leading supplement companies
W: www.highernature.co.uk
T: 0800 4584747

Revital
A mail order and retail company selling high-quality supplements, foods, books and CDs
W: www.revital.com
T: 0800 252875

Nutrilink
A supplier of nutritional supplements to practitioners
W: www.nutri-linkltd.co.uk
T: 0870 4054002

Supplement companies – worldwide

Higher Nature
Delivers products worldwide
W: www.highernature.co.uk

Australia

Blackmores
W: www.blackmores.com.au
T: 02 9951 0111

South Africa

Bioharmony
W: www.bioharmony.co.za
T: (021) 762 8803

New Zealand

Aurora Natural Therapies
W: www.aurora.org.nz
T: (03) 578 1236

USA

Nature's Plus
W: www.naturesplus.com
T: (800) 6459500

Solgar
W: www.solgar.com
T: (800) 6452246

Diagnostic testing – UK

Genova Diagnostics Europe
W: www.gdx.uk.net
T: 0208 336 7750

Cambridge Nutritional Sciences
W: www.cambridge-nutritional.com
T: 01353 863279

Diagnostic testing – worldwide

Australia

Nutritional Laboratory Services
W: www.nlabs.com.au
T: 03 96631554

New Zealand

Ideal Health
W: www.healthyonline.co.nz
T: 09 4432584

South Africa

Molecular Diagnostic Services
W: www.mdsafrica.net
T: (31) 267 7000

USA

Genova Diagnostics
W: www.genovadiagnostics.com
T: 800 522 4762

Complementary medical approaches recommended in parts 4 and 5

Acceptance and Commitment Therapy (ACT) is a unique and creative model for both therapy and coaching, based on the innovative use of mindfulness. The aim of ACT is to create a rich, full and meaningful life, cultivating vitality and wellbeing through mindfulness and values-guided action. For more information visit the website of the Association for Contextual Behavioural Science: www.contextualpsychology.org

Acupuncture is an ancient oriental healing technique based on the theoretical concept of balanced *qi* (pronounced 'chee') or vital energy that flows throughout the body via certain pathways (meridians) that are accessed by puncturing the skin with hair-thin needles at particular locations called acupuncture points. Stimulation of acupuncture points is believed to stimulate the brain and spinal cord to release chemicals that change the experience of pain or cause biochemical changes that may stimulate healing and promote general wellbeing. For more information visit the website of the British Acupuncture Council: www.acupuncture.org.uk

Aromatherapy is the systematic use of essential oils in holistic treatments to improve physical and emotional wellbeing. Essential oils, extracted from plants, possess distinctive therapeutic properties, which can be utilised to improve health and prevent disease. For more information visit the website of the Aromatherapy Council: www.aromatherapycouncil.co.uk

Art therapy is a form of psychotherapy that uses art media as its primary mode of communication. For more information visit the website of the British Association of Art Therapists: www.baat.org

Ayurveda is the ancient Indian philosophy of health and wellbeing. It means the 'art of living wisely'. In simple terms, Ayurveda is a holistic system which guides us so that we can live a healthier and more balanced lifestyle. It recognises that we are all unique and focuses on food, lifestyle, massage, yoga and herbal remedies to suit our individual make-up. For more information visit the website of the Ayurvedic Company of Great Britain: www.ayurvedagb.com

Bach Flower Remedies are dilutions of flower material developed by Edward Bach, an English physician and homeopath. The remedies are used primarily for emotional and spiritual conditions. For more information visit the website of the Bach Flower Remedy Centre: www.bachcentre.com

Breathwork is a simple, gentle, yet powerful technique which allows you to access, release and integrate memories, emotions and patterns stored in your body, mind and soul that hinder you from living to your full potential, physically, emotionally and mentally. For more information visit the website of Inbreath: www.inbreath.info

Colon hydrotherapy, which is also known as colonic irrigation, colonics or colonic lavage, uses filtered water to help remove waste from the bowels. For more information visit the website of the Association and Register of Colon Hydrotherapists: www.colonic-association.org

Core energetics is a powerful therapeutic approach that seeks the integration of all aspects of our being – body, mind, emotions, will and spirit. It is a supportive process enabling you to explore past and present issues. For more information visit the website of Core Energetics UK: www.core-energetics.co.uk

Counselling, while varying in its approach, is usually designed to help you explore ways in which you can experience a more healthy and fulfilling life. For more information visit the website of the British Association for Counselling and Psychotherapy: www.bacp.co.uk

Ear acupuncture is an ancient oriental therapy that uses acupuncture points on different parts of the ear to trigger healing in the body. For more information visit the website of the Society of Auricular Acupuncture: www.auricularacupuncture.org.uk

Guided imagery involves the guided use of images in order to bring about a specific goal, relaxation, healing or insight. For more information visit the website of the Mindfields College: www.mindfields.org.uk

Homeopathy is a term derived from the Greek words *homoios*, meaning 'similar', and *pathos*, meaning 'suffering'. Homeopathy is an alternative medical system that treats the symptoms of a disease with minute doses of a natural substance or remedy. For more information visit the website of the Society of Homeopaths: www.homeopathy-soh.org

Hypnotherapy is the application of hypnotic techniques in such a way as to bring about therapeutic changes and realistic goals. For more information visit the website of the National Council for Hypnotherapy: www.hypnotherapists.org.uk

The Journey is an emotional healing technique developed by Brandon Bays, one of the world's leading mind–body experts. You can either attend a workshop or a one-to-one consultation with a trained 'journey' therapist. For more information visit www.thejourney.com

Life coaching aims to help you unlock your potential for a healthy, happy, successful and fulfilling life. For more information visit the website of the Association for Coaching: www.associationforcoaching.com

Massage is a form of therapy in which the soft tissues are made more pliable, promoting increased blood flow and healing. For more information visit the website of the British Massage Therapy Council: www.bmtc.co.uk

Motivational interviewing is a focused, goal-directed approach to counselling that is designed to explore and resolve ambivalence to change. For more information visit the website of the Motivational Interviewing Network of Trainers: www.motivationalinterview.org

Music therapy is the use of music in order to promote healing and enhance quality of life. Music therapy may be used to encourage emotional expression, promote social interaction, relieve symptoms and for other purposes. For more information visit the website of the British Society for Music Therapy: www.bsmt.org

Osteopathy is a way of detecting and treating damaged parts of the body such as muscles, ligaments, nerves and joints. For more information visit the website of the Osteopathic Council: www.osteopathy.org.uk

Rebounding involves performing a series of exercises on a mini-trampoline. I recommend the PT Rebounder from www.bouncyhappypeople.co.uk

Reflexology is a complementary therapy that works on the feet or hands, unblocking vital energy pathways and restoring a state of balance. For more information visit the website of the Association of Reflexologists: www.aor.org.uk

Reiki is an original method of healing, developed by Mikao Usui in Japan, early in the 20th century, which is activated by intention. Reiki's natural healing energy works on every level, not just the physical, and promotes the body's regenerative self-healing ability. For more information visit the website of the UK Reiki Federation: www.reikifed.co.uk

Solution-focused brief therapy is a brief future-focused approach to counselling that works with the strengths of those who come by making the best use of their resources. It can bring about lasting change precisely because it aims to build solutions rather than solve problems. For more information visit the website of the Brief Therapy Practice: www.brieftherapy.org.uk

Spiritual counselling is designed to help you discover the truth of who you are and to help resolve the blocks or barriers to you thriving and flourishing as a human being. I can recommend any of the following spiritual counsellors: Catherine Lucas (UK) www.catherinelucas.co.uk, Leo Hawkins (UK) www.globalalchemy.com or Stephan Bodian (USA) www.stephanbodian.org

Spiritual healing is a natural energy therapy which treats the whole person – mind, body and spirit. Spiritual healers act as a conduit for healing energy, often described as 'love and light', which relaxes the body, releases tensions and stimulates self-healing. For more information visit the website of the National Federation of Healers: www.nfsh.org.uk

Tibetan medicine is a natural and holistic medical science, which addresses the individual's needs of body, mind and spirit, in an integrated way. Dating back to antiquity, Tibetan medicine has a genesis, history and development of its own, rooted in the Tibetan landscape, the indigenous culture and the spirit of the Tibetan people. For more information visit the website of the Kailash Centre of Oriental Medicine: www.kailashcentre.org

Traditional Chinese medicine is an ancient and comprehensive approach to health and healing that embraces a wide variety of theories, diagnoses and treatments, such as herbal medicine, acupuncture, massage and qi gong. For more information visit the website of the Chinese Medical Institute: www.cmir.org.uk

Western herbal medicine is a healthcare system practised by professionals called 'herbalists' that uses the healing properties of plants to combat illness. For more information visit the website of the National Institute of Medical Herbalists: www.nimh.org.uk

Yoga is translated as 'union' between mind, body and spirit. In the West, the most widely taught form of yoga is hatha yoga, with classes offering students exercises to stretch and flex the body, develop breath awareness, relaxation and sometimes meditation. For more information visit the website of the British Wheel of Yoga: www.bwy.org.uk

Recommended supplements, products and websites

Part One: You are unique

Section One: Women and the New Medicine

Websites
Society for Women's Health Research:
www.womenshealthresearch.org
Alternative and Complementary Health and Wellbeing:
www.healthy.net

National Center for Complementary and Alternative Medicine
www.nccam.nih.gov

Section Two: Your Personal Health, Healing and Happiness Programme

Websites
General information on women's health: www.womens-health-concern.org
News and advice on health issues: www.netdoctor.co.uk
UK patient information: www.patient.co.uk
Medical encyclopaedia: www.gpnotebook.co.uk
UK National Health Service: www.nhsdirect.nhs.uk
To check for supplement/medication interactions: www.wholehealthmd.com

Part Two: The five secrets of health, healing and happiness

Secret One: Nurture Your Physical Body

Websites
Details of women's health screening recommendations: www.library.nhs.uk/screening
Eating disorders help: www.eating-disorders.org.uk
GI and GL information: www.nutritiondata.com

Rest and sleep
Alphastim SCS and Guided Imagery CD: www.mindbodyproducts.com

Healthy eating and supplements
Multivitamin-mineral: Advanced Nutrition Complex (from Higher Nature) or Formula VM-75 Tablets (from Solgar) or if you have adrenal fatigue Dr Wilson's Adrenal Powder (from Nutrilink) or if your immune system needs supporting Wholly Immune (from Nutrilink)
Vitamin C: Allergy Research Group Buffered Vitamin C (from Nutrilink) or True Food C (from Higher Nature)
Fish oil: Nordic Naturals Arctic Omega – Liquid (from Nutrilink) or Lemon Fish Oil (from Higher Nature) or Organic Flaxseed Oil if

vegetarian (from Higher Nature) or Organic Omega 3:6:9 Balance Oil (from Higher Nature)

Antioxidant: Super-Antioxidant Protection (from Higher Nature) or Advanced Antioxidant Formula (Solgar)

Wholefood supplement: Easy-3 (from Higher Nature)

Cordyceps, Maitake, Reishi, Shiitake and Trametes Complex (from Fruiting Bodies: www.fruiting-bodies.co.uk/01550 740306)

Rhodiola and Ashwagandha (from Higher Nature)

Healthy environment and sunlight

Natural cleaning products: from Natural House (www.natural-house.co.uk) and 21st Century Health (www.21stcenturyhealth.co.uk)

Personal care products: Absolutely Pure (www.absolutelypure.com), Neways (www.neways.com) and Goodness Direct (www.goodnessdirect.co.uk). Natracare (www.natracare.com) produce a range of 100 per cent cotton tampons that do not produce the toxin associated with toxic shock.

Water filters: a wellness filter system (www.highernature.co.uk) or a reverse osmosis system (www.freshlysqueezedwater.com) will provide you with clean water, free from contaminants.

Negative air ioniser: www.elanra.co.uk

Mercury-free dentistry: www.mercuryfreedentistry.org.uk

Secret Two: De-Stress and Relax

Recommended test: Comprehensive Adrenal Stress Profile (from Genova Diagnostics)

Recommended CDs:

Richard Miller, *Yoga Nidra*, Sounds True

Rod Stryker, *Relax into Greatness*, Pure Yoga

Andrew Weil and Martin Rossman, *Self-Healing with Guided Imagery*, Sounds True

Puran and Susanna Bair, *Energizing Heart Rhythm Meditation* (from www.iamheart.org)

Secret Three: Face and Embrace Your Emotions

Recommendations for resolving trauma

Significant trauma needs to be dealt with by a professional who is trained to do so. This is especially so if you are suffering distressing or debilitating symptoms as a result of the trauma. While there are many different approaches to treating trauma, including trauma incident reduction (www.tir.org), somatic experiencing (www.traumahealing.com) and core energetics (www.core-energetics.co.uk), the two that I am most familiar with are the rewind technique (www.hgi.org.uk/register) and EMDR (www.emdrassociation.org.uk)

Secret Four: Accept Yourself

Inner child workshops: www.clairehershman.com, www.innerchildhealing.com and www.ppfoundation.org
Inner child CD: Shaina Noll, *Songs for the Inner Child*, Singing Heart

Secret Five: Develop and Deepen Your Relationships

The Freedom Process is a workshop that teaches a psychological approach to transforming barriers to intimacy: www.thefreedomprocess.com
Recovering Couples Anonymous: www.recovering-couples.org

Part Three: Holistic health tools

Tool One: Mindfulness

Recommended CDs:
Guided Meditations: For Calmness, Awareness and Love by Bodhipaska
Guided Mindfulness Meditation by Jon Kabat-Zinn

Tool Two: Emotional Freedom Technique

For information about how EFT works, and also a course in EFT, visit the website of Gary Craig: www.emofree.com. See also Dr Patricia Carrington's website: www.eftupdate.com

Tool Three: EmoTrance

For more information or to find a practitioner visit: www.EmoTrance.com

Tool Four: The Work

For more information visit Byron Katie's website: www.thework.com

Part Four: Women's health solutions

PMS
For more information on PMS visit The National Association for Premenstrual Syndrome: www.pms.org.uk

Painful periods
Recommended products
Menastil: www.menastil.co.uk
MagnoPulse MN8: www.magno-pulse.com
Pain Ease: www.lifes2good.com

Fibroids
For more information on natural progesterone cream visit: www.npis.info

Endometriosis
For more information on natural progesterone cream visit: www.npis.info
Pain Ease microcurrent patches visit: www.lifes2good.com

Support groups
The support group Endometriosis UK has got a lot of information: http://www.endometriosis-uk.org/. Another good website is: www.endometriosis.org/support.html

Cystitis
Recommended supplements (in addition to the foundation programme):
Biotech D-Mannose (from Nutrilink) or D-Mannose Plus (from Vitamin Research Products)
AlkaClear (alkaline mineral salts) (from Higher Nature)
DLPA Complex (contains bromelain, astaxanthin and DLPA) (from Higher Nature) or Ultra Bromelain (150mg) (Nature's Plus)
Cranberry Extract (from Solgar) or Cranberry Complex (from Solgar)

Fibrocystic breast disease
Liv Kit visit: www.livkit.com
For more information on digital infra-red thermal imaging visit:
www.wholisticmedical.co.uk and www.chironclinic.com
For more information on breast care visit:
www.breastcancercare.org.uk
For more information on natural progesterone cream visit:
www.npis.info

Infertility
The Human Fertilisation and Embryology Authority (HFEA):
www.hfea.gov.uk
For more information on infertility treatment visit Foresight:
www.foresight-preconception.org.uk and the Infertility Network:
www.infertilitynetworkuk.com

Infertility treatment clinics – UK
There are many different clinics in the UK designed to improve a
couple's chances of conceiving. Here are just some of those that I am
aware of:
The Life Fertility Care Programme: www.lifefertilitycare.co.uk
The Zita West Clinic: www.zitawest.com
Dr Marilyn Glenville: www.marilynglenville.com
The Endometriosis and Fertility Clinic: www.makingbabies.com

Menopause
Recommended supplements (in addition to the foundation programme):
True Food Super Potency Soyagen (fermented soya) (from Higher
Nature) or Red Clover (from Revital)
For more information on natural progesterone cream visit:
www.npis.info

Recommended tests
Home menopause test: www.checkmybody.co.uk
Essence Menopause: www.gdx.uk.net

Part Five: Integrated medical solutions

Acne
For more information about the Sher System visit: www.sher.co.uk

Addictions
Addictive tendency questionnaire: www.s-p-q.com.
Information on the 12 steps: www.12step.org
Alcoholics Anonymous: www.alcoholics-anonymous.org.uk
For information on the SMART recovery programme visit:
www.smartrecovery.org

UK treatment centres
LifeWorks: www.lifeworkscommunity.com
Promis Clinics: www.promis.co.uk
Western Counselling: www.westerncounselling.co.uk
Action on Addiction: www.actiononaddiction.org.uk

US treatment centres
The Bridge to Recovery: www.thebridgetorecovery.com
The Meadows Institute: www.themeadows.org
Bridging the Gaps: www.bridgingthegaps.com
The Betty Ford Center: www.bettyfordcenter.org

Adrenal fatigue
Recommended test
Comprehensive Adrenal Stress Profile: www.gdx.uk.net
I start most of my patients with adrenal fatigue on Dr Wilson's
Adrenal Powder, a specially formulated supplement (from Nutrilink)

Anxiety and panic disorders
Recommended supplements (in addition to the foundation programme):
Zen (from Nutrilink) or Balance for Nerves (from Higher Nature)
Online anxiety management course: www.moodgym.anu.edu.au
Alphastim SCS: www.mindbodyproducts.com

Support groups/more information
Social Anxiety UK: http://www.social-anxiety.org.uk
Anxiety Care: www.anxietycare.org.uk
MIND: www.mind.org.uk

For a therapist to support you in treating your anxiety
Human Givens therapist: www.hgi.org.uk
Cognitive behavioural therapist: www.babcp.com
Solution-focused brief therapy: www.brieftherapy.org.uk
Acceptance and commitment therapist:
www.contextualpsychology.org

Cancer
Recommended self-help books/reports
The Cancer Lifeline Kit from Health Creation:
www.healthcreation.co.uk
Self-help starter pack from the Penny Brohn Cancer Centre:
www.pennybrohncancercare.org
The Moss Reports from: www.cancerdecisions.com

Supplements
Organic mushroom tinctures: www.fruiting-bodies.co.uk

Recommended cancer websites
www.canceractive.com
www.annieappleseedproject.org
www.cancer.gov

Recommended products
The Magnessage from Vitalia Health: www.vitalia-health.co.uk
Guided imagery for cancer from: www.mindbodyproducts.com

Cardiovascular disease
Recommended supplements
Cardiovascular Support (from Solgar)
Cardio Heart Nutrients (from Higher Nature)

Recommended test
Comprehensive Cardiovascular Risk Assessment 2.0: www.gdx.uk.net

For further information about heart disease visit the website of the British Heart Foundation: www.bhf.org.uk and the Stroke Association: www.stroke.org.uk
For more information on stopping smoking visit: www.quit.org.uk and www.gosmokefree.nhs.uk

Cellulite
AlkaClear (from Higher Nature)
Phytotec Cellulite System: www.treatmentgels.co.uk
The Anti-Cellulite Body Blitz: www.urbanretreat.co.uk

CFS/Fibromyalgia
Recommended workshops/therapists
The Freedom Process: www.thefreedomprocess.com
Neurostructural Integration Technique: www.nsthealth.com
The Lightening Process: www.lighteningprocess.com
Reverse Therapy: www.reverse-therapy.com
The Perrin Technique: www.theperrinclinic.com

Codependency
Treatment programmes
The Bridge to Recovery in Bowling Green, Kentucky, USA: www.thebridgetorecovery.com
The Survivors Workshop at The Meadows in Wickenburg, Arizona, USA: www.themeadows.com
12-step group: Codependants Anonymous (CODA): www.codependents.org
Workshops/consultations with Barry and Janae Weinhold: www.weinholds.org
Emotionally focused therapy: www.eft.ca

Constipation
Oxytech (oxygenated magnesium): www.dulwichhealth.co.uk

Depression
For a therapist to support you in treating your depression
Human Givens therapist: www.hgi.org.uk
Cognitive behavioural therapist: www.babcp.com
Solution-focused brief therapy: www.brieftherapy.org.uk
Acceptance and commitment therapist:
www.contextualpsychology.org

For depression products
Alphastim and CDs: www.mindbodyproducts.com
SAD light boxes: www.sadbox.co.uk
Positive Outlook (from Higher Nature)

For more information
The charity Depression Alliance has a lot of useful information on its
website: www.depressionalliance.org

For free self-help depression programmes
The two that my patients like most and the two that I regard most
highly are: www.clinical-depression.co.uk and
www.moodgym.anu.edu.au

Diabetes
For more information on diabetes visit: www.diabetes.org.uk

Dysbiosis
Recommended test
Comprehensive Digestive Stool Analysis with Parasitology (CDSAP)
2.0: www.gdx.uk.net

Recommended supplements (in addition to the foundation programme):
Oxytech (oxygenated magnesium): www.dulwichhealth.co.uk
AlkaClear (from Higher Nature)
To prevent infection while travelling, Paraclens: (from Higher Nature)

Eczema
Elenas Nature Collection: www.elenasnaturecollection.co.uk

Food intolerances
Recommended tests
The Food Detective – Cambridge Nutritional Laboratories:
www.food-detective.com
FACT: www.gdx.uk.net

Hypothyroidism
Recommended test
Total Thyroid Screen: www.gdx.uk.net

Metabolic syndrome
Recommended test
Metabolic Syndrome Profile: www.gdx.uk.net

Osteoporosis
Recommended test
Osteoporosis Risk Assessment: www.gdx.uk.net

Recommended supplements (in addition to the foundation programme):
AlkaClear (from Higher Nature)
For more information on natural progesterone visit: www.npis.info

Rheumatoid arthritis
For more information on the idea of an infection causing rheumatoid arthritis visit www.mercola.com

Recommended supplements (in addition to the foundation programme):
Bromelain (from Lamberts @ Revital)
AlkaClear (from Higher Nature)
DLPA Complex (contains bromelain, DLPA and astaxanthin) (from Higher Nature)

Recommended products
Magnessage: www.vitalia-health.co.uk
Pain Ease microcurrent patch: www.lifes2good.com

TMS

For the TMS Workbook visit: www.tmsbackpain.com
For the Freedom Process Workshop visit: www.freedomprocess.com
For more information on TMS and TMS Practitioners visit:
www.tmsrecovery.com

Vaginal thrush
Recommended supplements (in addition to the foundation programme):

VagiClear (probiotic pessary) (from Higher Nature)

Weight loss

BMI calculator: www.nhsdirect.nhs.uk/interactiveTools/bmi
Full? Stop! (potato protein powder supplement) (from Higher Nature)
For details of my weight loss consultations and workshops visit:
www.drmarkatkinson.com

Recommended reading

Part 1: You are unique

Section One: Women and the New Medicine
Andrew Weil, *Spontaneous Healing*, Sphere, 2008
Christiane Northrup, *Women's Bodies, Women's Wisdom: The Complete Guide to Women's Health and Well-being*, Piatkus Books, 1998
Tracy Gaudet, *Consciously Female*, Bantam Books, 2004

Section Two: Your Personal Health, Healing and Happiness Programme
Steve Bratman, *Complementary and Alternative Health*, Collins, 2007
David Peters, *The New Medicine*, DK Publishing, 2007

Part 2: The five secrets of health, healing and happiness

Secret One: Nurture Your Physical Body
Patrick Holford, *The Optimum Nutrition Bible*, Piatkus Books, 2004
William Wolcott and Trish Fahey, *The Metabolic Typing Diet*, Broadway Books, 2002
Paula Baillie-Hamilton, *Stop the 21st Century Killing You: Toxic Chemicals Have Invaded Our Life. Fight Back! Eliminate Toxins, Tackle Illness, Get Healthy and Live Longer*, Vermilion, 2005
Paul Glovinsky, *The Insomnia Answer: A Personalized Drug-free Program for Identifying and Overcoming the Three Types of Insomnia*, Perigee Books, 2006

Secret Two: De-Stress and Relax

Sonja Lyubomirsky, *The How of Happiness*, Sphere, 2007

Robert Emmons, *Thanks!*, Houghton Mifflin Company, 2007

Robert L. Leahy, *The Worry Cure*, Piatkus Books, 2006

Secret Three: Face and Embrace Your Emotions

Darlene Minnini, *The Emotional Toolkit*, Piatkus Books, 2006

Joe Griffin and Ivan Tyrrell, *Human Givens: A New Approach to Emotional
    Health and Clear Thinking*, Human Givens Publishing, 2004

Peter Levine, *Healing Trauma*, Sounds True, 2005

Ruth King, *Healing Rage*, Gotham Books, 2007

Secret Four: Accept Yourself

Cheri Huber, *There is Nothing Wrong with You: Going Beyond Self-Hate, A
    Compassionate Process for Learning to Accept Yourself Exactly as You
    Are*, Keep it Simple Books, 2001

Michael Brown, *The Presence Process,* Beaufort Books, 2005

Lucia Capacchione, *Recovery of Your Inner Child,* Simon and Schuster, 1991

John Bradshaw, *Homecoming: Reclaiming and Championing Your Inner
    Child,* Piatkus Books, 1991

Secret Five: Develop and Deepen Your Relationships

Dr Sue Johnson, *Hold Me Tight*, Little, Brown and Company, 2008

Harville Hendrix, *Getting the Love You Want*, Pocket Books, 2005

Pia Mellody, *Intimacy Factor: The Ground Rules for Overcoming the
    Obstacles to Truth, Respect, and Lasting Love,* HarperCollins, 2003

Part 3: Holistic health tools

Tool One: Mindfulness

Jon Kabat-Zinn, *Full Catastrophe Living*, Piatkus Books, 2001

Thich Nhat Hanh, *The Miracle of Mindfulness: The Classic Guide to
    Meditation by the World's Most Revered Master,* Rider and Co, 2008

Tool Two: Emotional Freedom Technique

David Feinstein, *The Healing Power of EFT and Energy Psychology:
    Revolutionary Methods for Dramatic Personal Change*, Piatkus Books,
    2006

Silvia Hartman, *Adventures in EFT: The Essential Field Guide to Emotional Freedom Techniques*, Dragon Rising, 2000

Tool Three: EmoTrance
Silvia Hartmann, *Oceans of Energy*, Dragon Rising, 2003

Tool Four: The Work
Bryon Katie, *Loving What Is*, Rider and Co, 2002
Bryon Katie, *I Need Your Love – Is It True?*, Rider and Co, 2005

Tool Five: Values-based Goal Setting
Brian Mayne, *Goal Mapping*, Watkins Publishing, 2006
Brian Tracy, *Goals! How to Get Everything You Want – Faster Than You Ever Thought Possible*, Berrett-Koehler, 2004

Part 4: Women's health solutions

Premenstrual Syndrome
Marilyn Glenville, *Overcoming PMS the Natural Way: How to Get Rid of Those Monthly Symptoms for Ever*, Piatkus Books, 2006

Fibroids
Allan Warshowsky and Ellen Oumano, *Healing Fibroids: A Doctor's Guide to a Natural Cure*, Simon and Schuster, 2002

Endometriosis
Michael Vernon and Dian Shepperson Mills, *Endometriosis: A Key to Healing Through Nutrition*, Thorsons, 2002

Polycystic Ovary Syndrome
Colette Harris and Theresa Cheung, *The Ultimate PCOS Handbook: Lose Weight, Boost Fertility, Clear Skin and Restore Self-esteem*, Thorsons, 2006

Cystitis
Larrian Gillespie, *You Don't Have to Live with Cystitis*, Ebury Press, 1988

Infertility

Marilyn Glenville, *Natural Solutions to Infertility: How to Increase Your Chances of Conceiving and Preventing Miscarriage*, Piatkus Books, 2000

Menopause

Christiane Northrup, *The Wisdom of Menopause*, Piatkus Books, 2001

Clarissa Pinkola Estes, *Women Who Run with the Wolves: Contacting the Power of the Wild Woman*, Rider and Co, 2008

Part 5: Integrated medical solutions

Acne

Nicholas Perricone, *The Acne Prescription: The Perricone Program for Clear and Healthy Skin at Every Age*, HarperResource, 2003

Addictions

Charlotte Davis Kasl, *Women, Sex and Addiction: A Search for Love and Power*, HarperPerennial, 1990

Pia Mellody, *Facing Love Addiction*, HarperSanFrancisco, 2003

Adrenal fatigue

James L. Wilson, *Adrenal Fatigue: The 21st Century Stress Syndrome*, Smart Publications, 2001

Richard L. Shames and Karilee Halo Shames, *Feeling Fat, Fuzzy, or Frazzled?: A 3-Step Program To: Beat Hormone Havoc, Restore Thyroid, Adrenal, and Reproductive Balance, and Feel Better Fast!*, Hudson Street Press, 2005

Anxiety and panic disorders

Edmund J. Bourne, *The Anxiety and Phobia Workbook*, New Harbinger Publications, 2005

Joe Griffin and Ivan Tyrrell, *How to Master Anxiety: All You Need to Know to Overcome Stress, Panic Attacks, Trauma, Phobias, Obsessions and More*, HG Publishing, 2006

Cancer
Chris Wollams, *Everything You Need To Know To Help You Beat Cancer,* Health Issues, 2002
Rosy Daniel, *The Cancer Directory,* HarperThorsons, 2005

Cardiovascular disease
Dean Ornish, *Dr. Dean Ornish's Programme for Reversing Heart Disease,* Ivy Books, 1997
Stephen Sinatra, *Reverse Heart Disease Now: Stop Deadly Cardiovascular Plaque Before It's Too Late,* John Wiley and Sons, 2008

Cellulite
Howard Murad, *The Cellulite Solution: A Doctor's Programme for Losing Lumps, Bumps, Dimples and Stretch Marks,* Piatkus Books, 2006

Chronic fatigue syndrome/fibromyalgia
Raymond Perrin, *The Perrin Technique: How to Beat Chronic Fatigue Syndrome/ME,* Hammersmith Press, 2007
John Eaton, *M.E., Chronic Fatigue Syndrome and Fibromyalgia – The Reverse Therapy Approach,* authorsonline.co.uk, 2005

Codependency
Barry and Janae Weinhold, *Breaking Free of the Codependency Trap,* New World Library, 2008
Rokelle Lerner, *Boundaries for Codependents,* Hazelden Information and Educational Services, 1988
John Bradshaw, *Healing the Shame That Binds You,* Health Communications, 2006

Constipation
Kathryn Marsden, *Good Gut Healing: The No-nonsense Guide to Bowel and Digestive Disorders,* Piatkus Books, 2003

Depression
Joe Griffin and Ivan Tyrell, *How to Lift Depression Fast,* HG Publishing, 2004
Bob Murray and Alicia Fortinberry, *Creating Optimism,* McGraw-Hill Contemporary, 2005

Diabetes
Richard K. Bernstein, *Dr Bernstein's Diabetes Solution: Complete Guide to Achieving Normal Blood Sugars,* Sphere, 2007
Sarah Brewer, *Natural Approaches to Diabetes*, Piatkus Books, 2005

Dysbiosis
Leon Chaitow, *Candida Albicans: The Non-drug Approach to the Treatment of Candida Infection,* HarperCollins, 2003
Erica White, *Beat Candida Cookbook: Over 250 Recipes with a 4-point Plan for Attacking Candidiasis,* HarperCollins, 1999

Eczema
Sue Armstrong-Brown, *The Eczema Solution*, Vermilion, 2002
Carolyn Charman, *Eczema: What Really Works,* Robinson Publishing, 2006

Food intolerances
Antoinette Savill and Antony Haynes, *The Food Intolerance Bible: A Nutritionist's Plan to Beat Food Cravings, Fatigue, Mood Swings, Bloating, Headaches and IBS,* HarperThorsons, 2005
Linda Gamlin and Jonathan Brostoff, *The Allergy Bible: Understanding, Diagnosing, Treating Allergies and Intolerance*, Quadrille Publishing, 2005

Headaches and migraines
Claire Houlding, *Managing Migraines: Dealing with Migraines from All Perspectives,* AuthorHouse, 2007
Alexander Mauskop, *What Your Doctor May Not Tell You about Migraines,* Warner Books, 2001

Hypothyroidism
Karilee Shames, *Thyroid Power: Ten Steps to Total Health*, HarperCollins, 2002

Irritable bowel syndrome
John Hunter, *Irritable Bowel Solutions: The Essential Guide to IBS, Its Causes and Treatments*, Vermilion, 2007

William B Salt, *Irritable Bowel Syndrome and the Mindbodyspirit Connection: 7 Steps for Living a Healthy Life With a Functional Bowel*, ebrandedbooks.com, 2002

Metabolic syndrome
Antony Haynes, *The Insulin Factor*, HarperCollins, 2004
Karlene Karst, *The Metabolic Syndrome Program: How to Lose Weight, Beat Heart Disease, Stop Insulin Resistance and More*, John Wiley and Sons, 2006

Osteoporosis
Marilyn Glenville, *Osteoporosis: The Silent Epidemic*, Kyle Cathie, 2005
Jane Plant, *Understanding, Preventing and Overcoming Osteoporosis*, Virgin Books, 2004

Rheumatoid arthritis
Arthritis Foundation, *The Arthritis Foundation's Guide to Good Living with Rheumatoid Arthritis*, Arthritis Foundation, 2005
Barbara D Allan, *Conquering Arthritis*, Shining Prairie Flower Productions, 2002

TMS
John Sarno, *The Divided Mind*, Gerald Duckworth and Co, 2008
John Sarno, *The Mindbody Prescription,* Little, Brown and Company, 1999

Varicose veins
Christine Craggs-Hinton, *Coping Successfully with Varicose Veins*, Sheldon Press, 2008

Weight loss
Patrick Holford, *The Holford Low-GL Diet Made Easy*, Piatkus Books, 2007
Fedon Alexander Lindberg, *The Greek Doctor's Diet*, Rodale International, 2006

References

Introduction

1. Weil, A., *Spontaneous Healing: How to Discover and Enhance Your Body's Natural Ability to Maintain and Heal Itself,* Sphere, 2008

Part 1: You are unique

Section One: Women and the new medicine

1. Summerfield, D., 'Depression: epidemic or pseudo-epidemic?', *Journal of The Royal Society of Medicine*, Vol. 99(3) (2006), pp. 161–2.
2. Gallup Poll, 'The Happiness Formula Poll', *BBC 2 Series*, Wednesday 3 May 2006.
3. Eaton, S.B., Konner, M., Shostak, M., 'Stone agers in the fast lane: chronic degenerative diseases in evolutionary perspective', *American Journal of Medicine*, Vol. 84 (1988), pp. 739–49.
4. Beral, V., Banks, E., Reeves, G., 'Evidence from randomised trials on the long-term effects of hormone replacement therapy', *Lancet*, Vol. 360 (2002), pp. 942–4.
5. Merkatz, R.B., Junod, S.W., 'Historical background of changes in FDA policy on the study and evaluation of drugs in women', *Academic Medicine*, Vol. 69 (1994), pp. 703–7.
6. Derman, R.J., 'Effects of sex steroids on women's health: implications for practitioners', *The American Journal of Medicine*, Vol. 98(1A) (16 January 1995), pp. 137S–43S.
7. Gan, S.C., Beaver, S.K., Houck, P.M., MacLehose, R.F., Lawson, H.W., Chan, L., 'Treatment of acute myocardial infarction and 30-day mortality among women and men', *New England Journal of Medicine*, Vol. 343(1) (6 July 2000), pp. 8–15.
8. Silverstein, B., 'Gender differences in the prevalence of somatic versus pure depression: a replication', *The American Journal of Psychiatry*, Vol. 159(6) (2002), pp. 1051–2.

9. Holbrook, T.L., Hoyt, D.B., Stein, M.B., et al., 'Gender differences in long-term posttraumatic stress disorder outcomes after major trauma: women are at higher risk of adverse outcomes than men', *The Journal of Trauma: Injury, Infection & Critical Care*, Vol. 53 (November 2002), pp. 882–8.

10. Bolego, C., Poli, A., Paoletti, R., 'Smoking and gender', *Cardiovascular Research*, Vol. 53(3) (2002), pp. 568–76.

11. Pogun, S., 'Sex differences in brain and behavior: emphasis on nicotine, nitric oxide and place learning', *International Journal of Psychophysiology*, Vol. 42(2) (2001), pp. 195–208.

12. Rademaker, M., 'Do women have more adverse drug reactions?', *American Journal of Clinical Dermatology*, Vol. 2(6) (2001), pp. 349–51.

13. Gallup Poll, 'Coronary Heart Disease: Women's Heart Health Initiative', *American Medical Women's Association* (1995), http://www.amwa-doc.org/Education/gallup.htm.

14. Mosca, L., et al., 'National study of physician awareness and adherence to cardiovascular disease prevention guidelines', *Circulation*, Vol. 111(4) (2005), pp. 499–510.

15. Erik J. Giltay, Johanna M. Geleijnse, Frans G. Zitman, Tiny Hoekstra, Evert G. Schouten, 'Dispositional Optimism and All-Cause and Cardiovascular Mortality in a Prospective Cohort of Elderly Dutch Men and Women', *Archives of General Psychiatry*, Vol. 61 (2004), pp. 1126–35.

16. Lyubomirsky, S., et al., 'The Benefits of Frequent Positive Affect: Does Happiness Lead to Success?', *Psychological Bulletin*, Vol. 131(6) (2005), pp. 803–55.

17. Davidson, R., et al., 'Alterations in Brain and Immune Function Produced by Mindfulness Meditation', *Psychosomatic Medicine*, Vol. 65 (2003), pp. 564–70.

18. Ernst, E., *The Desktop Guide to Complementary and Alternative Medicine: An Evidence-Based Approach*, Mosby, 2006.

Part 2: The five secrets of health, healing and happiness

Secret One: Nurture your physical body

1. National Statistics Website, http://www.statistics.gov.uk/cci/nugget.asp?id=1894.

2. 'Fresh Thinking – Re:fresh Report' (May 2006), www.freshproduce.org.uk.

3. Economic & Social Research Council Diet & Obesity in the UK Fact Sheet, http://www.esrcsocietytoday.ac.uk/ESRCInfoCentre/facts/index55.aspx.

4. Emslie, C., Hunt, K., Macintyre, S., 'Perceptions of body image amongst working men and women', *Journal of Epidemiology & Community Health*, Vol. 55 (2001), pp. 406–7.

5. Ipsos Mori, 'The Laughing Cow Extra Light Dieting Survey' (December 2006), http://www.laughingcowdietreport.co.uk/.

6. Institute of Medicine, www.ion.edu/sleep.

7. Lauderdale et al., 'Respond to "How Much Do We Really Sleep?" ', *American Journal of Epidemiology*, Vol. 164(1) (1 July 2006), pp. 19–20.

8. Johnson, E., 'Sleep in America 2000', National Sleep Foundation, www.sleepfoundation.org.

9. Institute of Medicine, www.ion.edu/sleep.

10. Johnson, E., 'Sleep in America 2000', National Sleep Foundation, www.sleepfoundation.org.

11. Castillo, Alvaro, 'Why Women Have Insomnia More Frequently Than Men' (13 March 2008), www.EzineArticles.com.

12. Donath, F., Quispe, S., Diefenbach, K., et al., 'Critical evaluation of the effect of valerian extract on sleep structure and sleep quality', *Pharmacopsychiatry*, Vol. 33 (2000), pp. 47–53.

13. Garfinkel, D., Laudon, M., Nof, D., Zisapel, N., 'Improvement of sleep quality in elderly people by controlled-release melatonin', *Lancet*, Vol. 346 (1995), pp. 541–4.

14. Hornyak, M., Voderholzer, U., Hohagen, F., et al., 'Magnesium therapy for periodic leg movements-related insomnia and restless legs syndrome: an open pilot study', *Sleep*, Vol. 21 (1998), pp. 501–5.

15. Puttini, P.S., Caruso, I., 'Primary fibromyalgia syndrome and 5-hydroxy-L-tryptophan: a 90 day open study', *Journal of International Medical Research*, Vol. 20 (1992), pp. 182–9.

16. Cade, J., et al., 'Dietary fibre and risk of breast cancer in the UK Women's Cohort Study', *International Journal of Epidemiology*, Vol. 36(2) (2007), pp. 431–8.

17. Gilhooly, C.H., Das, S.K., Golden, J.K., McCrory, M.A., Dallal, G.E., Saltzman, E., Kramer, F.M., Roberts, S.B., 'Food cravings and energy regulation: the characteristics of craved foods and their relationship with eating behaviors and weight change during 6 months of dietary energy restriction, *International Journal of Obesity*; advance electronic version 26 June 2007; doi: 10.1038/sj.ijo.0803672.

18. Corby, M., et al. 'Changes in Food Cravings during Low-Calorie and Very-Low-Calorie Diets', *Obesity*, Vol. 14 (2006), pp. 115–121.

19. Beat eating disorders website, www.b-eat.co.uk/.

20. Challem, J., *The Inflammation Syndrome: The Complete Nutritional Program to Prevent and Reverse Heart Disease, Arthritis, Diabetes, Allergies and Asthma*, John Wiley & Sons Inc., 2004.

21. Oomen, C., et al., 'Association between trans fatty acid intake and 10-year risk of coronary heart disease in the Zutphen Elderly Study: a prospective population-based study', *Lancet*, Vol. 357(9258), pp. 746–51.

22. Watkins, B.A., and Seifert, M.F., 'Food Lipids and Bone Health', in R.E. McDonald and D.B. Min (eds), *Food Lipids and Health*, Marcel Dekker Inc., 1996, p. 101.

23. Meyer, K., et al., 'Carbohydrates, dietary fibre, and incident type 2 diabetes in older women', *American Journal of Clinical Nutrition*, Vol. 71(4) (April 2000), pp. 921–30.

24. Larsson, S., et al., 'Consumption of sugar and sugar-sweetened foods and the risk of pancreatic cancer in a prospective study', *American Journal of Clinical Nutrition*, Vol. 84(5) (November 2006), pp. 1171–6.

25. Walton, R.G., et al., 'Adverse reactions to aspartame: double blind challenge in patients from a vulnerable population', *Journal of Biological Psychiatry*, Vol. 34(1–2) (1993), p. 13.

26. Joosens, J.V., et al., 'Dietary salt, nitrate and stomach cancer mortality in 24 countries', European Cancer Prevention (ECP) and the INTERSALT Cooperative Research Group, *International Journal of Epidemiology*, Vol. 3 (1996), pp. 494–504.

27. US Environmental Protection Agency, www.epa.gov/mercury/advisories.

28. Barzel, U., et al., 'Excess Dietary Protein Can Adversely Affect Bone', *The Journal of Nutrition*, Vol. 128(6) (June 1998), pp. 1051–3.

29. Grodstein, F., Goldman, M.B., Ryan, L., Cramer, D.W., 'Relation of female infertility to consumption of caffeinated beverages', *American Journal of Epidemiology*, Vol. 137 (1993), pp. 1353–60.

30. Worthington, V., 'Effect of agricultural methods on nutritional quality: a comparison of organic with conventional crops', *Alternative Therapies*, Vol. 4(1), pp. 58–69.

31. Singletary, K.W., Gapstur, S.M., 'Alcohol and Breast Cancer: Review of Epidemiologic and Experimental Evidence and Potential Mechanisms', *The Journal of the American Medical Association,* Vol. 286 (2001), pp. 2143–51.

32. Food Standards Agency, 'National Diet & Nutrition Survey: Adults aged 19 to 64', Vol. 5 (2004). See http://www.food.gov.uk/science/dietarysurvey/ndnsdocuments/ndnsvd52004.

33. ibid.

34. 'Meat and dairy, where have the minerals gone?', *Food Magazine,* Vol. 72 (Jan/March 2006), p. 10.

35. Gaby, A.R., Wright, J.V. 'Diabetes', *Nutritional Therapy in Medical Practice: Reference Manual and Study Guide* (1996), pp. 54–64 [review].

36. Cover, C.M., et al., 'Indole-3-carbinol inhibits the expression of cyclin-dependent kinase-6 and induces a G1 cell cycle arrest of human breast cancer cells independent of estrogen receptor signaling', *Journal of Biological Chemistry,* Vol. 273 (1998), pp. 3838–47.

37. Tan, B.K., Vanitha, J., 'Immunomodulatory and antimicrobial effects of some traditional Chinese medicinal herbs: a review', *Current Medicinal Chemistry,* Vol. 11(11) (2004), pp. 1423–30.

38. Hobbs, C., *Medicinal Mushrooms: An exploration of tradition, healing and culture,* Botanica Press, 1995.

39. Farnsworth, N.R., Kinghorn, A.D., Soejarto, D.D., Waller, D.P., 'Siberian ginseng (*Eleutherococcus senticosus*): Current status as an adaptogen', H. Wagner, H.Z. Hikino, N.R. Farnsworth (eds), *Economic and Medicinal Plant Research,* Academic Press, Vol. 1 (1985), pp. 155–215 [review].

40. Brown, R.P., Gerbarg, P.L., Ramazanov, Z., 'Rhodiola rosea: a phytomedicinal overview', *Herbalgram,* Vol. 56 (2002), pp. 40–52.

41. Wagner, H., Nörr, H., Winterhoff, H., 'Plant adaptogens', *Phytomedicine,* Vol. 1 (1994), pp. 63–76.

42. Crespo, C.J., et al., 'The relationship of physical activity and body weight with all-cause mortality: results from The Puerto Rico Heart Health Program', *Annals of Epidemiology,* Vol. 12(8) (November 2002), pp. 543–52.

43. Wessel, T., et al., 'Relationship of Physical Fitness vs Body Mass Index with Coronary Artery Disease and Cardiovascular Events in Women', *The Journal of the American Medical Association,* Vol. 292(10) (8 September 2004), pp. 1179–1187.

44. 'Medical aspects of exercise: benefits and risks', Summary of a Report of the Royal College of Physicians, *Journal of the College of Physicians, London,* Vol. 25(3) (July 1991), pp. 193–6.

45. Bernstein, L. et al., 'Physical exercise and reduced risk of breast cancer in young women', *Journal of the National Cancer Institute,* Vol. 86(18), (1994), pp. 1403–8.

46. Hammar, M., et al., 'Does Physical Exercise Influence the Frequency of Postmenopausal Hot Flushes?', *Acta Obstetricia et Gynecologica Scandinavica,* Vol. 69(5) (1990), pp. 409–12.

47. Kim, T., Shin, Y., White-Traut, R., 'Multisensory intervention improves physical growth and illness rates in Korean orphaned newborn infants', *Research In Nursing And Health,* Vol. 26(6) (2003), pp. 424–33.

48. Wood, D., Craven, R., Whitney, J., 'The effect of therapeutic touch on behavioral symptoms of persons with dementia', *Alternative Therapies in Health and Medicine,* Vol. 11(1) (2005), pp. 66–74.

49. Islam, T., et al., 'Childhood sun exposure influences risk of multiple sclerosis in monozygotic twins', *Neurology,* Vol. 69 (2007), pp. 381–8.

50. Zipitis, C.S., et al., 'Vitamin D Supplementation in Early Childhood and Risk of Type I Diabetes: a Systematic Review and Meta-analysis', *Archives of Disease in Childhood* [e-pub 13 March 2008], doi:10.1136/adc.2007.128579.

51. Baille-Hamilton, P., *Stop the 21st Century Killing You*, Vermilion, 2005.

52. Scott Davis, Dana K. Mirick, Richard G. Stevens, 'Night Shift Work, Light at Night, and Risk of Breast Cancer', *Journal of the National Cancer Institute*, Vol. 93(20) (2001), pp. 1557–62.

53. Kaiser, J., 'Air pollution: evidence mounts that tiny particles can kill', *Science*, Vol. 289(54767) (7 July 2000), pp. 22–3.

54. World Resources Institute, www.wri.org.

55. 'Mothers milk: Record levels of toxic fire retardants found in American mothers' breast milk', EWG (Environmental Working Group), Washington, DC (2003). Available online at http://www.ewg.org/reports/mothersmilk.

56. Wollams, C., 'Oestrogen: The Killer in Our Midst', Health Issues Ltd, 2006.

57. Augood, C., et al., 'Smoking and female infertility: a systematic review and meta-analysis', *Human Reproduction,* Vol. 13 (1998), pp. 1532–9.

58. Robbins, R., et al., 'Production of toxic shock syndrome toxin 1 by Staphylococcus aureus as determined by tampon disk-membrane-agar method', *Journal of Clinical Microbiology*, Vol. 25(8) (August 1987), pp. 1446–9.

59. Environmental Protection Agency, www.epa.gov/airnow.

60. Grinshpun, S.A., Adhikari, A., Lee, B.U., Trunov, M., Mainelis, G., Yermakov, M., and Reponen, T., Brebbia, C.A. (ed.), 'Indoor Air Pollution Control Through Ionization', in *Air Pollution: Modeling, Monitoring and Management of Air Pollution*, WIT Press, 2004, pp. 689–704.

61. Groves, B., *The Fluoride Deception*, Seven Stories Press, 2006.

62. Huggins, H., *Uninformed Consent: Hidden Dangers in Dental Care*, Hampton Roads Publishing Co., 1999.

63. Wenstrup, D., Ehmann, W., Markesbery, W., 'Trace element imbalances in isolated subcellular fractions of Alzheimer's disease brains', *Brain Research*, Vol. 533 (1990), pp. 125–30.

64. Lorscheider, F., Vimy, M., 'Evaluation of the safety issue of mercury release from dental fillings', *FASEB Journal*, Vol. 7 (December 1993), pp. 1432–3.

Secret Two: De-stress and relax

1. Selye, H., *The Stress of Life*, McGraw-Hill Publishing Co., 1978.

2. 'Are Women Hardwired for Worry?', Gallup Poll (2005), http://www.gallup.com/poll/16219/Women-Hardwired-Worry.aspx.

3. Taylor, S., 'Tend and Befriend: Biobehavioral Bases of Affiliation Under Stress', *Current Directions in Psychological Science,* Vol. 15(6) (December 2006), pp. 273–7.

4. Reported in the 27 November, 2006 issue of *Archives of Internal Medicine*. A report on the study can be seen at http://www.medicalnewstoday.com/articles/57687.php.

5. Emmons, R., *Thanks!: How the New Science of Gratitude Can Make You Happier*, Houghton Mifflin Company, 2007.

Secret Three: Face and embrace your emotions

1. Mininni, D., *The Emotional Toolkit*, Piatkus, 2006.

2. Hutson-Comeaux, S., Kelly, J., 'Gender stereotypes of emotional reactions: how we judge an emotion as valid', *Sex Roles: A Journal of Research* (July 2002).

3. Harasty, J., Double, K.L., Halliday, G.M., Kril, J.J., McRitchie, D.A., 'Language-

associated cortical regions are proportionally larger in the female brain', *Archives of Neurology*, Vol. 54(2) (February 1997), pp. 171–6.

4. Graham, S., 'Study Shows That, for Women, Suppressing Emotions Increases Anger' *Scientific America*, (15 January 2002).

5. Ellsberg, M., 'Violence against women and the Millennium Development Goals: Facilitating women's access to support', *International Journal of Gynecology & Obstetrics*, Vol. 94(3), pp. 325–32.

Secret Five: Develop and deepen your relationships

1. Gilligan, C., *In a Different Voice: Psychological Theory and Women's Development*, Harvard University Press; Reissue edition, 1990.

2. Brown, M., *The Presence Process*, Beaufort Books, 2005.

3. Orth-Gomer, K., Johnson, J.V. 'Social network interaction and mortality. A six year follow-up study of a random sample of the Swedish population', *Journal of Chronic Diseases,* Vol. 40(10) (1987), pp. 949–57.

4. Ornish, D., *Love and Survival*, Vermilion, 2001.

5. ibid.

6. Seeman, T., Syme, S.L., 'Social Networks and Coronary Artery Disease: A Comparison of the Structure and Function of Social Relations as Predictors of Disease', *Psychosomatic Medicine,* Vol. 49 (1987), pp. 341–54.

7. Medalie, J.H., et al., 'The Importance of Biopsychosocial Factors in the Development of Duodenal Ulcer in a Cohort of Middle-Aged Men', *American Journal of Epidemiology,* Vol. 136 (1992), pp. 1280–7.

8. Berkman, L.F., Syme, S.L., 'Social networks, host resistance, and mortality: a nine-year follow-up study of Alameda County residents', *American Journal of Epidemiology*, Vol. 109(2) (1979), pp. 186–205.

9. Bowlby, J., *A secure base: Parent-child attachment and healthy human development*, Basic Books, 1988.

Part 3: Holistic health tools

Tool One: Mindfulness

1. Kabat-Zinn, J., *Full Catastrophe Living: How to Cope with Stress, Pain and Illness Using Mindfulness Meditation*, Piatkus Books, 2001.

2. Teasdale, John D., et al., 'Prevention of Relapse/Recurrence in Major Depression by Mindfulness-Based Cognitive Therapy', *Journal of Consulting and Clinical Psychology*, Vol. 68(4) (2000), pp. 615–23.

Part 4: Women's health solutions

Premenstrual syndrome

1. London, R.S., Bradley, L., Chiamori, N.Y., 'Effect of a nutritional supplement on premenstrual symptomatology in women with premenstrual syndrome: a double-blind longitudinal study', *Journal of the American College of Nutrition,* Vol. 10 (1991), pp. 494–9.

2. Wyatt, K.M., Dimmock, P.W., Jones, P.W., Shaughn O'Brien, P.M., 'Efficacy of vitamin B-6 in the treatment of premenstrual syndrome: systematic review', *British Medical Journal*, Vol. 318 (1999), pp. 1375–81.

3. Walker, A.F., De Souza, M.C., Vickers, M.F., et al., 'Magnesium supplementation alleviates premenstrual symptoms of fluid retention', *Journal of Women's Health*, Vol. 7 (1998), pp. 1157-65.
4. Ockerman, P.A., Bachrack, I., Glans, S., Rassner, S., 'Evening primrose oil as a treatment of the premenstrual syndrome', *European Journal of Clinical Nutrition*, Vol. 2 (1986), pp. 404-5.
5. Werbach, M.R., 'Premenstrual syndrome: magnesium', *International Journal of Alternative & Complementary Medicine*, Vol. 29 (February 1994) [review].
6. Thys-Jacobs, S., Ceccarelli, S., Bierman, A., et al., 'Calcium supplementation in premenstrual syndrome', *Journal of General Internal Medicine*, Vol. 4 (1989), pp. 183-9.
7. Loch, E.G., Selle, H., Boblitz, N., 'Treatment of premenstrual syndrome with a phytopharmaceutical formulation containing Vitex agnus castus', *Journal of Women's Health Gender Based Medicine*, Vol. 9(3) (2000), pp. 315-20.

Heavy menstrual bleeding

1. Lithgow, D.M., Politzer, W.M., 'Vitamin A in the treatment of menorrhagia', *South African Medical Journal*, Vol. 51 (1977), pp. 191-3.
2. Cohen, J.D., Rubin, H.W., 'Functional menorrhagia: treatment with bioflavonoids and vitamin C', *Current Therapeutic Research, Clinical and Experimental*, Vol. 2 (1960), pp. 539-42.
3. Bone, K., 'Vitex agnus-castus: Scientific studies and clinical applications', *European Journal of Herbal Medicine*, Vol. 1 (1994), pp. 12-15.

Painful periods

1. Marjoribanks, J., Proctor, M.L., Farquhar, C., 'Nonsteroidal anti-inflammatory drugs for primary dysmenorrhoea', *Cochrane Review*, in: The Cochrane Library, Issue 2, 2006. Wiley, Chichester, UK.
2. Proctor, M.L., Murphy, P.A., 'Herbal and dietary therapies for primary and secondary dysmenorrhoea', *Cochrane Review*, in: The Cochrane Library, Issue 2, 2006. Wiley, Chichester, UK.
3. Benassi, L., Barletta, F.P., Baroncini, L., et al., 'Effectiveness of magnesium pidolate in the prophylactic treatment of primary dysmenorrhea', *Clinical and Experimental Obstetrics & Gynecology*, Vol. 19 (1992), pp. 176-9.
4. Butler, E.B and McKnight, E., 'Vitamin E in the primary treatment of dysmenorrhoea', *Lancet*, Vol. 1 (1955), pp. 844-7.
5. Hudgins, A.P., 'Vitamins P, C and niacin for dysmenorrhea therapy', *Western Journal of Surgery, Obstetrics, and Gynecology* (December 1994), pp. 610-11.
6. Harel, Z., Biro, F.M., Kottenhahn, R.K., Rosenthal, S.L., 'Supplementation with omega-3 polyunsaturated fatty acids in the management of dysmenorrhea in adolescents', *American Journal of Obstetrics and Gynecology*, Vol. 174 (1996), pp. 1335-8.

Fibroids

1. Rossetti, A., Sizzi, O., Soranna, L., et al., 'Long-term results of laparoscopic myomectomy: recurrence rate in comparison with abdominal myomectomy', *Human Reproduction*, Vol. 16 (2001), pp. 770-4.
2. Cohen, J.D., Rubin, H.W., 'Functional menorrhagia: treatment with bioflavonoids and vitamin C', *Current Therapeutic Research, Clinical and Experimental*, Vol. 2 (1960), pp. 539-42.

3. Michnovicz, J., et al., 'Induction of Estradiol Metabolism by Dietary Indole-3-carbinol in Humans', *Journal of the National Cancer Institute*, Vol. 82(11) (1990), pp. 947–9.
4. Bone, K., 'Vitex agnus-castus: Scientific studies and clinical applications', *European Journal of Herbal Medicine*, Vol. 1 (1994), pp. 12–15.

Endometriosis

1. The National Endometriosis Society, http://www.endometriosis-uk.org.
2. Giudice, L.C., Kao, L.C., 'Endometriosis', *Lancet*, Vol. 364 (2004), pp. 1789–99.
3. http://clinicalevidence.bmj.com/ceweb/conditions/woh/0802/0802_16.jsp.
4. Abbott, J., Hawe, J., Hunter, D., et al. 'Laparoscopic excision of endometriosis: a randomized, placebo-controlled trial', *Fertility and Sterility*, Vol. 82 (2004), pp. 878–84.
5. Johnson, K., 'Antioxidant therapy quickly improves endometriosis pain', *Family Practice Management*, Vol. 75 (15 March 2004) [News report].
6. Covens, A.L., Christopher, P., Casper, R.F., 'The effect of dietary supplementation with fish oil fatty acids on surgically induced endometriosis in the rabbit', *Fertility & Sterility*, Vol. 49 (1988), pp. 698–703.
7. Michnovicz, J., et al., 'Induction of Estradiol Metabolism by Dietary Indole-3-carbinol in Humans', *Journal of the National Cancer Institute*, Vol. 82(11) (1990), pp. 947–9.
8. Blumenthal, M., Busse, W.R., Goldberg, A., et al. (eds), *The Complete Commission E Monographs: Therapeutic Guide to Herbal Medicines,* Integrative Medicine Communications, 1998, p. 108.

Polycystic ovary syndrome

1. The Rotterdam ESHRE/ASRM, 'Consensus on diagnostic criteria and long-term health risks related to polycystic ovary syndrome (PCOS)', http://humrep.oxfordjournals.org/cgi/content/short/19/1/41 (accessed on 4 December 2006).
2. Hill, K.M., 'Update: The pathogenesis and treatment of PCOS', *The Nurse Practitioner*, Vol. 28 (2003), pp. 8–23.
3. Patel, S.M, Nestler, J.E., 'Fertility in Polycystic Ovary Syndrome', *Endocrinology and Metabolism Clinics of North America*, Vol. 35 (2005), pp. 137–55.
4. Rychlik, D., 'Pharmacological treatment of polycystic ovary syndrome', *Seminars in Reproductive Medicine,* Vol. 3 (2003), p. 21.
5. Moghetti, P., Castello, R., Negri, C., et al., 'Metformin effects on clinical features, endocrine and metabolic profiles, and insulin sensitivity in polycystic ovary syndrome: a randomized, double-blind, placebo-controlled 6-month trial, followed by open, long-term clinical evaluation', *Journal of Clinical Endocrinology and Metabolism*, Vol. 85 (2000), pp. 139–46.
6. Nadler, J.L., Buchanan, T., Natarajan, R., et al., 'Magnesium deficiency produces insulin resistance and increased thromboxane synthesis', *Hypertension*, Vol. 21 (1993), pp. 1024–9.
7. Anderson, R.A., 'Chromium, glucose intolerance and diabetes', *Journal of the American College of Nutrition*, Vol. 17 (1998), pp. 548–55 [review].
8. Blumenthal, M., Busse, W.R., Goldberg, A., et al. (eds), *The Complete Commission E Monographs: Therapeutic Guide to Herbal Medicines,* Integrative Medicine Communications (1998), p. 108.
9. Di Silverio, F., Monti, S., Sciarra, A., et al., 'Effects of long-term treatment with

Serenoa repens (Permixon®) on the concentrations and regional distribution of androgens and epidermal growth factor in benign prostatic hyperplasia', *Prostate*, Vol. 37 (1998), pp. 77–83.

Cystitis

1. Hooton, T.M., Scholes, D., Hughes, J.P., et al., 'A prospective study of risk factors for symptomatic urinary tract infection in young women', *New England Journal of Medicine*, Vol. 335 (1996), pp. 468–74.
2. Albert, X., Huertas, I., Pereiro, I., et al., 'Antibiotics for preventing recurrent urinary tract infection in non-pregnant women', *Cochrane Review,* in: The Cochrane Library, Issue 2, 2005. Wiley, Chichester, UK.
3. ibid.
4. Ofek, I., Goldhar, J., Esltdat, Y., Sharon, N., 'The importance of mannose specific adhesins (lectins) in infections caused by Escherichia coli', *Scandinavian Journal of Infectious Diseases*, Vol. 33 (1982), pp. 61–7.
5. Mori, S., Ojima, Y., Hirose, T., et al., 'The clinical effect of proteolytic enzyme containing bromelain and trypsin on urinary tract infection evaluated by double blind method', *Acta Obstetrica et Gynaecologica Japonica*, Vol. 19 (1972), pp. 147–53.
6. Axelrod, D.R., 'Ascorbic acid and urinary pH', *Journal of The American Medical Association,* Vol. 254 (1985), pp. 1310–11.
7. Jepson, R.G., Mihaljevic, L., Craig, J., 'Cranberries for preventing urinary tract infections', *Cochrane Review,* in: The Cochrane Library, Issue 3, 2002. Update Software, Oxford, UK.

Fibrocystic breast disease

1. Boyle, C.A., Berkowitz, G.S., LiVolsi, V.A., Ort, S., Merino, M.J., White, C., Kelsey, J.L., 'Caffeine consumption and fibrocystic breast disease: a case-control epidemiologic study', *Journal of the National Cancer Institute*, Vol. 72(5) (1984), pp. 1015–19.
2. London, R., et al., 'Mammary dysplasia: endocrine parameters and tocopherol therapy', *Nutrition Research*, Vol. 7 (1982), p. 243.
3. Michnovicz, J., et al., 'Induction of Estradiol Metabolism by Dietary Indole-3-carbinol in Humans', *Journal of the National Cancer Institute,* Vol. 82(11) (1990), pp. 947–9.
4. Blumenthal, M., Busse, W.R., Goldberg, A., et al. (eds), *The Complete Commission E Monographs: Therapeutic Guide to Herbal Medicines,* Integrative Medicine Communications, 1998, p. 108.

Infertility

1. National Institute for Clinical Excellence, 'Fertility: assessment and treatment for people with fertility problems' (August 2003), http://www.nice.org.uk/pdf/ CG011niceguideline.pdf (accessed on 13 June 2008).
2. Beck, J.J., Boothroyd, C., Proctor, M., et al., 'Oral anti-oestrogens and medical adjuncts for subfertility associated with anovulation', *Cochrane Review,* in: The Cochrane Library, Wiley, Chichester, UK.
3. Lord, J.M., Flight, I.H., Norman, R.J., 'Insulin-sensitising drugs (metformin, troglitazone, rosiglitazone, pioglitazone, D-chiro-inositol) for polycystic ovary syndrome', *Cochrane Review,* in: The Cochrane Library, Wiley, Chichester, UK.
4. Human Fertilisation and Embryology Authority, 'Facts and figures' (April 2008), http://www.hfea.gov.uk (accessed on 16 June 2008).

5. Czeizel, A.E., Metneki, J., Dudas, I., 'The effect of preconceptional multivitamin supplementation on fertility', *International Journal for Vitamin & Nutrition Research,* Vol. 66 (1996), pp. 55–8.

6. Dawson, E.B., Harris, W.A., Powell, L.C., 'Relationship between ascorbic acid and male fertility', in: *Aspects of Some Vitamins, Minerals and Enzymes in Health and Disease,* ed. G.H. Bourne, *World Review of Nutrition & Dietitics,* Vol. 62 (1990), pp. 1–26 [review].

7. Scibona, M., Meschini, P., Capparelli, S., et al., 'L-arginine and male infertility', *Minerva urologica e nefrologica,* Vol. 46 (1994), pp. 251–3.

8. Costa, M., Canale, D., Filicori, M., et al., 'L-carnitine in idiopathic asthenozoospermia: a multicenter study', *Andrologia,* Vol. 26 (1994), pp. 155–9.

9. Omu, A.E., Dashti, H., Al-Othman, S., 'Treatment of asthenozoospermia with zinc sulphate: andrological, immunological and obstetric outcome', *European Journal of Obstetrics & Gynecology and Reproductive Biology,* Vol. 79 (1998), pp. 179–84.

10. Propping, D., Katzorke, T., 'Treatment of corpus luteum insufficiency', *Zeitschr Allgemeinmedizin,* Vol. 63 (1987), pp. 932–3.

Menopause

1. Al-Azzawi, F., 'The menopause and its treatment in perspective', *Postgraduate Medical Journal,* Vol. 77 (2001), pp. 292–304.

2. Porter, M., Penney, G.C., Russell, D., et al., 'A population based survey of women's experience of the menopause', *British Journal of Obstetrics and Gynaecology,* Vol. 103 (1996), pp. 1025–8.

3. Guyton, A.C., Hall, J.E., *Textbook of Medical Physiology,* WB Saunders, 2001.

4. MacLennan, A.H., Broadbent, J.L., Lester, S., et al., 'Oral oestrogen and combined oestrogen/progestogen therapy versus placebo for hot flushes', *Cochrane Review,* in: The Cochrane Library, Issue 4, 2006. Wiley, Chichester, UK.

5. Hays, J., Ockene, J.K., Brunner, R.L., et al., 'Effects of estrogen plus progestin on health-related quality of life', *New England Journal of Medicine,* Vol. 348 (2003), pp. 1839–54.

6. Writing Group for the Women's Health Initiative Investigators, 'Risks and Benefits of Estrogen Plus Progestin in Healthy Postmenopausal Women', *The Journal of the American Medical Association,* Vol. 288(3) (17 July 2002), pp. 321–33.

7. Beral, V., Banks, E., Reeves, G., 'Evidence from randomised trials on the long-term effects of hormone replacement therapy', *Lancet,* Vol. 360 (2002), pp. 942–4.

8. Beral, V., et al., 'Breast cancer and hormone-replacement therapy in the Million Women Study', *Lancet,* Vol. 362(9382) (2003), pp. 419–27.

9. Beral, V., et al., 'Endometrial cancer and hormone-replacement therapy in the Million Women Study', *Lancet,* Vol. 365(9470) (30 April–6 May 2005), pp. 1543–51.

10. Shumaker et al., 'Estrogen Plus Progestin and the Incidence of Dementia and Mild Cognitive Impairment in Postmenopausal Women', *The Journal of the American Medical Association,* Vol. 289(20) (28 May 2003), pp. 650–52.

11. Dale, E., Vessey, M.P., Hawkins, M.M., et al., 'Risk of venous thromboembolism in users of hormone replacement therapy', *Lancet,* Vol. 348 (1996), pp. 977–80.

12. Mosca, L., Collins, P., Herrington, D.M., et al., 'Hormone replacement therapy and cardiovascular disease: a statement for healthcare professionals from the American Heart Association', *Circulation,* Vol. 104 (2001), pp. 499–503.

13. Gozan, H.A., 'The use of vitamin E in treatment of the menopause', *New York State Journal of Medicine,* Vol. 52 (1952), pp. 1289–91.

14. Smith, C.J., 'Non-hormonal control of vaso-motor flushing in menopausal patients', *The Chicago Medical Journal,* Vol. 67 (1964), pp. 193–5.

15. Lieberman, S., 'A review of the effectiveness of *Cimicifuga racemosa* (black cohosh) for the symptoms of menopause', *The Journal of Women's Health*, Vol. 7 (1998), pp. 525–9.

16. Newton, K.M., Reed, S.D., LaCroix, A.Z., et al., 'Treatment of vasomotor symptoms of menopause with black cohosh, multibotanicals, soy, hormone therapy, or placebo: a randomized trial', *Annals of Internal Medicine*, Vol. 145 (2006), pp. 869–79.

17. Han, K.K., Soares, J.M. Jr, Haidar, M.A., et al., 'Benefits of soy isoflavone therapeutic regimen on menopausal symptoms', *Obstetrics & Gynecology*, Vol. 99 (2002), pp. 389–94.

18. Leonetti, H.B., Long, S., Anasti, J.M., 'Transdermal progesterone cream for vasomotor symptoms and postmenopausal bone loss', *Obstetrics & Gynecology*, Vol. 95 (1999), pp. 225–8.

Part 5: Integrated medical health solutions

Acne

1. Chu, T.C., 'Acne and other facial eruptions', *Medicine*, Vol. 25 (1997), pp. 30–3.

2. Lookingbill, D.P., Chalker, D.K., Lindholm, J.S., et al.'Treatment of acne with a combination clindamycin/benzoyl peroxide gel compared with clindamycin gel, benzoyl peroxide gel and vehicle gel: combined results of two double-blind investigations', *Journal of the American Academy of Dermatology*, Vol. 37 (1997), pp. 590–5.

3. Haider, A., Shaw, J.C. 'Treatment of acne vulgaris' *Journal of the American Medical Association*, Vol. 292 (2004), pp. 726–35.

4. Snider, B., Dietman, D.F., 'Pyridoxine therapy for premenstrual acne flare', *Archives of Dermatology*, Vol. 110 (1974), pp. 130–1 [letter].

5. Michaelsson, G., Juhlin, L., Ljunghall, K., 'A double blind study of the effect of zinc and oxytetracycline in acne vulgaris', *British Journal of Dermatology*, Vol. 97 (1977), pp. 561–6.

6. Loch, E.G., Selle, H., Boblitz, N., 'Treatment of premenstrual syndrome with a phytopharmaceutical formulation containing Vitex agnus castus', *Journal of Women's Health Gender Based Medicine*, Vol. 9(3) (2000), pp. 315–20.

7. Bassett, I.B., Pannowitz, D.L., Barnetson, R.S., 'A comparative study of tea-tree oil versus benzoyl peroxide in the treatment of acne', *The Medical Journal of Australia*, Vol. 53 (1990), pp. 455–8.

Addictions

1. Guenther, R.M., 'Role of nutritional therapy in alcoholism treatment', *International Journal of Biosocial and Medical Research*, Vol. 4(1) (1983), pp. 5–18.

2. Glen, I., Skinner, F., Glen, E., MacDonell, L., 'The role of essential fatty acids in alcohol dependence and tissue damage', *Alcoholism, Clinical and Experimental Research*, Vol. 11 (1987), pp. 37–41.

3. Anderson, R.A., 'Chromium, glucose intolerance and diabetes', *Journal of The American College of Nutrition*, Vol. 7 (1998), pp. 548–55 [review].

4. Rogers, L.L., Pelton, R.B., 'Glutamine in the treatment of alcoholism', *Quarterly Journal of Studies on Alcohol*, Vol. 18 (1957), pp. 581–7.

5. Birmingham, C.L., Goldner, E.M., Bakan, R., 'Controlled trial of zinc supplementation in anorexia nervosa', *International Journal of Eating Disorders*, Vol. 15 (1994), pp. 251–5.

6. Nolen, W.A., van de Putte, J.J., Dijken, W.A., Kamp, J.S., 'L-5-HTP in depression resistant to re-uptake inhibitors. An open comparative study with tranylcypromine', *The British Journal of Psychiatry*, Vol. 147 (1985), pp. 16–22.
7. Juneja, L.R., Chu, D.C., Okubo, T., et al., 'L-theanine a unique amino acid of green tea and its relaxation effect in humans', *Trends in Food Science & Technology*, Vol. 10 (1999), pp. 199–204.
8. Ferenci, P., Dragosics, B., Dittrich, H., et al., 'Randomized controlled trial of silymarin treatment in patients with cirrhosis of the liver', *Journal of Hepatology*, Vol. 9 (1989), pp. 105–13.
9. Allen, S.S., et al., 'Menstrual phase effects on smoking relapse', *Addiction*, Vol. 103(5) (May 2008), pp. 809–21.

Adrenal fatigue

1. Brown, R.P., Gerbarg, P.L., Ramazanov, Z., 'Rhodiola rosea: a phytomedicinal overview', *Herbalgram*, Vol. 56 (2002), pp. 40–52.
2. Wagner, H., Nörr, H., Winterhoff, H., 'Plant adaptogens', *Phytomed*, Vol. 1 (1994), pp. 63–76.
3. Asano, K., Takahashi, T., Miyashita, M., et al. 'Effect of *Eleutherococcus senticosus* extract on human working capacity', *Planta Medica*, Vol. 37 (1986), pp. 175–7.
4. Duke, J., *Ginseng: A Concise Handbook*, Algonac, MI: Reference Publications, 1989, p. 36.

Anxiety and panic disorders

1. Wittchen, H.U., Hoyer, J. 'Generalized anxiety disorder: nature and course', *Journal of Clinical Psychiatry*, Vol. 62(11) (2001), pp. 15–19.
2. Tyrer, P., 'Current problems with the benzodiazepines', in: D. Wheatly (ed), *The Anxiolytic Jungle: Where Next?* Wiley, Chichester, UK, 1990.
3. Rickels, K., Downing, R., Schweizer, E., et al., 'Antidepressants for the treatment of generalised anxiety disorder: a placebo-controlled comparison of imipramine, trazodone and diazepam', *Archives of General Psychiatry*, Vol. 50 (1993), pp. 884–95.
4. Carroll, D., Ring, C., Suter, M., Willemsen, G., 'The effects of an oral multivitamin combination with calcium, magnesium, and zinc on psychological well-being in healthy young male volunteers: a double-blind placebo-controlled trial', *Psychopharmacology (Berl)*, Vol. 150 (2000), pp. 220–5.
5. Buydens-Branchey, L., Branchey, M., 'n-3 polyunsaturated fatty acids decrease anxiety feelings in a population of substance abusers', *Journal of Clinical Psychopharmacology*, Vol. 26 (2006), pp. 661–5.
6. Weston, P.G., et al., 'Magnesium sulfate as a sedative', *The American Journal of Medical Sciences*, Vol. 165 (1923), pp. 431–3.
7. Wong, A.H.C., Smith, M., Boon, H.S., 'Herbal remedies in psychiatric practice', *Archives of General Psychiatry*, Vol. 55 (1998), pp. 1033–44.
8. Juneja, L.R., Chu, D.-C., Okubo, T., et al., 'L-theanine a unique amino acid of green tea and its relaxation effect in humans', *Trends in Food Science & Technology*, Vol. 10 (1999), pp. 199–204.
9. Akhondzadeh, S., Naghavi, H.R., Vazirian, M., et al., 'Passionflower in the treatment of generalized anxiety: a pilot double-blind randomized controlled trial with oxazepam', *Journal of Clinical Pharmacy and Therapeutics*, Vol. 26 (2001), pp. 363–7.

Cancer

1. Michnovicz, J., et al., 'Induction of Estradiol Metabolism by Dietary Indole-3-carbinol in Humans', *Journal of the National Cancer Institute,* Vol. 82(11) (1990), pp. 947–9.
2. Gao, Y., et al., 'Effects of ganopoly (a Ganoderma lucidum polysaccharide extract) on the immune functions in advanced-stage cancer patients', *Immunological Investigations,* Vol. 32(3) (August 2003), pp. 201–15.
3. Ghoneum, M., Jewett, A., 'Production of tumor necrosis factor-alpha and interferon-gamma from human peripheral blood lymphocytes by MGN-3, a modified arabinoxylan from rice bran, and its synergy with interleukin-2 in vitro', *Cancer Prevention,* Vol. 24 (2000), p. 314.
4. Harkey, M.R., et al., 'Variability in commercial ginseng products: an analysis of 25 preparations', *American Journal of Clinical Nutrition,* Vol. 73 (2001), pp. 1101–6.
5. Chlebowski, R.T., Bulcavage, L., Grosvenor, M., et al., 'Hydrazine sulfate in cancer patients with weight loss. A placebo-controlled clinical experience', *Cancer,* Vol. 59(3) (1987), pp. 406–10.
6. Lau, C.B., et al., 'Cytotoxic activities of Coriolus versicolor (Yunzhi) extract on human leukemia and lymphoma cells by induction of apoptosis', *Life Sciences,* Vol. 75(7) (2004), pp. 797–808.
7. Taixiang, W., et al., 'Chinese medical herbs for chemotherapy side effects in colorectal cancer patients', *Cochrane Database Systematic Review,* Vol. 1 (25 January 2005), CD004540.
8. Hobbs, C., *Medicinal Mushrooms,* Interweave Press, 1996.

Cardiovascular disease

1. British Heart Foundation, 'European Cardiovascular Disease Statistics' (2000 Edition), www.bhf.org.uk.
2. British Heart Foundation, 'Women & Heart Disease' (British Heart Foundation 2005), www.bhf.org.uk.
3. The Stroke Association, 'Facts and figures about stroke', http://www.stroke.org.uk.
4. Ornish, D., *Dr. Dean Ornish's Programme for Reversing Heart Disease,* Ivy Books, 1997.
5. Singh, S., 'Long term double blind evaluation of amlodipine and nadolol in patients with stable exertional angina pectoris', *Clinical Cardiology,* Vol. 16 (1993), pp. 54–8.
6. Dargie, H.J., Ford, I., Fox, K.M., et al., 'Total Ischaemic Burden European Trial (TIBET): effects of ischaemia and treatment with atenolol, nifedipine SR and their combination on outcome in patients with chronic stable angina', *European Heart Journal,* Vol. 17 (1996), pp. 104–12.
7. Singh, S., 'Long term double blind evaluation of amlodipine and nadolol in patients with stable exertional angina pectoris', *Clinical Cardiology,* Vol. 16 (1993), pp. 54–8.
8. Hall, R., Chong, C., 'A double-blind parallel group study of amlodipine versus long acting nitrate in the management of elderly patients with stable angina', *Cardiolog,* Vol. 96 (2001), pp. 72–7.
9. Simpson, D., Wellington, K., 'Nicorandil: a review of its use in the management of stable angina pectoris, including high-risk patients', *Drugs,* Vol. 64 (2004), pp. 1941–55.
10. Antiplatelet Trialists' Collaboration, 'Collaborative overview of randomised trials of antiplatelet therapy—I: Prevention of death, myocardial infarction, and stroke by

prolonged antiplatelet therapy in various categories of patients', *British Medical Journal,* Vol. 308 (1994), pp. 81–106.

11. Fibrinolytic Therapy Trialists (FTT), 'Indications for fibrinolytic therapy in suspected acute myocardial infarction: collaborative overview of early mortality and major morbidity results of all randomized trials of more than 1000 patients', *Lancet,* Vol. 343 (1994), pp. 311–22.

12. Keeley, E.C., Boura, J.A., Grines, C.L., 'Primary angioplasty versus intravenous thrombolytic therapy for acute myocardial infarction: a quantitative review of 23 randomised trials', *Lancet,* Vol. 361 (2003), pp. 13–20.

13. Freemantle, N., Cleland, J., Young, P., et al., 'Beta blockade after myocardial infarction: systematic review and meta regression analysis', *British Medical Journal,* Vol. 318 (1999), pp. 1730–7.

14. Domanski, M.J., Exner, D.V., Borkowf, C.B., et al., 'Effect of angiotensin converting enzyme inhibition on sudden cardiac death in patients following acute myocardial infarction: a meta-analysis of randomized clinical trials', *Journal of the American College of Cardiology,* Vol. 33 (1999), pp. 598–604.

15. Indredavik, B., Bakke, F., Slordahl, S.A., et al., 'Stroke unit treatment: 10-year follow-up', *Stroke,* Vol. 30 (1999), pp. 1524–7.

16. Gubitz, G., Sandercock, P., Counsell, C., 'Antiplatelet therapy for acute ischaemic stroke', *Cochrane Review,* in: The Cochrane Library, Issue 2, 2006. Wiley, Chichester, UK.

17. Wardlaw, J.M., del Zoppo, G., Yamaguchi, T., 'Thrombolysis for acute ischaemic stroke', *Cochrane Review,* in: The Cochrane Library, Issue 2, 2006. Wiley, Chichester, UK.

18. Tegos, T.J., Kalodiki, E., Sabetai, M.M., et al., 'Stroke: pathogenesis, investigations, and prognosis: Part II of III', *Angiology,* Vol. 51 (2000), pp. 885–94.

19. Antithrombotic Trialists' Collaboration, 'Collaborative meta-analysis of randomised trials of antiplatelet therapy for prevention of death, myocardial infarction, and stroke in high risk patients', *British Medical Journal,* Vol. 324 (2002), pp. 71–86.

20. National Institute for Health and Clinical Excellence, 'Clopidrogel and modified-release dipyridamole in the prevention of occlusive vascular events', www.nice.org.uk.

21. Sanchez-Moreno, C., Dashe, J.F., Scott, T., Thaler, D., Folstein, M.F., Martin, A., 'Decreased Levels of Plasma Vitamin C and Increased Concentrations of Inflammatory and Oxidative Stress Markers After Stroke', *Stroke,* Vol. 35 (2004), pp. 163–8.

22. Saynor, R., Verel, D., Gillott, T., 'The long-term effect of dietary supplementation with fish lipid concentrate on serum lipids, bleeding time, platelets and angina', *Atherosclerosis,* Vol. 50 (1984), pp. 3–10.

23. Spagnoli, L.G., Orlandi, A., et al., 'Propionyl-L-carnitine prevents the progression of atherosclerotic lesions in aged hyperlipemic rabbits', *Atherosclerosis,* Vol. 114(1) (7 April 1995), pp. 29–44.

24. Kamikawa, T., Kobayashi, A., Yamashita, T., et al., 'Effects of coenzyme Q10 on exercise tolerance in chronic stable angina pectoris', *The American Journal of Cardiology,* Vol. 56 (1985), p. 247.

25. Koscielny, J., Klüendorf, D., Latza, R., et al., 'The antiatherosclerotic effect of Allium sativum', *Atherosclerosis,* Vol. 144 (1999), pp. 237–49.

26. Hanack, T., Brückel, M.-H., 'The treatment of mild stable forms of angina pectoris using Crataegutt (R) Novo', *Therapiewoche,* Vol. 33 (1983), pp. 4331–3 [in German].

Chronic fatigue syndrome/fibromyalgia

1. Sharpe, M., Hawton, K., Simkin, S., et al., 'Cognitive behaviour therapy for chronic fatigue syndrome: a randomised controlled trial', *British Medical Journal*, Vol. 312 (1996), pp. 22–6.
2. O'Malley, P.G., Balden, E., Tomkins, G., Santoro, J., Kroenke, K., Jackson, J.L., 'Treatment of fibromyalgia with antidepressants: a meta-analysis', *Journal of General Internal Medicine*, Vol. 15 (2000), pp. 659–66.
3. Gray, J.B., Martinovic, A.M., 'Eicosanoids and essential fatty acid modulation in chronic disease and the chronic fatigue syndrome', *Medical Hypothesis*, Vol. 43(1) (1994), pp. 31–42.
4. Teitelbaum, J.E., 'The use of D-ribose in chronic fatigue syndrome and fibromyalgia: a pilot study', *Journal of Alternative and Complementary Medicine*, Vol. 12(9) (November 2006), pp. 857–62.
5. Plioplys, A.V., Plioplys, S., 'Amantadine and L-carnitine treatment of chronic fatigue syndrome', *Neuropsychobiology*, Vol. 35 (1997), pp. 16–23.
6. Howard, J.M., Davies, S., Hunnisett, A., 'Magnesium and chronic fatigue syndrome', *Lancet*, Vol. 34 (1992), p. 426.
7. Overvad, K., Diamant, B., Holm, L., Holmer, G., Mortensen, S.A., Stender, S., 'Review coenzyme Q10 in health and disease', *European Journal of Clinical Nutrition*, Vol. 53 (1999), pp. 764–70.
8. Caruso, I., Sarzi Puttini, P., Cazzola, M., Azzolini, V., 'Double-blind study of 5-hydroxytryptophan versus placebo in the treatment of primary fibromyalgia syndrome', *Journal of International Medical Research*, Vol. 18 (1990), pp. 201–9.

Constipation

1. Heaton, K.W., 'Cleave and the fibre story', *Journal of the Royal Naval Medical Service*, Vol. 66 (1980), pp. 5–10.
2. Probert, C.S., Emmett, P.M., Heaton, K.W., 'Some determinants of whole-gut transit time: a population-based study', *Quarterly Journal of Medicine*, Vol. 88 (1995), pp. 311–15.
3. Attar, A., Lemann, M., Ferguson, A., et al., 'Comparison of a low dose polyethylene glycol electrolyte solution with lactulose for treatment of chronic constipation', *Gut*, Vol. 44 (1999), pp. 226–30.
4. Tarpila, S., Tarpila, A., Grohn, P., Silvennoinen, T., Lindberg, L., 'Efficacy of ground flaxseed on constipation in patients with irritable bowel syndrome', *Current Topics in Nutraceutical Research*, Vol. 2 (2004), pp. 119–25.
5. Hamilton-Miller, J., 'Probiotics and prebiotics in the elderly', *Postgraduate Medical Journal*, Vol. 80 (2004), pp. 447–51.
6. Ashraf, W., Park, F., Lof, J., Quigley, E.M., 'Effects of psyllium therapy on stool characteristics, colon transit and anorectal function in chronic idiopathic constipation', *Alimentary Pharmacology and Therapeutic*, Vol. 9 (1995), pp. 639–47.

Depression

1. Kirsch, I., Deacon, B.J., Huedo-Medina, T.B., Scoboria, A., Moore, T.J., et al., 'Initial Severity and Antidepressant Benefits: A Meta-Analysis of Data Submitted to the Food and Drug Administration', *PLoS Med*, Vol. 5(2) (2008), e45 doi:10.1371/journal.pmed.0050045.

2. Sugden, D., 'One carbon metabolism in psychiatric illness', *Nutrition Reviews*, Vol. 19 (2006), pp. 117–36.
3. Coppen, A., et al., 'Enhancement of the antidepressant action of fluoxetine by folic acid', *Journal of Affective Disorders*, Vol. 60 (2000), pp. 121–30.
4. Docherty, J., et al., 'A double blind, placebo-controlled, exploratory trial of chromium picolinate in atypical depression', *Journal of Psychiatric Practice*, Vol. 11(5) (2005), pp. 302–14.
5. Adams, P.B., Lawson, S., Sanigorski, A., Sinclair, A.J., 'Arachidonic acid to eicosapentaenoic acid ratio in blood correlates positively with clinical symptoms of depression', *Lipids*, Vol. 31 (1996), pp. S157–S161.
6. Poldinger, W., et al., 'A functional-dimensional approach to depression: serotonin deficiency and target syndrome in a comparison of 5-HTP and fluvoxamine', *Psychopathology*, Vol. 24(2) (1991), pp. 53–81.
7. Harrer, G., Schmidt, U., Kuhn, U., Biller, A., 'Comparison of equivalence between the St. John's wort extract LoHyp-57 and fluoxetine', *Arzneimittelforschung*, Vol. 49 (1999), pp. 289–96.

Diabetes

1. Diabetes UK, 'What is diabetes?', http://www.diabetes.org.uk.
2. Department of Health, 'Health Survey for England' (2003), http://www.dh.gov.uk.
3. Department of Health, 'National Service Framework for Diabetes: Delivery Strategy' (2003), http://www.diabetes.org.uk.
4. Johansen, K., 'Efficacy of metformin in the treatment of NIDDM: meta-analysis', *Diabetes Care*, Vol. 22 (1999), pp. 33–7.
5. Inzucchi, S.E., 'Oral antihyperglycemic therapy for type 2 diabetes: scientific review', *Journal of the American Medical Association*, Vol. 287 (2002), pp. 360–72.
6. National Institute for Clinical Excellence, 'NICE issues national guidelines for the management of blood glucose levels in people with type 2 diabetes' (2002), http://www.nice.org.uk/36734 (accessed on 3 March 2008).
7. Barringer, T.A., Kirk, J.K., Santaniello, A.C., et al., 'Effect of a multivitamin and mineral supplement on infection and quality of life. A randomized, double-blind, placebo-controlled trial', *Annals of Internal Medicine*, Vol. 138 (2003), pp. 365–71.
8. Paolisso, G., Balbi, V., Volpe, C., et al., 'Metabolic benefits deriving from chronic vitamin C supplementation in aged non-insulin dependent diabetics', *Journal of the American College of Nutrition*, Vol. 14 (1995), pp. 387–92.
9. Jamal, G.A., Carmichael, H., 'The effect of gamma-linolenic acid on human diabetic peripheral neuropathy: a double-blind placebo-controlled trial', *Diabetes Medicine*, Vol. 7 (1990), pp. 319–23.
10. Martin, J., Wang, Z.Q., Zhang, X.H., et al., 'Chromium picolinate supplementation attenuates body weight gain and increases insulin sensitivity in subjects with type 2 diabetes', *Diabetes Care*, Vol. 29 (2006), pp. 1826–32.
11. Baskaran, K., Ahmath, B.K., Shanmugasundaram, K.R., Shanmugasundaram, E.R.B., 'Antidiabetic effect of a leaf extract from *Gymnema sylvestre* in non-insulin-dependent diabetes mellitus patients', *Journal of Ethnopharmacology*, Vol. 30 (1990), pp. 295–305.
12. Ziegler, D., Ametov, A., Barinov, A., et al., 'Oral treatment with alpha-lipoic acid improves symptomatic diabetic polyneuropathy: the SYDNEY 2 trial', *Diabetes Care*, Vol. 29 (2006), pp. 2365–70.

Headaches and migraines

1. Schwartz, B.S., Stewart, W.F., Simon, D., et al., 'Epidemiology of tension-type headache', *Journal of the American Medical Association,* Vol. 279 (1998), pp. 381–3.
2. Steiner, T.J., Scher, A.L., Stewart, W.F., et al., 'The prevalence and disability burden of adult migraine in England and their relationships to age, gender and ethnicity', *Cephalalgia,* Vol. 23 (2003), pp. 519–27.
3. Ferrari, M.D., Goadsby, P.J., Roon, K.I., et al., 'Triptans (serotonin, 5-HT1B/1D agonists) in migraine: detailed results and methods of a meta-analysis of 53 trials', *Cephalalgia,* Vol. 22 (2002), pp. 633–58.
4. Peikert, A., Wilimzig, C., Kohne-Volland, R., 'Prophylaxis of migraine with oral magnesium: results from a prospective, multi-center, placebo-controlled and double-blind randomized study', *Cephalalgia,* Vol. 16 (1996), pp. 257–63.
5. McCarren, T., Hitzemann, R., Allen, C., et al., 'Amelioration of severe migraine by fish oil (omega-3) fatty acids', *American Journal of Clinical Nutrition,* Vol. 41 (1985), p. 874 [abstract].
6. Diener, H.C., Rahlfs, V.W., Danesch, U., 'The first placebo-controlled trial of a special butterbur extract for the prevention of migraine: reanalysis of efficacy criteria', *European Neurology,* Vol. 51 (2004), pp. 89–97.
7. Murphy, J.J., Hepinstall, S., Mitchell, J.R., 'Randomized double-blind placebo controlled trial of feverfew in migraine prevention', *Lancet,* Vol. 2 (1988), pp. 189–92.
8. De Benedittis, G., Massei, R., '5-HTP precursors in migraine prophylaxis: A double-blind cross-over study with L-5-hydroxytryptophan versus placebo', *The Clinical Journal of Pain,* Vol. 3 (1986), pp. 123–9.

Hypothyroidism

1. Vanderpump, M.P., Tunbridge, W.M., French, J.M., et al., 'The incidence of thyroid disorder in the community: a twenty-year follow-up of the Whickham survey', *Clinical Endocrinology,* Vol. 43 (1995), pp. 55–68.
2. Faber, J., Galloe, A.M., 'Changes in bone mass during prolonged subclinical hyperthyroidism due to L-thyroxine treatment: a meta-analysis', *European Journal of Endocrinology,* Vol. 130 (1994), pp. 350–6.
3. Clark, C.D., Bassett, B., Burge, M.R., 'Effects of kelp supplementation on thyroid function in euthyroid subjects', *Endocrine Practice,* Vol. 9(5) (2003), pp. 363–9.

Irritable bowel syndrome

1. Kennedy, T.M., Jones, R.H., 'Epidemiology of cholecystectomy and irritable bowel syndrome in a UK population', *British Journal of Surgery,* Vol. 87 (2000), pp. 1658–63.
2. Quartero, A.O., Meineche-Schmidt, V., Muris, J., et al., 'Bulking agents, antispasmodic and antidepressant medication for the treatment of irritable bowel syndrome', *Cochrane Review,* The Cochrane Library: Issue 2, 2006. Wiley, Chichester, UK.
3. Lesbros-Pantoflickova, D., Michetti, P., Fried, M., et al., 'Meta-analysis: the treatment of irritable bowel syndrome', *Alimentary Pharmacology and Therapeutics,* Vol. 20 (2004), pp. 1253–69.
4. Bijkerk, C.J., Muris, J.W., Knottnerus, J.A., et al., 'Systematic review: the roles of different types of fibre in the treatment of irritable bowel syndrome', *Alimentary Pharmacology and Therapeutics,* Vol. 19 (2004), pp. 245–51.

5. Jackson, J.L., O'Malley, P.G., Tomkins, G., et al., 'Treatment of functional gastrointestinal disorders with antidepressant medications: a meta-analysis', *American Journal of Medicine*, Vol. 108 (2000), pp. 65–72.
6. Bohmer, C.J., Tuynman, H.A., 'The clinical relevance of lactose malabsorption in irritable bowel syndrome', *European Journal of Gastroenterology & Hepatology*, Vol. 8 (1996), pp. 1013–16.
7. Maupas, J., Champemont, P., Delforge, M., 'Treatment of irritable bowel syndrome with *Saccharomyces boulardii*: a double blind, placebo controlled study', *Medicine Chirurgie Digestives*, Vol. 12(1) (1983), pp. 77–9.
8. Prior, A., Whorwell, P.J., 'Double blind study of ispaghula irritable bowel syndrome', *Gut*, Vol. 11 (1987), pp. 1510–13.
9. Pittler, M.H., Ernst, E., 'Peppermint oil for irritable bowel syndrome: a critical review and metaanalysis', *American Journal of Gastroenterology*, Vol. 93 (1998), pp. 1131–5.

Metabolic syndrome

1. British Nutrition Foundation, BNF in Europe, 'Ob-Age, Report 2: The metabolic syndrome', http://www.nutrition.org.uk.
2. Third Report of the National Cholesterol Education Program (NCEP) Expert Panel on Detection, 'Evaluation, and Treatment of High Blood Cholesterol in Adults (Adult Treatment Panel III) final report', *Circulation*, Vol. 106(25) (17 December 2002), pp. 3143–421.
3. Cucheret, M., Lievre, M., Gueyffier, F., 'Clinical benefits of cholesterol lowering treatments: meta-analysis of randomized therapeutic trials', *Presse Medicale*, Vol. 29 (2000), pp. 965–76.
4. Anderson, R.A., Cheng, N., Bryden, N.A., et al., 'Elevated intakes of supplemental chromium improve glucose and insulin variables in individuals with type 2 diabetes', *Diabetes*, Vol. 46(11) (November 1997), pp. 1786–91.
5. Ebbesson, S.O., Risica, P.M., et al., 'Omega-3 fatty acids improve glucose tolerance and components of the metabolic syndrome in Alaskan Eskimos: The Alaska Siberia project', *International Journal of Circumpolar Health*, Vol. 64(4) (September 2005), pp. 396–408.
6. Liu, J., et al., 'Memory loss in old rats is associated with brain mitochondrial decay and RNA/DNA oxidation: partial reversal by feeding aceyl-l-carnitine and/or R-alpha-lipoic acid', *The Proceedings of the National Academy of Sciences*, Vol. 19(4) (February 2002), pp. 2356–61.
7. Hodgson, J.M., Watts, G.F., et al., 'Coenzyme Q10 improves blood pressure and glycaemic control: A controlled trial in subjects with type 2 diabetes', *European Journal of Clinical Nutrition*, Vol. 56(11) (November 2002), pp. 1137–42.
8. Silagy, C., Neil, A.W., 'A meta-analysis of the effect of garlic on blood pressure', *Journal of Hypertension*, Vol. 12 (1994), pp. 463–8.
9. Singh, R.B., Niaz, M.A., Rastogi, S.S., et al., 'Effect of hydrosoluble coenzyme Q10 on blood pressures and insulin resistance in hypertensive patients with coronary artery disease', *Journal of Human Hypertension*, Vol. 13 (1999), pp. 203–8.
10. Walker, A.F., Marakis, G., Simpson, E., et al., 'Hypotensive effects of hawthorn for patients with diabetes taking prescription drugs: a randomised controlled trial', *British Journal of General Practice*, Vol. 56 (2006), pp. 437–43.
11. Pezza, V., Bernardini, F., Pezza, E., et al., 'Study of supplemental oral l-arginine in hypertensives treated with enalapril + hydrochlorothiazide', *American Journal of Hypertension*, Vol. 11 (1998), pp. 1267–70 [letter].
12. Murray, M., 'Lipid-lowering drugs vs. Inositol hexaniacinate', *American Journal of Natural Medicine*, Vol. 2 (1995), pp. 9–12 [review].

13. Blair, S.N., Capuzzi, D.M., Gottlieb, S.O., et al., 'Incremental reduction of serum total cholesterol and low-density lipoprotein cholesterol with the addition of plant stanol ester-containing spread to statin therapy', *The American Journal of Cardiology*, Vol. 86 (2000), pp. 46–52.

Osteoporosis

1. Royal College of Physicians, 'Osteoporosis: clinical guidelines for prevention and treatment', http://www.rcplondon.ac.uk/pubs/wp_osteo_update.htm.
2. Cranney, A., Wells, G., Willan, A., et al., 'Meta-analysis of alendronate for the treatment of postmenopausal women', *Endocrine Reviews*, Vol. 23 (2002), pp. 508–16.
3. Reid, I.R., Ames, R.W., Evans, M.C., et al., 'Long-term effects of calcium supplementation on bone loss and fractures in postmenopausal women: a randomized controlled trial', *American Journal of Medicine*, Vol. 98 (1995), pp. 331–5.
4. Brot, C., Jorgensen, N., Madsen, O.R., et al., 'Relationships between bone mineral density, serum vitamin D metabolites and calcium: phosphorus intake in healthy perimenopausal women', *Journal of Internal Medicine*, Vol. 245 (1999), pp. 509–16.
5. Lydeking-Olsen, E., Beck-Jensen, J.E., Setchell, K.D., Holm-Jensen, T., 'Soymilk or progesterone for prevention of bone loss: a 2 year randomized, placebo-controlled trial', *European Journal of Clinical Nutrition*, Vol. 43 (2004), pp. 246–57.

Rheumatoid arthritis

1. Symmons, D., Turner, G., Webb, R., et al., 'The prevalence of rheumatoid arthritis in the United Kingdom: new estimates for a new century', *Rheumatology*, Vol. 41 (2002), pp. 793–800.
2. Felson, D.T., Anderson, J.J., Meenan, R.F., 'The comparative efficacy and toxicity of second-line drugs in rheumatoid arthritis: results of two metaanalyses', *Arthritis and Rheumatism*, Vol. 33 (1990), pp. 1449–61.
3. Kremer, J.M., Lawrence, D.A., Petrillow, G.F., et al., 'Effects of high dose fish oil on rheumatoid arthritis after stopping nonsteroidal antiinflammatory drugs', *Arthritis & Rheumatism*, Vol. 38 (1995), pp. 1107–14.
4. Zurier, R.B., Rossetti, R.G., Jacobson, E.W., et al., 'Gamma-linolenic acid treatment of rheumatoid arthritis. A randomized, placebo-controlled trial', *Arthritis & Rheumatism*, Vol. 39 (1996), pp. 1808–17.
5. Cohen, A., Goldman, J., 'Bromelain therapy in rheumatoid arthritis', *The Pennsylvania Medical Journal*, Vol. 67 (1964), pp. 27–30.

Vaginal thrush

1. Sobel, J.D., Faro, S., Force, R.W., et al., 'Vulvovaginal candidiasis: epidemiologic, diagnostic, and therapeutic considerations', *American Journal of Obstetrics and Gynecology*, Vol. 178 (1998), pp. 203–11.
2. Hilton, E., Isenberg, H.D., Alperstein, P., et al., 'Ingestion of yogurt containing Lactobacillus acidophilus as prophylaxis for candidal vaginitis', *Annals of Internal Medicine*, Vol. 116 (1992), pp. 353–7.

Varicose veins

1. Evans, C.J., Fowkes, F.G., Ruckley, C.V., et al., 'Prevalence of varicose veins and chronic venous insufficiency in men and women in the general population:

Edinburgh Vein Study', *Journal of Epidemiology and Community Health,* Vol. 53 (1999), pp. 149–53.

2. Goldman, M.P., 'Treatment of varicose and telangiectatic leg veins: double-blind prospective comparative trial between aethoxyskerol and sotradecol', *Dermatologic Surgery,* Vol. 28 (2002), pp. 52–5.

3. Belcaro, G., Cesarone, M.R., Di Renzo, A., et al., 'Foam-sclerotherapy, surgery, sclerotherapy, and combined treatment for varicose veins: a 10-year, prospective, randomized, controlled, trial', *Angiology,* Vol. 54 (2003), pp. 307–15.

4. Einarsson, E., Eklof, B., Neglen, P., 'Sclerotherapy or surgery as treatment for varicose veins: a prospective randomized study', *Phlebology,* Vol. 8 (1993), pp. 22–6.

5. Vascular Surgical Society of Great Britain and Ireland, 'Patient Information: varicose veins – general information' (March 2006), http://www.vascularsociety.org.uk/patient/vv.html (accessed on 13 November 2007).

6. Einarsson, E., Eklof, B., Neglen, P., 'Sclerotherapy or surgery as treatment for varicose veins: a prospective randomized study', *Phlebology,* Vol. 8 (1993), pp. 22–6.

7. Sohn, C., Jahnichen, C., Bastert, G., 'Effectiveness of beta-hydroxyethylrutoside in patients with varicose veins in pregnancy', *Zentralbl Gynakol,* Vol. 117 (1995), pp. 190–7 [in German].

8. Blumenthal, M., Busse, W.R., Goldberg, A., et al. (eds), *The Complete German Commission E Monographs: Therapeutic Guide to Herbal Medicines,* Integrative Medicine Communications, 1998, p. 149.

9. Gaby, A.R., 'The story of bromelain', *Nutritional Healing,* Vol. 3 (May 1995), pp. 4, 11.

Weight loss

1. Ipsos Mori., 'The Laughing Cow Extra Light Dieting Survey' (December 2006), http://www.laughingcowdietreport.co.uk.

2. Department of Health, 'Health survey for England 2004: updating of trend tables to include 2004 data' (December 2005), http://www.dh.gov.uk.

3. National Heart, Lung, and Blood Institute, 'Clinical guidelines on the identification, evaluation and treatment of overweight and obesity in adults', http://www.nhlbi.nih.gov/guidelines.

4. Hutton, B., Fergusson, D., 'Changes in body weight and serum lipid profile in obese patients treated with orlistat in addition to a hypocaloric diet: a systematic review of randomized clinical trials', *American Journal of Clinical Nutrition,* Vol. 80 (2004), pp. 1461–8.

5. Medicines and Healthcare Products Regulatory Agency, 'New advice concerning the use of Acomplia (rimonabant) for weight loss in patients taking antidepressants or those with major depression' (July 2007), http://www.mhra.gov.uk (accessed on 7 July 2008).

6. Arterburn, D.E., Crane, P.K., Veenstra, D.L., 'The efficacy and safety of sibutramine for weight loss: a systematic review', *Archives of Internal Medicine,* Vol. 164 (2004), pp. 994–1003.

7. Blundell, J.E., Hill, A.J., Peikin, S.R., Ryan, C.A., 'Oral administration of proteinase inhibitor II from potatoes reduces energy intake in man', *Physiology & Behaviour,* Vol. 48 (1990), pp. 241–6, *Research Center* (1999).

8. Anderson, R.A., Cheng, N., Bryden, N.A., et al., 'Elevated intakes of supplemental chromium improve glucose and insulin variables in individuals with type 2 diabetes', *Diabetes,* Vol. 46(11) (November 1997), pp. 1786–91.

9. Tardif, J.C., et al., 'Lipoic acid supplementation and endothelial function', *British Journal of Pharmacology,* Vol. 153 (2008), pp. 1587–8.

Index